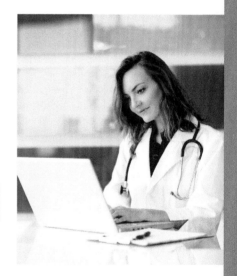

Contemporary Antibiotic Management for Urologic Procedures and Infections

Editors

SARAH C. FLURY
ANTHONY J. SCHAEFFER

UROLOGIC CLINICS
OF NORTH AMERICA

www.urologic.theclinics.com

Consulting Editor
SAMIR S. TANEJA

November 2015 • Volume 42 • Number 4

ELSEVIER

1600 John F. Kennedy Boulevard • Suite 1800 • Philadelphia, Pennsylvania, 19103-2899

http://www.theclinics.com

UROLOGIC CLINICS OF NORTH AMERICA Volume 42, Number 4
November 2015 ISSN 0094-0143, ISBN-13: 978-0-323-41356-5

Editor: Kerry Holland
Developmental Editor: Alison Swety

Urologic Clinics of North America (ISSN 0094-0143) is published quarterly by Elsevier Inc., 360 Park Avenue South, New York, NY 10010-1710. Months of issue are February, May, August, and November. Business and Editorial Offices: 1600 John F. Kennedy Blvd., Suite 1800, Philadelphia, PA 19103-2899. Periodicals postage paid at New York, NY and additional mailing offices. Subscription prices are $355.00 per year (US individuals), $602.00 per year (US institutions), $415.00 per year (Canadian individuals), $752.00 per year (Canadian institutions), $515.00 per year (foreign individuals), and $752.00 per year (foreign institutions). Foreign air speed delivery is included in all *Clinics* subscription prices. All prices are subject to change without notice. **POSTMASTER:** Send address changes to *Urologic Clinics of North America*, Elsevier Health Sciences Division, Subscription Customer Service, 3251 Riverport Lane, Maryland Heights, MO 63043. **Customer Service: 1-800-654-2452 (US). From outside the United States, call 1-314-447-8871. Fax: 1-314-447-8029. E-mail: JournalsCustomerServiceusa@elsevier.com (for print support)** and **JournalsOnlineSupport-usa@elsevier.com (for online support).**

Reprints. For copies of 100 or more, of articles in this publication, please contact the Commercial Reprints Department, Elsevier Inc., 360 Park Avenue South, New York, New York 10010-1710. Tel.: 212-633-3874; Fax: 212-633-3820; E-mail: reprints@elsevier.com.

Urologic Clinics of North America is covered in MEDLINE/PubMed (*Index Medicus*), *Excerpta Medica, Current Contents/ Clinical Medicine, Science Citation Index,* and *ISI/BIOMED.*

PROGRAM OBJECTIVE
The goal of *Urologic Clinics of North America* is to keep practicing urologists and urology residents up to date with current clinical practice in urology by providing timely articles reviewing the state of the art in patient care.

TARGET AUDIENCE
Practicing urologists, urology residents and other health care professionals practicing in the discipline of urology.

LEARNING OBJECTIVES
Upon completion of this activity, participants will be able to:
1. Review the epidemiology and management of infections due to drug-resistant bacteria.
2. Discuss hazards and complications of urinary tract infections in children, the elderly, during pregnancy, and in patients with compromised bladder control.
3. Recognize methods of contemporary antibiotic treatment for conditions such as sexually transmitted infections, bacteriuria, and sepsis.

ACCREDITATION
The Elsevier Office of Continuing Medical Education (EOCME) is accredited by the Accreditation Council for Continuing Medical Education (ACCME) to provide continuing medical education for physicians.

The EOCME designates this enduring material for a maximum of 15 *AMA PRA Category 1 Credit*(s)™. Physicians should claim only the credit commensurate with the extent of their participation in the activity.

All other health care professionals requesting continuing education credit for this enduring material will be issued a certificate of participation.

DISCLOSURE OF CONFLICTS OF INTEREST
The EOCME assesses conflict of interest with its instructors, faculty, planners, and other individuals who are in a position to control the content of CME activities. All relevant conflicts of interest that are identified are thoroughly vetted by EOCME for fair balance, scientific objectivity, and patient care recommendations. EOCME is committed to providing its learners with CME activities that promote improvements or quality in healthcare and not a specific proprietary business or a commercial interest.

The planning committee, staff, authors and editors listed below have identified no financial relationships or relationships to products or devices they or their spouse/life partner have with commercial interest related to the content of this CME activity:
Travis O. Abicht, MD; Michael P. Angarone, DO; Kristy M. Borawski, MD; Daniel P. Boyle, MD; Amanda C. Chi, MD; Hillary L. Copp, MD, MS; Keri Detweiler, DO; Matthew Ferroni, MD; Sophie G. Fletcher, MD; Sarah C. Flury, MD; Daniel J. Fuchs, MD; Alexander P. Glaser, MD; Matthias D. Hofer, MD; Tracy Marien, MD; Daniel Mayers, DO; Daniel J. Mazur, MD; Barry M. McGuire, MD; Maxim J. McKibben, MD; Nicole L. Miller, MD; Adam Bryant Murphy, MD, MBA, MSCI; Robert B. Nadler, MD; Terrance D. Peabody, MD; Sherry S. Ross, MD; Bogdana Schmidt, MD, MPH; Patrick Seed, MD, PhD; Lindsay Smith, MD; Aisha Khalali Taylor, MD; Lewis Thomas, MD; Chad R. Tracy, MD; Teresa R. Zembower, MD.

The planning committee, staff, authors and editors listed below have identified financial relationships or relationships to products or devices they or their spouse/life partner have with commercial interest related to the content of this CME activity:
Chris M. Gonzalez, MD has research support from American Medical Systems, LLC and Coloplast Corp.
Anthony J. Schaeffer, MD is a consultant/advisor for KLJ Associates, Inc.; ClearView Healthcare Partners; Navigant Consulting, Inc.; and has royalties/patents from UpToDate, Inc.
Samir S. Taneja, MD is a consultant/advisor for Bayer Pharma AG, Eigen Pharma LLC, GTx, Inc., HealthTronics, Inc. and Hitachi, Ltd.

UNAPPROVED/OFF-LABEL USE DISCLOSURE
The EOCME requires CME faculty to disclose to the participants:
1. When products or procedures being discussed are off-label, unlabelled, experimental, and/or investigational (not US Food and Drug Administration [FDA] approved); and
2. Any limitations on the information presented, such as data that are preliminary or that represent ongoing research, interim analyses, and/or unsupported opinions. Faculty may discuss information about pharmaceutical agents that is outside of FDA-approved labelling. This information is intended solely for CME and is not intended to promote off-label use of these medications. If you have any questions, contact the medical affairs department of the manufacturer for the most recent prescribing information.

TO ENROLL
To enroll in the *Urologic Clinics of North America* Continuing Medical Education program, call customer service at 1-800-654-2452 or sign up online at http://www.theclinics.com/home/cme. The CME program is available to subscribers for an additional annual fee of USD $270.

METHOD OF PARTICIPATION

In order to claim credit, participants must complete the following:

1. Complete enrolment as indicated above.
2. Read the activity.
3. Complete the CME Test and Evaluation. Participants must achieve a score of 70% on the test. All CME Tests and Evaluations must be completed online.

CME INQUIRIES/SPECIAL NEEDS

For all CME inquiries or special needs, please contact elsevierCME@elsevier.com.

Contributors

CONSULTING EDITOR

SAMIR S. TANEJA, MD
The James M. Neissa and Janet Riha Neissa
Professor of Urologic Oncology; Professor of
Urology and Radiology; Director, Division of
Urologic Oncology; Co-Director, Department
of Urology, Smilow Comprehensive Prostate
Cancer Center, NYU Langone Medical Center,
New York, New York

EDITORS

SARAH C. FLURY, MD
Assistant Professor, Department of Urology,
Northwestern University Feinberg School of
Medicine, Chicago, Illinois

ANTHONY J. SCHAEFFER, MD
Chair, Department of Urology,
Herman L. Kretschmer Professor of Urology,
Northwestern University Feinberg School of
Medicine, Chicago, Illinois

AUTHORS

TRAVIS O. ABICHT, MD
Assistant Professor, Department of
Surgery-Cardiac Surgery, Northwestern
University Feinberg School of Medicine,
Chicago, Illinois

MICHAEL P. ANGARONE, DO
Division of Infectious Diseases, Northwestern
University Feinberg School of Medicine,
Chicago, Illinois

KRISTY M. BORAWSKI, MD
Department of Urology, University of North
Carolina at Chapel Hill, Chapel Hill, North
Carolina

DANIEL P. BOYLE, MD
Clinical Instructor, Division of Infectious
Diseases, Department of Medicine,
Northwestern University Feinberg School of
Medicine, Chicago, Illinois

AMANDA C. CHI, MD
Chief Resident, Department of Urology,
Northwestern University Feinberg School of
Medicine, Chicago, Illinois

HILLARY L. COPP, MD, MS
Associate Professor of Urology, University of
California – San Francisco, San Francisco,
California

KERI DETWEILER, DO
Touro University College of Osteopathic
Medicine – California, Vallejo, California

MATTHEW FERRONI, MD
PGY-5, Physician Resident, Department of
Urology, University of Pittsburgh Medical
Center, Pittsburgh, Pennsylvania

SOPHIE G. FLETCHER, MD
Kaiser Permanente Northern California, Santa
Rosa, California

DANIEL J. FUCHS, MD
Department of Orthopedic Surgery,
Northwestern University Feinberg School of
Medicine, Chicago, Illinois

ALEXANDER P. GLASER, MD
Department of Urology, Northwestern
University Feinberg School of Medicine,
Chicago, Illinois

CHRIS M. GONZALEZ, MD
Department of Urology, Northwestern
University Feinberg School of Medicine,
Chicago, Illinois

MATTHIAS D. HOFER, MD
Department of Urology, Northwestern
University Feinberg School of Medicine,
Chicago, Illinois

TRACY MARIEN, MD
Department of Urologic Surgery, Vanderbilt
University Medical Center, Nashville,
Tennessee

DANIEL MAYERS, DO
Touro University College of Osteopathic
Medicine – California, Vallejo, California

DANIEL J. MAZUR, MD
Department of Urology, Northwestern
University Feinberg School of Medicine,
Chicago, Illinois

BARRY B. McGUIRE, MD
Endourology Fellow, Department of Urology,
Northwestern University Feinberg School of
Medicine, Chicago, Illinois

MAXIM J. McKIBBEN, MD
Department of Urology, University of North
Carolina at Chapel Hill, Chapel Hill, North
Carolina

NICOLE L. MILLER, MD
Associate Professor, Department of Urologic
Surgery, Vanderbilt University Medical Center,
Nashville, Tennessee

ADAM BRYANT MURPHY, MD, MBA, MSCI
Assistant Professor, Department of Urology,
Northwestern Memorial Hospital, Chicago,
Illinois

ROBERT B. NADLER, MD
Professor and Vice Chair, Department of
Urology, Northwestern University Feinberg
School of Medicine, Chicago, Illinois

TERRANCE D. PEABODY, MD
Professor and Chair, Department of
Orthopedic Surgery, Northwestern University
Feinberg School of Medicine, Chicago,
Illinois

SHERRY S. ROSS, MD
Department of Urology, University of North
Carolina at Chapel Hill, Chapel Hill, North
Carolina

ANTHONY J. SCHAEFFER, MD
Chair, Department of Urology,
Herman L. Kretschmer Professor of Urology,
Northwestern University Feinberg School of
Medicine, Chicago, Illinois

BOGDANA SCHMIDT, MD, MPH
Urology Resident, University of
California – San Francisco, San Francisco,
California

PATRICK SEED, MD, PhD
Division of Infectious Disease, Department of
Pediatrics, Duke University Medical Center,
Durham, North Carolina

LINDSAY SMITH, MD
Division of Infectious Diseases, Northwestern
University Feinberg School of Medicine,
Chicago, Illinois

AISHA KHALALI TAYLOR, MD
Assistant Professor; Physician, Department of
Urology, University of Pittsburgh Medical
Center, Pittsburgh, Pennsylvania

LEWIS THOMAS, MD
Department of Urology, University of Iowa
Hospitals and Clinics, Iowa City, Iowa

CHAD R. TRACY, MD
Associate Professor, Department of Urology,
University of Iowa Hospitals and Clinics,
Iowa City, Iowa

TERESA R. ZEMBOWER, MD
Associate Professor, Division of Infectious
Diseases, Department of Medicine,
Northwestern University Feinberg School of
Medicine, Chicago, Illinois

Contents

Mechanical bowel preparation (MBP) and antibiotics (oral and/or intravenous) have historically been used to decrease infectious complications in surgeries that involve manipulation of bowel or potential risk of injury. The use of MBP has recently been challenged in the colorectal surgery literature, thus inspiring similar critical evaluation of our practices in urology. This review gives a brief overview of the history of mechanical and oral antibiotic bowel preparation, as well as the evolution of the practice trends in colorectal surgery and urology. We also examine contemporary guidelines in skin preparation as well as antimicrobial prophylaxis before surgery.

Infection of artificial joint replacements and heart valves is an uncommon but serious complication encountered anytime after the implantation of these prostheses. It is known that bacteremia can lead to infection of a prosthetic device. However, there is no strong evidence to correlate urologic procedures with the development of periprosthetic joint infection or prosthetic valve endocarditis. Therefore, antibiotic prophylaxis for the prevention of endocarditis is not recommended in patients undergoing urologic procedures. However, guidelines regarding prophylaxis to prevent infection of an artificial joint in the setting of a genitourinary procedure are more varied.

Transrectal ultrasound-guided biopsy of the prostate (TRUSP) remains the primary procedure for the accurate histologic diagnosis of prostate cancer. Fluoroquinolones (FQs) are still recommended as the agents of choice for antimicrobial prophylaxis for TRUSP despite the alarming increasing incidence of FQ-resistant organisms among men undergoing TRUSP. This article reviews the current TRUSP antimicrobial prophylaxis guidelines, antimicrobial resistance and its implications for these guidelines, the incidence of post-TRUSP infectious complications including urosepsis, the seminal data supporting pre-TRUSP rectal swab (RS), RS technique and protocol, and the current available literature surrounding the efficacy of RS in reducing post-TRUSP infectious complications.

Infected kidney stones refer to stones that form because of urinary tract infections with urease-producing bacteria, secondarily infected stones of any composition, or stones obstructing the urinary tract leading to pyelonephritis. The mainstay of treatment of infection stones is complete stone removal. Kidney stones that obstruct the urinary tract and cause obstructive pyelonephritis are also frequently referred to as infected stones. Obstructive pyelonephritis is a urologic emergency as it can result in sepsis and even death. Infection stones and obstructive stones causing pyelonephritis are different disease processes, and their workup and management are described separately.

Funguria, and particularly candiduria, is an increasingly common problem encountered by the practicing urologist and is associated with high-acuity care, indwelling catheters, diabetes mellitus, antibiotic and steroid use, and urinary tract disease. In most cases, candiduria is asymptomatic and follows a benign clinical course with antifungal therapy only required in symptomatic or high-risk cases, because spontaneous resolution is common in patients with asymptomatic colonization. Rarely, invasive infections can occur (such as fungus balls or renal abscesses) and may require percutaneous and endoscopic interventions. This article highlights the workup and treatment of funguria and its related urologic manifestations.

Implantation of penile prostheses and artificial urinary sphincters have gained widespread acceptance for the treatment of refractory erectile dysfunction and incontinence, respectively. In the past 3 decades, improved device design and an increased understanding of the pathophysiology of device infections have contributed to a decrease in infection rates. However, understanding the concepts related to infection prevention and management remains critical. In this article, the authors review and discuss these concepts and provide outlines for the practicing urologists for both infection prevention and treatment.

Worldwide prevalence of antimicrobial resistance is rapidly increasing, primarily a result of antibiotic misuse in the medical community. Resistant infections involving the urinary tract are typically caused by gram-negative bacteria. When treating these infections, clinicians have few effective antimicrobials to choose from and many are associated with significant adverse effects. There are now situations when clinicians are tasked with managing infections from pan-resistant organisms; thus, it is of paramount importance that spread of resistance be controlled. This review discusses common gram-negative resistance classes, highlighting the mechanisms of resistance, risk factors, type of infections, treatment, and outcomes associated with each class.

antimicrobial overuse. This article reviews definitions of ASB, epidemiology of ASB, literature surrounding ASB in diabetic patients, risk factors of ASB, microbiologic data regarding bacterial virulence, use of ASB strains for treatment of symptomatic urinary tract infection, and approaches to addressing translational barriers to implementing IDSA recommendations regarding diagnosis and management of ASB.

Bacteriuria during pregnancy may be classified as asymptomatic bacteriuria, infections of the lower urinary tract (cystitis), or infections of the upper urinary tract (pyelonephritis). Lower tract bacteriuria is associated with an increased risk of developing pyelonephritis in pregnancy, which is itself associated with adverse maternal and fetal outcomes. Pregnant women should be screened for the presence of bacteriuria early in pregnancy. All bacteriuria in pregnancy should be treated, and antimicrobial choice in pregnancy should reflect safety for both the mother and the fetus. After treatment of bacteriuria, patients should be followed closely due to risk of recurrent bacteriuria.

Both urinary tract infection (UTI) and asymptomatic bacteriuria (ASB) are common problems among elderly adults and represent a significant health care burden. Despite their frequency, differentiating between ASB and true UTI remains controversial among health care providers. Several challenges exist in the evaluation of urinary symptoms in the elderly patient. Symptoms of UTI are variable; problems are encountered in the collection, testing, and interpretation of urine specimens; and results of urinalysis are often misinterpreted and mishandled. Multiple studies have shown no morbidity or mortality benefit to antibiotic therapy in either community or long-term care facility residents with ASB.

UROLOGIC CLINICS OF NORTH AMERICA

RELATED INTEREST

Infectious Disease Clinics of North America, March 2014 (Vol. 28, Issue 1)
Urinary Tract Infections: Diagnostic and Management Issues
Kalpana Gupta, *Editor*

THE CLINICS ARE AVAILABLE ONLINE!
Access your subscription at:
www.theclinics.com

Foreword

Contemporary Antibiotic Management for Urologic Procedures and Infections

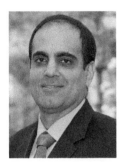

Samir S. Taneja, MD
Consulting Editor

Infection is a problem ubiquitous to medicine, but antisepsis carries a unique role in the evolution of Urology as a medical specialty. Prior to the emergence of Urology as a surgical discipline, urologic procedures (cystolithalopaxy) were carried out by traveling barbers. Bladder stones were removed through a largely blind transperineal extraction procedure with high rates of mortality due to bleeding and perineal sepsis. Those who survived did so because of the rich vascularity of the perineum allowing for clearance of infection. With the emergence of antisepsis (and anesthesia), urologic procedures transitioned to more methodical, deliberate procedures requiring formal training and medical basis.

The management of urologic disease requires consideration of infections pre-existing within the urinary tract, those emerging from urologic disease (obstruction, stones, and stasis), and those introduced through urologic procedures. With the widespread use and overuse of antibiotics in medicine, the emergence of antibiotic-resistant strains of bacteria and fungi has further complicated the management of our patients. In particular, recently, the performance of routine procedures, such as cystoscopy, prostate biopsy, or nephrostomy placement, utilizing recommended antibiotic prophylaxis, has resulted in near-fatal infectious complications.

The rate of infectious complications in the United States is rising, resulting in a need for standardized approaches to antibiotic prophylaxis and individualized approaches to address antibiotic resistance. In this issue of *Urologic Clinics*, Drs Sarah C. Flury and Anthony J. Schaeffer have created a comprehensive overview of antibiotic strategies in contemporary urologic practice, including anticipating and dealing with drug resistance. Each of the authors has done a fantastic job in presenting the latest recommendations for managing infectious problems in a variety of settings. This is one issue that I have no doubt will be of value to every practicing urologist as there are topics that impact every type of urologic practice. I am deeply indebted to our guest editors and authors for a fantastic issue.

Samir S. Taneja, MD
Division of Urologic Oncology
Smilow Comprehensive Prostate Cancer Center
Department of Urology
NYU Langone Medical Center
150 East 32nd Street, Suite 200
New York, NY 10016, USA

E-mail address:
samir.taneja@nyumc.org

Urol Clin N Am 42 (2015) xiii
http://dx.doi.org/10.1016/j.ucl.2015.09.001
0094-0143/15/$ – see front matter © 2015 Published by Elsevier Inc.

urologic.theclinics.com

Preface

Contemporary Antibiotic Management for Urologic Procedures and Infections

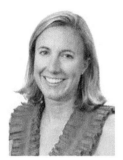 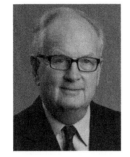

Sarah C. Flury, MD   Anthony J. Schaeffer, MD

Editors

The challenge to tailor antibiotic choices to the individual patient as well as the specific procedure is ever increasing in the modern era of multi-drug-resistant organisms and increasingly complex patients and surgeries. The urologist faces decisions every day in both clinical practice and the operating room setting on how to effectively utilize antibiotics while taking into account individual patient factors as well as procedural factors. The goals of minimizing the incidence of infections and limiting morbidity from infections are shared by clinicians across the specialties ranging from Cardiology, to Orthopedics, to Infectious Disease, to Obstetrics, to Pediatrics, to Internal Medicine. Collaboration on the part of the physicians is key to managing individual patients with infections that require treatment and in procedures that necessitate prophylaxis. Judicious use of antibiotics in the appropriate doses for the indicated duration helps to limit the development of resistant organisms and to maintain the efficacy of broad spectrum antibiotics for the continued treatment of patients in the future.

In this issue of *Urologic Clinics*, we focus on antibiotic management in cases specific to the urologist, including penile prosthesis and artificial urinary sphincters, transrectal prostate biopsy, and stone treatment, as well as general open and laparoscopic urologic surgeries. We also address antibiotic management for urologic infections in multiple specific patient scenarios, including UTI in pregnancy, UTI in patients with neurogenic bladder, and infections in the elderly, as well as the workup of pediatric UTI. Sexually transmitted infections and fungal infections are also covered in detail. Our goal is for this issue to provide guidance to physicians in urology as well as other specialties as we all work to effectively treat urologic infections and provide appropriate prophylaxis prior to procedures in order to minimize incidence of infections. Maintaining efficacy of antibiotics, minimizing morbidity from infection, and managing complex patients in the setting of increasingly resistant organisms are challenges best met by a multidisciplinary approach.

Thank you to all who contributed their time and expertise to this issue. We appreciate all the work that went into assembling this comprehensive review and anticipate that it will serve as

Urol Clin N Am 42 (2015) xv–xvi
http://dx.doi.org/10.1016/j.ucl.2015.08.014
0094-0143/15/$ – see front matter © 2015 Published by Elsevier Inc.

urologic.theclinics.com

a guide for clinicians across the specialties as they manage urologic infections in the modern era.

Sarah C. Flury, MD
Department of Urology
Feinberg School of Medicine
Northwestern University
675 North Saint Clair Street
Suite 20-150
Chicago, IL 60611, USA

Anthony J. Schaeffer, MD
Department of Urology
Tarry 16-715
Feinberg School of Medicine
Northwestern University
303 East Chicago Avenue
Chicago, IL 60611, USA

E-mail addresses:
sflury@nm.org (S.C. Flury)
ajschaeffer@northwestern.edu (A.J. Schaeffer)

Modern Guidelines for Bowel Preparation and Antimicrobial Prophylaxis for Open and Laparoscopic Urologic Surgery

Amanda C. Chi, MD, Barry B. McGuire, MD,
Robert B. Nadler, MD*

KEYWORDS

- Bowel preparation • Antimicrobial prophylaxis • Oral antibiotic bowel preparation

KEY POINTS

- Evidence would suggest that mechanical bowel preparation can be safely omitted in cystectomy with ileal urinary diversion.
- Use of oral antibiotic bowel preparation in urology has not been well studied, although colorectal literature shows that it is associated with decreased rate of infective complications.
- Intravenous antibiotic prophylaxis should be given within 1 hour before incision and discontinued 24 hours after termination of surgery unless patient has risk factors.

INTRODUCTION

Historically, preoperative mechanical bowel preparation (MBP) has been considered the standard of care in patients undergoing colorectal and urologic surgeries involving bowel.[1,2] In recent years, the routine preoperative MBP has been questioned, with a shift away from use in both colorectal[3,4] and urology literature.[5] In this review, we examine the evidence behind MBP, antimicrobial prophylaxis (AMP), and skin preparation for open and laparoscopic urologic surgeries.

MECHANICAL BOWEL PREPARATION
Rationale

The main concerns of a surgeon performing bowel anastomosis include infectious complications, bowel leak, and anastomotic dehiscence. Additionally, quick recovery of bowel function and reduction of the hospital length of stay are other important goals. These objectives spurred many historical prophylaxis regimens, which continue to a large extent today. Ironically, recent evidence would suggest that these practices may not serve these goals.

Mechanical cleansing of the bowel was thought to be associated with a lower complication rate by decreasing intestinal microflora; however, even early studies reported that MBP did not reduce the concentration of intestinal microflora in the ileum, colon, and stool.[2] In fact, a more contemporary study showed that patients who received MBP actually have more bacteria at the anastomosis compared with those who did not received MBP.[6]

Disclosure: The authors of this paper have nothing to disclose.
Department of Urology, Northwestern University Feinberg School of Medicine, Chicago, IL 60611, USA
* Corresponding author. Department of Urology, Northwestern University Feinberg School of Medicine, 675 North Saint Clair Street, Suite 20-150, Chicago, IL 60611.
E-mail address: r-nadler@northwestern.edu

Urol Clin N Am 42 (2015) 429–440
http://dx.doi.org/10.1016/j.ucl.2015.05.007
0094-0143/15/$ – see front matter © 2015 Elsevier Inc. All rights reserved.

Another perception is that MBP decreases intestinal contents, thereby limiting spillage into the peritoneal cavity at the time of bowel resection, thus potentially decreasing infective complication rates; however, evidence would suggest the contrary. A prospective trial of MBP versus none in 333 patients undergoing colorectal surgery showed a higher spillage rate in patients with liquid bowel contents, which was associated with MBP.[7] Although this study demonstrated a trend toward higher surgical and overall complication rates when spillage occurred, this did not achieve statistical significance.

Last, concerns with regard to anastomotic leak and wound infections have been extensively reviewed in colorectal literature. A recent Cochrane review of 18 trials evaluating a role of MBP in elective colorectal surgery demonstrated that there was no difference between anastomotic leakage or wound infection when MBP is compared with none or compared with rectal enema alone.[8] In a more recent review by the Agency for Healthcare Research and Quality of 60 studies, there was no difference in all-cause mortality, anastomotic leakage, wound infection, and peritonitis for patients undergoing elective colorectal surgery.[9]

Types of Mechanical Bowel Preparation

MBP has evolved since first popularized by Nichols and colleagues[10] in the early 1970s. The Nichols-Condon preparation has been used for colorectal surgery and often adopted by urologists. Freiha[1] also described a mechanical and antibiotic preparation regimen for urologic surgery in 1977 (**Table 1**). Since then, different agents and regimens have emerged. Current literature of MBP agents primarily come from gastroenterology exploring the efficacy of various regimens in the setting of colonoscopy.[11] Contemporary practices

are usually less extensive than those of the Nichols-Condon or Freiha regimens. The different types of MBP are reviewed in **Table 2**.

Oral Antibiotics in Combination with Mechanical Bowel Preparation

Although the routine administration of parenteral antibiotics is recommended in nearly all patients, the use of oral antibiotics has largely fallen out of favor. Similar to the use of MBP, the practice of using oral antimicrobials to decrease intraluminal bacterial load has decreased over time, from 87% to 92% routine use in colorectal surgery in the 1990s[3,12] to 36% in a 2010 survey.[4] However, there is recent renewed interest in evaluating the effect of oral antibiotic use.[13] Using oral antibiotics to decrease intraluminal microbial burden began in 1940[14] and was popularized in the early 1970s by Nichols and colleagues.[10,15] They showed that use of oral neomycin and erythromycin (see **Table 1**) in combination with MBP decreased bacterial concentration from intraluminal aspirates of ileum, cecum, and transverse colon, and was superior in MBP alone in preventing wound infections.[10,15]

More recently, a large retrospective analysis in 9940 patients found that the use of oral antibiotics, with or without MBP, was associated with 67% decrease in surgical site infection (SSI) in colorectal surgeries.[16] The reduction of SSI maintained even if MBP was not performed. Similarly, a prospective, multi-institution study demonstrated that patients undergoing colorectal surgery and receiving oral antibiotics with MBP are less likely to have SSI (4.5% vs 11.8%), organ space infection (1.8% vs 4.2%), and superficial SSI (2.6% vs 7.6%) when compared with MBP alone. They also had lower rate of prolonged ileus of 3.9% versus 8.6%, and a similar rate of *Clostridium difficile* infection.[17] Meta-analysis of randomized controlled trials

| Table 1 Traditional mechanical bowel preparation regimens | |
Author	Regimen
Nichols et al,[10] 1972	• *Pre-Op Day 3*: low-residue diet; bisacodyl 5 mg orally at 6 PM • *Pre-Op Day 2*: low-residue diet; magnesium sulfate, 30 mL of 50% solution (15 g) orally at 10 AM, 2 PM, and 6 PM; saline enemas in the evening until returns clear • *Pre-Op Day 1*: clear-liquid diet; magnesium sulfate; 30 mL of 50% at 10 AM, 2 PM, no enemas; neomycin 1 g and erythromycin base 1 g at 1, 2, and 11 PM
Freiha,[1] 1977	• *Pre-Op Day 2*: clear liquid diet, 30 g magnesium citrate and 2 tablets bisacodyl, cleansing soap suds enemas until clear • *Pre-Op Day 1*: clear liquid diet; 1 g neomycin every hour × 4 h, then 1 g every 4 h for total of 7 g. Erythromycin base orally 4 times daily (4 g), neomycin enema in the evening. No oral food or drink after midnight • Gentamicin (80 mg), intramuscular with induction of anesthesia

Table 2
Mechanical bowel preparation agents

Agent	Dosage and Precautions
Polyethylene glycol-3350 (PEG) electrolyte solution (GoLYTELY and NuLYTELY: Braintree Laboratories, Braintree, MA)	• Dosage: reconstitute in 4 L solution • Contraindications: gastrointestinal obstruction, ileus, or • Gastric retention, bowel perforation, toxic colitis, toxic megacolon, or known hypersensitivity[74,75]
PEG alone	• Dosage: 238 g PEG in combination with ~2 L carbohydrate electrolyte solution, such as Gatorade (PepsiCo Inc [Purchase, New York]) and bisacodyl • Shown in population undergoing colonoscopy to be as effective as GoLYTELY or NuLYTELY[76] • Contraindications: same as PEG electrolyte solutions
Magnesium citrate	• Dosage: 150–300 mL • Electrolytes should be monitored in patients with renal disease and magnesium intake of >50 mEq, as magnesium citrate can cause hyponatremia and hypermagnesemia in susceptible populations[77] • Contraindications: hypersensitivity, acute abdomen, gastrointestinal obstruction, appendicitis
Oral sodium phosphate solution	• Dosage: 45 mL × 2 • Tolerability and efficacy is generally better than PEG[78] • Induces hyperphosphatemia, hypocalcemia, and hypokalemia • Elderly patients and those with compromised renal function are at risk for significant electrolyte disturbances[79]

showed that nonabsorbable oral antibiotic in addition to an intravenous antibiotic versus intravenous antibiotic alone had reduced risk of wound infections with relative risk of 0.57. No difference was seen between the groups with regard to risk of anastomotic leak or intra-abdominal abscess.[18] The 1999 Centers for Disease Control and Prevention guidelines for prevention of SSIs continue to advocate for nonabsorbable oral antimicrobials administered in divided doses the day before colorectal surgeries.[19]

There is a paucity of studies evaluating the effect of the use of oral antibiotic bowel preparation for urologic surgeries. The use of oral antibiotics has traditionally been advocated for urinary diversion using bowel segment,[5,20] although the use of oral antibiotics has been eliminated in various contemporary series evaluating MBP in cystectomy and urinary diversion. These oral antibiotic regimens are described in **Table 3**.

Disadvantages of Mechanical and Antibiotic Bowel Preparation

Although the complications associated with MBP and/or oral antibiotic ingestion are low, risks are acceptable if offset against perceived benefit. Urologic operations that incorporate bowel are usually operations associated with increased operative duration, or in patients with more risk factors. For instance, radical cystectomies with urinary diversion are often performed in patients older than

Table 3
Oral antibiotic bowel preparation regimens

Antibiotic	Regimen
Kanamycin	• *Pre-Op Day 3*: 1 g orally every h × 4 h, then every 4 h • *Pre-Op Days 2 and 1*: 1 g orally 4 times daily
Neomycin + erythromycin base	• *Pre-Op Day 1*: 1 g erythromycin base + 1 g neomycin at 1 PM, 2 PM, and 11 PM
Neomycin + metronidazole	• *Pre-Op days 2 and 1*: 1 g neomycin 4 times daily + 750 mg metronidazole 4 times daily

Data from Dahl D, McDougal WS. Use of intestinal segments in urinary diversion. In: Wein A, Kavoussi L, Novick A, et al, editors. Campbell-Walsh urology. 10th edition. Philadelphia: Saunders; 2012. p. 2411–49.

70 years with extensive smoking history, and as such have other respiratory or cardiovascular co-morbidities. Additionally, bladder augmentations are performed in patients with neurogenic blad-ders who often have other comorbidities also, including hypoalbuminemia. Therefore, if MBP and/or oral antibiotic ingestion offers no distinct advantage, then 1 to 2 days of fasting or clear fluids, diarrhea, and potential for dehydration would be best avoided.

MBP adverse effects are largely associated with electrolyte disturbances, which would be normally tolerated except in those with renal dysfunction, or the elderly. There also have been case reports of electrolyte abnormalities and seizures with use of sodium picosulfates/magnesium citrate for bowel preparation in patients without history of sei-zures.[21] Histologic studies have revealed loss of superficial mucus with epithelial cells, as well as inflammatory changes within the bowel wall in patients undergoing MBP.[22]

The use of oral antibiotics to alter intestinal flora raises the question of whether patients are placed at higher risk for C difficile infection. Retrospective case-controlled study of patients receiving elective colon surgery who underwent MBP showed that the rate of C difficile infection within 30 days was 7.4% in those who received oral antibiotics versus 2.6% in those who did not receive oral antibiotics.[23] However, several recent studies have shown no increased rate of C difficile infection in those who received oral antibiotics (1.3% vs 1.8%),[17,24] but there also is no increased rate in those who received MBP versus those who did not.[24]

Bowel Preparation in Urology

Although colorectal surgery experience can guide practices, urologic surgery may have different re-quirements; most commonly small bowel is used, which has different microbiota from large bowel. Bacterial density increases in the distal small bowel (duodenum 10^1–10^3 colony-forming units [CFU]/mL, jejunum/ileum 10^4–10^7 CFU/mL), but it is still at markedly lower concentration than large bowel contents of 10^6–10^{12} CFU/mL.[2,25–27] Furthermore, bowel segments are typically incor-porated into the urinary tract, exposing sterile en-vironments to bowel contents.

Cystectomy with urinary diversion

Routine MBP before cystectomy and urinary diver-sion has recently been challenged and the evi-dence would suggest that MBP confers no distinct advantage. Although the reference uro-logic textbook Campbell-Walsh Urology 2012 rec-ommends 4 L polyethylene glycol 3350 and electrolytes starting noon the day before surgery,

along with intravenous hydration and oral antibi-otic preparation when using intestinal segments for urinary diversion,[20,28] many studies have concluded that there is no difference between mortality, infection rate, and bowel leakage rate.[26,27,29–33] In fact, a meta-analysis of 2 ran-domized controlled trials and 5 cohort studies looking at the impact of MBP on cystectomy with ileal urinary diversion showed no difference be-tween MBP versus none with regard to bowel leak, obstruction, or mortality rate.[34] One retro-spective review showed that there was increased length of stay and higher incidence of prolonged ileus in the MBP group.[32] Furthermore, in patients undergoing MBP in combination with oral antibi-otics, there is a higher frequency of mucosal edema and submucosal congestion on histopath-ological examination of ileum, and ironically a higher rate of bacterial overgrowth of Escherichia coli.[26] Although there are no American guidelines on the use of bowel preparation, European Associ-ation of Urology guidelines suggested that preop-erative bowel preparation is not mandatory before radical cystectomy.[35]

Enhanced recovery protocols

Recent emergence of enhanced recovery after sur-gery (ERAS) protocols for radical cystectomy and urinary diversion, which eliminate MBP and oral antibiotic preparation, have further corroborated evidence in support of abandoning MBP. In fact, evidence from these studies would suggest that MBP is possibly doing more harm than good. For example, in a retrospective series published by Daneshmand and colleagues,[36] excellent periop-erative, infective, and readmission rate outcomes were demonstrated in 110 patients receiving ERAS without MBP. When compared with a histor-ical group of matched patients, a significantly shorter hospital stay of 4 versus 8 days was observed in the ERAS group. Similarly, another ERAS study that eliminated the use of sodium pi-cosulfate MBP in cystectomy with patients receiving ileal urinary diversion demonstrated no differences in morbidity or mortality between groups, and again significantly reduced hospital stay in those receiving ERAS without MBP.[37] In 2013, a systematic review of the literature of cur-rent ERAS after radical cystectomy did not demon-strate any improvement in outcomes with MBP.[38]

Enterocystoplasty

The role of MBP in patients undergoing enterocys-toplasty, who commonly have concomitant neuro-genic bowel, has not been well studied. A study in children with myelomeningocele and constipation showed that 39% of children in the study have small intestinal bacterial overgrowth confirmed by H_2/CH_4 lactulose breath tests.[39] The increased bacterial load in small bowel in this population can potentially expose the augmented urinary tract to different bacterial concentration when compared with patients without neurogenic bowel or constipation undergoing the same surgery. Despite that, case series in the pediatric literature shows no difference in outcomes between children who underwent cystoplasty using ileum with preoperative MBP versus those who did not undergo MBP.[40] A retrospective review of 162 children undergoing enterocystoplasty without preoperative MBP, where colonic segments were used in more than 85% of the patients, showed no increased rate of complications.[41] Expert opinion in the field continues to be divided and questions whether or not omission of MBP can be adopted widely to those with constipation or neurogenic bowel, where large fecal bolus distal to the anastomotic site might become a source of obstruction. Suggestions have been made to consider abdominal radiography to determine if there is large fecal bolus distal to the future anastomotic site to prompt use of preoperative MBP.[40]

Radical prostatectomy

Because of the intimate anatomic relationship between the prostate and rectum, intraoperative rectal injury can occur, at a rate of 0% to 8.2% for open prostatectomy[42] and 0.8% to 1.2% in robotic-assisted laparoscopic prostatectomy (RALP).[43] MBP traditionally has been used to decrease potential complications, such as infections and fistula formation, in the event of rectal injury and to avoid the need for diverting colostomy in a primary repair.[44,45] Older literature advocates diverting colostomy in the event of rectal injury in unprepared bowel given reports of higher complication rate after primary repair in patients who did not undergo MBP.[42,46] Now, some investigators advocate the use of diverting colostomy only for those with massive fecal spillage, previous radiotherapy, or a tense suture line.[47] Whether there is a need for full MBP versus modified protocols continues to be debated, especially in the modern era of RALP, which now accounts for the overwhelming majority of radical prostatectomies carried out currently in the United States.[48] In the senior author's (RBN) experience, during RALP, minor rectal injuries recognized intraoperatively can safely be repaired robotically, without the need for tissue interposition or diverting colostomy. However, experience of all of these to date occurred in patients who received MBP, and moving away from this practice is difficult without a high level of evidence to persuade otherwise. Published data are

nearly exclusively in open surgery, where other investigators describe successful primary repair of rectal injuries without MBP, but using omentum as interposition flap.[49] Another retrospective review of an open radical prostatectomy cohort in Japan demonstrated that, in those who sustained rectal injuries, there was no difference in outcomes between the MBP group and non-MBP group with regard to infectious complication, delayed colostomy rate, length of stay, or total cost.[50] Most contemporary series reviewing the outcomes of repair of intraoperative rectal injury still include preoperative MBP. The investigators in several studies noted that they have trended away from MBP, although they continue to advocate the use of MBP in select patients with high-grade disease and suggested that MBP should be considered for those with history of previous transurethral resection of the prostate or radiotherapy.[42,51] Evidence would suggest that many urologists find it difficult to move away from indoctrinated practices too. In a recent survey of US urologists, 35% of those who performed open prostatectomy use MBP, whereas 19% use enema alone; 55% of urologists who perform laparoscopic and/or RALP used MBP for these surgeries, whereas 16% use enema alone (Chi AC, McGuire BB, Nadler RB: Bowel preparation in urologic surgery: practice pattern amongst urologists, 2015. Submitted manuscript). For both open prostatectomy and RALP, many experts still recommend clear liquid diet and magnesium citrate on day before surgery, with an enema on the morning of surgery.[52,53]

Laparoscopic and robotic surgery

Little has been published assessing the need of MBP in laparoscopic surgeries. The Society of American Gastrointestinal and Endoscopic Surgeons guidelines recommended the use of MBP, recognizing the lack of evidence, before laparoscopic resection of curable colon and rectal cancer, to facilitate bowel manipulation and possibility for intraoperative endoscopy.[54] Expert opinion in urology agrees that although no MBP is necessary for laparoscopic and robotic operations that are extraperitoneal or retroperitoneal, MBP might be helpful to improve visualization and working space. For transperitoneal procedures not using bowel segments, a light MBP, such as clear liquid diet, Dulcolax suppository, or half dose of magnesium citrate can be used. Surgeries in which entry into the bowel lumen is anticipated, or if dense intra-abdominal adhesions are likely to be encountered, a full MBP is suggested.[55,56] However, more recent studies suggest that MBP in surgeries not involving bowel can be omitted. A retrospective study in Japan showed that for patients undergoing laparoscopic nephrectomy for T1-T3 tumor, the use of MBP did not affect operating room time, length of stay, or overall complications.[57] Another study, randomizing 308 patients undergoing laparoscopic gynecologic surgery to MBP versus none showed that although intraoperative surgical view and bowel handling was statistically better in the MBP group, the small difference was not clinically important.[58] In a survey conducted among adult urologists practicing in the United States, there is a wide range of frequency of MBP use across various urologic surgeries, shown in **Fig. 1** (Chi AC, McGuire BB, Nadler RB: Bowel preparation in urologic surgery: practice pattern amongst urologists, 2015. Submitted manuscript).

ANTIMICROBIAL PROPHYLAXIS
Before Skin Incision

The use of antibiotics shortly before incision for preventing wound infection was pioneered by Dr Seley in 1939.[59] Since then, it is accepted that the use of prophylactic antibiotics reduces surgical wound infection, when compared with placebo or no treatment. A Cochrane review of AMP in colorectal surgery showed a reduction in risk from 39% to 13% with AMP.[60] Importantly, the same review showed that combined oral and intravenous AMP was superior for prevention of wound infections when compared with either route alone (risk ratio (RR) 0.44 and RR 0.47, respectively).[60] Similar to other surgical specialties, urologic surgery is concerned with wound and organ space infections, but it is unique in that the manipulation of the urinary tract coinciding with catheter and stent placement make prevention of urinary tract infections an additional concern.

The timing of prophylactic antibiotics in elective clean and clean-contaminated surgical procedures is optimal when given within 2 hours before incision. The relative risk of infection is 6.7 higher when AMP is given 2 to 24 hours before incision, and 2.4 higher when it is given within 3 hours after incision.[61] The antimicrobial also should be maintained at therapeutic serum and tissue levels throughout the operation.[62] In the American Urologic Association (AUA)'s Best Practice Policy Statement on Antimicrobial Prophylaxis, AMP should begin within 1 hour of incision, or within 2 hours for intravenous fluoroquinolones and vancomycin.[63]

With the exception of transurethral resection of prostate and prostate biopsy, the use of AMP has not been extensively studied for urologic surgeries. Consequently, recommendations are generally offered based on surgical wound classification. AUA's Best Practice Policy Statement on Antimicrobial Prophylaxis for open and laparoscopic urologic surgery is summarized in **Table 4**. Due to lack of sufficient evidence for the benefit of

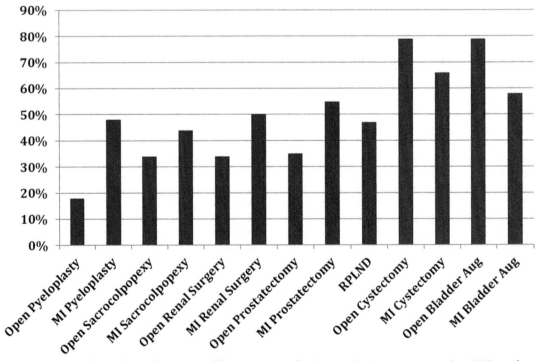

Fig. 1. Frequency of use of MBP for open and laparoscopic urologic surgeries. Aug, augmentation; MBP, mechanical bowel preparation; MI, minimally invasive; RPLND, retroperitoneal lymph node dissection.

Table 4
Recommended antimicrobial prophylaxis for urologic procedures: open or laparoscopic surgery, from 2008 AUA best practice policy statement

Procedure	Organisms	Prophylaxis Indicated	Antimicrobial(s) of Choice	Alternative Antimicrobial(s)	Duration of Therapy[a]
Vaginal surgery (includes urethral sling procedures)	GU tract[b], skin,[g] and Group B Streptococcus	All	• Vaginal surgery Aminoglycoside (aztreonam[c]) + Metronidazole or clindamycin	• Ampicillin/Sulbactam • Fluoroquinolone	≤24 h
Without entering urinary tract	Skin	If risk factors	• 1st gen. cephalosporin	• Clindamycin[d,e]	Single dose
Involving entry into urinary tract	GU tract and skin	All	• Involving entry into urinary tract Aminoglycoside (aztreonam[c]) + Metronidazole or clindamycin	• Ampicillin/Sulbactam • Fluoroquinolone	≤24 h
Involving intestine[h]	GU tract and skin and intestine[f]	All	• 2nd/3rd gen. cephalosporin • Aminoglycoside (aztreonam[c]) + Metronidazole or clindamycin	• Ampicillin/Sulbactam • Ticarcillin/Clavulanate • Piperacillin/Tazobactam • Fluoroquinolone	≤24 h
Involving implanted prosthesis	GU tract and skin	All	• Aminoglycoside (aztreonam[c]) + 1st/2nd gen. cephalosporin or vancomycin	• Ampicillin/Sulbactam • Ticarcillin/Clavulanate • Piperacillin/Tazobactam	≤24 h

Order of agents in each column is not indicative of preference. The absence of an agent does not preclude its appropriate use depending on specific situations.

Abbreviations: AUA, American Urologic Association; gen, generation; GU, genitourinary.

[a] Additional antimicrobial therapy may be recommended at the time of removal of an externalized urinary catheter.

[b] GU tract: Common urinary tract organisms are *Escherichia coli*, *Proteus sp*, *Klebsiella sp*, *Enterococcus*.

[c] Aztreonam can be substituted for aminoglycosides in patients with renal insufficiency.

[d] Clindamycin, or aminoglycoside + metronidazole or clindamycin, are general alternatives to penicillins and cephalosporins in patients with penicillin allergy, even when not specifically listed.

[e] Risk factors: as listed in text.

[f] Intestine: Common intestinal organisms are *E coli*, *Klebsiella sp*, *Enterobacter*, *Serratia sp*, *Serratia sp*, *Proteus sp*, *Enterococcus*, and anaerobes.

[g] Skin: Common skin organisms are *Staphylococcus aureus*, coagulase-negative *Staphylococcus sp*, Group A *Streptococcus sp*.

[h] For surgery involving the colon, bowel preparation with oral neomycin plus either erythromycin base or metronidazole can be added to or substituted for systemic agents.

Data from Wolf J Jr, Bennett C, Dmochowski R, et al. Best practice policy statement on urology surgery antimicrobial prophylaxis. J Urol 2008;179(4):1379–90.

AMP for clean operation, prophylaxis for surgeries such as open or laparoscopic nephrectomy is not indicated, except in patients with risk factors such as advanced age, anatomic anomalies of the urinary tract, poor nutritional status, smoking, chronic corticosteroid use, immunodeficiency, externalized catheters, colonized endogenous/exogenous material, distant coexistent infection, and prolonged hospitalization.[63–66]

Although AMP improves SSI rate, it is not without its consequences. Inappropriate use of antimicrobials can lead to the induction of bacterial resistance in the patient and in the community.[67] Hence, AMP should not extend beyond 24 hours after the procedure except in the following scenarios: placement of prosthetic material, presence of an existing infection, or manipulation of an indwelling tube. In cases in which an external urinary catheter is placed at the time of, or is present before the procedure, additional 24 hours or less of antimicrobial treatment is recommended in patients with risk factors as described previously.[63]

A retrospective cohort study of patients undergoing surgeries ranging from cardiac to gynecologic demonstrated AMP was commonly used beyond 24 hours and was discontinued within 24 hours of surgery end time for only 40.7% of the time.[68] Among US urologists, survey data showed that AMP is commonly continued beyond the 24-hour perioperative period, up to 26% to 36% in cystectomy and bladder augmentations (**Fig. 2**) (Chi AC, McGuire BB, Nadler RB: Bowel preparation in urologic surgery: practice pattern amongst urologists, 2015. Submitted manuscript). Recent study using a large collaborative health care database showed that the overall compliance (correct antibiotics class and therapy duration) rate of the 2008 AUA Best Practice Policy Statement among urologists was 53%, with a 57.8% noncompliance rate in radical prostatectomy, 99.4% in radical cystectomy, and 93.1% in nephrectomy. Average prophylaxis duration was 10.3 days after radical cystectomy.[69] Although these studies are unable to parse out the surgeon reasoning and patient characteristics that prompted deviation from guidelines, they illustrate the need to further investigate the outcomes associated with guideline adherence to determine if our practices or our guidelines need to be amended.

Preparation of Skin

Antiseptic agents are routinely used for preoperative preparation of skin at incision site and any potential incisions sites, with the most commonly used agents being chlorhexidine gluconate,

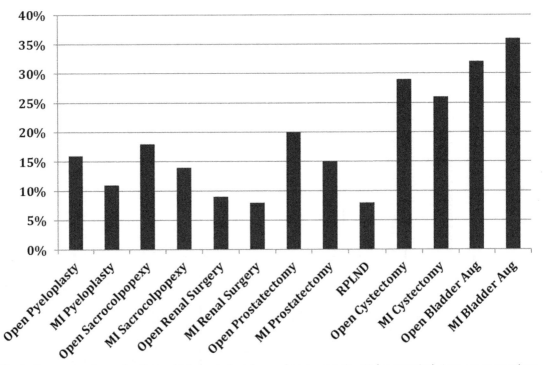

Fig. 2. Frequency of use of antimicrobial prophylaxis beyond peri-operative 24-hour period. Aug, augmentation; MI, minimally invasive; RPLND, retroperitoneal lymph node dissection.

alcohol-containing products, and iodophors such as povidone-iodine. Chlorhexidine gluconate and iodophors both have broad spectra of antimicrobial activity.[62] All are effective against a range of gram-positive and gram-negative bacteria, many fungi, and viruses. Both iodophors and alcohol also are effective against tubercle bacillus.[35] A recent Cochrane review comparing the effectiveness of various antiseptics concluded that even though one study showed weak evidence that 0.5% chlorhexidine in methylated spirits was associated with lower rates of SSIs when compared with an alcohol-based povidone-iodine solution (RR 0.47),[70] there was otherwise no difference in comparisons made between various concentrations of chlorhexidine, iodophors, or alcohol.[71]

Preparation for surgery usually also includes hair removal at site of surgery. Preoperative shaving of the surgical site the night before the operation is associated with higher rate of SSIs than the use of depilatory agents or no hair removal. The increased risk has been attributed to microscopic cuts that can later become nidus for bacterial colonization. Shaving more than 24 hours before operation was associated with more than 20% of SSIs. Shaving immediately before operation was associated with a lower rate of SSIs (3.1% vs 7.1%) when compared to within 24 hours.[72] With regard to methods of hair removal, a recent Cochrane review comparing various methods of hair removal showed that shaving is associated with significantly more SSIs than clipping, with relative risk of 2.09.[73]

SUMMARY

The use of mechanical and oral antibiotic bowel preparation as standard of practice in urology has recently been under scrutiny. Literature suggests that MBP can be safely omitted in RALP, as well as in cystectomy with ileal urinary diversion, prompting cystectomy ERAS protocols to abandon the use of MBP. Fewer studies have shown that MBP also can be safely omitted in enterocystoplasty, radical prostatectomy, and laparoscopic urologic surgeries, although more evidence is needed to change indoctrinated practice. The benefits of use of oral antibiotic bowel preparation in urologic surgeries has yet to be studied, but has been shown to decrease infectious complications in colorectal literature. AMP of appropriate antimicrobial class should be given within 1 hour before incision and stopped 24 hours after the end of the procedure. Although consideration can be given to patients with risk factors, manipulation of indwelling tubes, placement of prosthetic materials, and preexisting infections to extend the duration of AMP, the appropriate

duration has not yet been extensively studied. The low adherence to AMP practice guidelines and wide variation in MBP use present opportunities for future studies for evaluating outcomes associated with our practice patterns.

REFERENCES

1. Freiha FS. Preoperative bowel preparation in urologic surgery. J Urol 1977;118(6):955–6.
2. Nichols R, Gorbach S, Condon R. Alteration of intestinal microflora following preoperative mechanical preparation of the colon. Dis Colon Rectum 1971; 14(2):123–7.
3. Nichols R, Smith J, Garcia R, et al. Current practices of preoperative bowel preparation among North American colorectal surgeons. Clin Infect Dis 1997;24:609–19.
4. Markell KW, Hunt BM, Charron PD, et al. Prophylaxis and management of wound infections after elective colorectal surgery: a survey of the American Society of Colon and Rectal Surgeons membership. J Gastrointest Surg 2010;14(7):1090–8.
5. Ferguson K, McNeil J, Morey A. Mechanical and antibiotic bowel preparation for urinary diversion surgery. J Urol 2002;167:2352–6.
6. Fa-Si-Oen PR, Verwaest C, Buitenweg J, et al. Effect of mechanical bowel preparation with polyethylene-glycol on bacterial contamination and wound infection in patients undergoing elective open colon surgery. Clin Microbiol Infect 2005;11(2):158–60.
7. Mahajna A, Krausz M, Rosin D, et al. Bowel preparation is associated with spillage of bowel contents in colorectal surgery. Dis Colon Rectum 2005;48(8): 1626–31.
8. Güenaga K, Matos D, Wille-Jørgensen P. Mechanical bowel preparation for elective colorectal surgery. Cochrane Database Syst Rev 2011;(9):CD001544.
9. Dahabreh I, Steele D, Shah N, et al. Oral mechanical bowel preparation for colorectal surgery. Rockville (MD): Agency for Healthcare Research and Quality (US); 2014.
10. Nichols R, Condon R, Gorbach S, et al. Efficacy of preoperative antimicrobial preparation of the bowel. Ann Surg 1972;176(2):227–32.
11. Kelly N, Rodgers C, Patterson N, et al. A prospective audit of the efficacy, safety, and acceptability of low-volume polyethylene glycol (2 l) versus standard volume polyethylene glycol (4 L) versus magnesium citrate plus stimulant laxative as bowel preparation for colonoscopy. J Clin Gastroenterol 2012;46:595–601.
12. Solla JA, Rothenberger DA. Preoperative bowel preparation. A survey of colon and rectal surgeons. Dis Colon Rectum 1990;33(2):154–9.

13. Zelhart MD, Hauch AT, Slakey DP, et al. Preoperative antibiotic colon preparation: have we had the answer all along? J Am Coll Surg 2014;219(5):1070–7.

14. Poth E. Historical development of intestinal antisepsis. World J Surg 1982;6:153–9.

15. Nichols R, Broido P, Condon R, et al. Effect of preoperative neomycin-erythromycin intestinal preparation on the incidence of infectious complications following colon surgery. Ann Surg 1973;178:453–62.

16. Cannon JA, Altom LK, Deierhoi RJ, et al. Preoperative oral antibiotics reduce surgical site infection following elective colorectal resections. Dis Colon Rectum 2012;55(11):1160–6.

17. Englesbe MJ, Brooks L, Kubus J, et al. A statewide assessment of surgical site infection following colectomy: the role of oral antibiotics. Ann Surg 2010; 252(3):514–9 [discussion: 519–20].

18. Bellows CF, Mills KT, Kelly TN, et al. Combination of oral non-absorbable and intravenous antibiotics versus intravenous antibiotics alone in the prevention of surgical site infections after colorectal surgery: a meta-analysis of randomized controlled trials. Tech Coloproctol 2011;15(4):385–95.

19. Mangram A, Horan T, Pearson M, et al. Guideline for prevention of surgical site infection, 1999. Infect Control Hosp Epidemiol 1999;20(4):247–78.

20. Dahl D, McDougal WS. Use of intestinal segments in urinary diversion. In: Wein A, Kavoussi L, Novick A, et al, editors. Campbell-Walsh urology. 10th edition. Philadelphia: Saunders; 2012. p. 2411–49.

21. Frizelle FA, Colls BM. Hyponatremia and seizures after bowel preparation: report of three cases. Dis Colon Rectum 2005;48(2):393–6.

22. Bucher P, Gervaz P, Egger JF, et al. Morphologic alterations associated with mechanical bowel preparation before elective colorectal surgery: a randomized trial. Dis Colon Rectum 2006;49(1):109–12.

23. Wren S, Ahmed N, Jamal A, et al. Preoperative oral antibiotics in colorectal surgery increase the rate of Clostridium difficile colitis. Arch Surg 2005;140:752–6.

24. Krapohl GL, Phillips LR, Campbell DA Jr, et al. Bowel preparation for colectomy and risk of Clostridium difficile infection. Dis Colon Rectum 2011; 54(7):810–7.

25. Simren M, Barbara G, Flint H, et al. Intestinal microbiota in functional bowel disorders—a Rome foundation report. Gut 2012;62:159–76.

26. Hashad MM, Atta M, Elabbady A, et al. Safety of no bowel preparation before ileal urinary diversion. BJU Int 2012;110(11 Pt C):E1109–13.

27. Tabibi A, Simforoosh N, Basiri A, et al. Bowel preparation versus no preparation before ileal urinary diversion. Urology 2007;70(4):654–8.

28. Berglund R, Herr H. Surgery for bladder cancer. In: Wein A, Kavoussi L, Novick A, et al, editors. Campbell-Walsh urology. 10th edition. Philadelphia: Saunders; 2012. p. 2375–85.

29. Large MC, Kiriluk KJ, DeCastro GJ, et al. The impact of mechanical bowel preparation on postoperative complications for patients undergoing cystectomy and urinary diversion. J Urol 2012;188(5):1801–5.

30. Raynor MC, Lavien G, Nielsen M, et al. Elimination of preoperative mechanical bowel preparation in patients undergoing cystectomy and urinary diversion. Urol Oncol 2013;31(1):32–5.

31. Aslan G, Baltaci S, Akdogan B, et al. A prospective randomized multicenter study of Turkish Society of Urooncology comparing two different mechanical bowel preparation methods for radical cystectomy. Urol Oncol 2013;31(5):664–70.

32. Shafii M, Murphy D, Donovan M, et al. Is mechanical bowel preparation necessary in patients undergoing cystectomy and urinary diversion? BJU Int 2002;89: 879–81.

33. Xu R, Zhao X, Zhong Z, et al. No advantage is gained by preoperative bowel preparation in radical cystectomy and ileal conduit: a randomized controlled trial of 86 patients. Int Urol Nephrol 2010;42(4):947–50.

34. Deng S, Dong Q, Wang J, et al. The role of mechanical bowel preparation before ileal urinary diversion: a systematic review and meta-analysis. Urol Int 2014;92(3):339–48.

35. Witjes JA, Comperat E, Cowan NC, et al. EAU guidelines on muscle-invasive and metastatic bladder cancer: summary of the 2013 guidelines. Eur Urol 2014;65(4):778–92.

36. Daneshmand S, Ahmadi H, Schuckman AK, et al. Enhanced recovery protocol after radical cystectomy for bladder cancer. J Urol 2014;192(1):50–5.

37. Arumainayagam N, McGrath J, Jefferson KP, et al. Introduction of an enhanced recovery protocol for radical cystectomy. BJU Int 2008;101(6):698–701.

38. Cerantola Y, Valerio M, Persson B, et al. Guidelines for perioperative care after radical cystectomy for bladder cancer: enhanced recovery after surgery (ERAS) society recommendations. Clin Nutr 2013; 32(6):879–87.

39. Ojetti V, Bruno G, Paolucci V, et al. The prevalence of small intestinal bacterial overgrowth and methane production in patients with myelomeningocele and constipation. Spinal Cord 2014;52(1):61–4.

40. Gundeti MS, Godbole PP, Wilcox DT. Is bowel preparation required before cystoplasty in children? J Urol 2006;176(4 Pt 1):1574–6 [discussion: 1576–7].

41. Victor D, Burek C, Corbetta JP, et al. Augmentation cystoplasty in children without preoperative mechanical bowel preparation. J Pediatr Urol 2012;8(2):201–4.

42. McLaren R, Barrett D, Zincke H. Rectal injury occurring at radical retropubic prostatectomy for prostate cancer—etiology and treatment. Urology 1993; 42(4):401–5.

43. Wedmid A, Mendoza P, Sharma S, et al. Rectal injury during robot-assisted radical

prostatectomy: incidence and management. J Urol 2011;186(5):1928–33.

44. Igel TC, Barrett DM, Segura JW, et al. Perioperative and postoperative complications from bilateral pelvic lymphadenectomy and radical retropubic prostatectomy. J Urol 1987;137(6):1189–91.

45. Harpster LE, Rommel FM, Sieber PR, et al. The incidence and management of rectal injury associated with radical prostatectomy in a community based urology practice. J Urol 1995;154(4):1435–8.

46. Smith AM, Veenema RJ. Management of rectal injury and rectourethral fistulas following radical retropubic prostatectomy. J Urol 1972;108(5):778–9.

47. Shekarriz B, Upadhyay J, Wood DP. Intraoperative, perioperative, and long-term complications of radical prostatectomy. Urol Clin North Am 2001;28(3):639–53.

48. Pilecki MA, McGuire BB, Jain U, et al. National multi-institutional comparison of 30-day postoperative complication and readmission rates between open retropubic radical prostatectomy and robot-assisted laparoscopic prostatectomy using NSQIP. J Endourol 2014;28(4):430–6.

49. Borland RN, Walsh PC. The management of rectal injury during radical retropubic prostatectomy. J Urol 1992;147(3 Pt 2):905–7.

50. Sugihara T, Yasunaga H, Horiguchi H, et al. Does mechanical bowel preparation ameliorate damage from rectal injury in radical prostatectomy? Analysis of 151 rectal injury cases. Int J Urol 2014;21(6):566–70.

51. Kheterpal E, Bhandari A, Siddiqui S, et al. Management of rectal injury during robotic radical prostatectomy. Urology 2011;77(4):976–9.

52. Schaeffer E, Partin AW, Lepor H, et al. Radical retropubic and perineal prostatectomy. In: Wein A, Kavoussi L, Novick A, et al, editors. Campbell-Walsh urology. 10th edition. Philadelphia: Saunders; 2012. p. 2801–29.

53. Su L-M, Smith J. Campbell-Walsh urology. In: Wein A, Kavoussi L, Novick A, et al, editors. Laparoscopic and robotic-assisted laparoscopic radical prostatectomy and pelvic lymphadenectomy. 10th edition. Philadelphia: Saunders; 2012. p. 2830–49.

54. Zerey M, Hawver LM, Awad Z, et al. SAGES evidence-based guidelines for the laparoscopic resection of curable colon and rectal cancer. Surg Endosc 2013;27(1):1–10.

55. Kavoussi L, Schwartz M, Gill I. Laparoscopic surgery of the kidney. In: Wein A, Kavoussi L, Novick A, et al, editors. Campbell-Walsh urology. 10th edition. Philadelphia: Saunders; 2012. p. 1628–69.

56. Eichel L, McDougall E, Clayman R. Fundamentals of laparoscopic and robotic urologic surgery. In: Wein A, Kavoussi L, Novick A, et al, editors. Campbell-Walsh urology. 10th edition. Philadelphia: Saunders; 2012. p. 204–53.

57. Sugihara T, Yasunaga H, Horiguchi H, et al. Does mechanical bowel preparation improve quality of laparoscopic nephrectomy? Propensity score-matched analysis in Japanese series. Urology 2013;81(1):74–9.

58. Won H, Maley P, Salim S, et al. Surgical and patient outcomes using mechanical bowel preparation before laparoscopic gynecologic surgery: a randomized controlled trial. Obstet Gynecol 2013;121(3):538–46.

59. Wenzel R. Preoperative prophylactic antibiotics brief historical note. Infect Control 1993;14(3):121.

60. Nelson RL, Gladman E, Barbateskovic M. Antimicrobial prophylaxis for colorectal surgery. Cochrane Database Syst Rev 2014;(5):CD001181.

61. Classen DC, Evans RS, Pestotnik SL, et al. The timing of prophylactic administration of antibiotics and the risk of surgical-wound infection. N Engl J Med 1992;326(5):281–6.

62. Mangram A, Horan T, Pearson M, et al. Guideline for prevention of surgical site infection, 1999. Centers for Disease Control and Prevention (CDC) hospital infection control practices advisory committee. Am J Infect Control 1999;27(2):97–132.

63. Wolf J Jr, Bennett C, Dmochowski R, et al. Best practice policy statement on urology surgery antimicrobial prophylaxis. J Urol 2008;179(4):1379–90.

64. Grabe M. Antibiotic prophylaxis in urological surgery, a European viewpoint. Int J Antimicrob Agents 2011;38(Suppl):58–63.

65. Pessaux P, Atallah D, Lermite E, et al. Risk factors for prediction of surgical site infections in "clean surgery". Am J Infect Control 2005;33(5):292–8.

66. Bootsma AM, Laguna Pes MP, Geerlings SE, et al. Antibiotic prophylaxis in urologic procedures: a systematic review. Eur Urol 2008;54(6):1270–86.

67. Monroe S, Polk R. Antimicrobial use and bacterial resistance. Curr Opin Microbiol 2000;3(5):496–501.

68. Bratzler D, Houck P, Richards C, et al. Use of antimicrobial prophylaxis for major surgery: baseline results from the national surgical infection prevention project. Arch Surg 2005;140:174–82.

69. Mossanen M, Calvert JK, Holt SK, et al. Overuse of antimicrobial prophylaxis in community practice urology. J Urol 2015;193(2):543–7.

70. Berry AR, Watt B, Goldacre MJ, et al. A comparison of the use of povidone-iodine and chlorhexidine in the prophylaxis of postoperative wound infection. J Hosp Infect 1982;3(1):55–63.

71. Dumville JC, McFarlane E, Edwards P, et al. Preoperative skin antiseptics for preventing surgical wound infections after clean surgery. Cochrane Database Syst Rev 2013;(3):CD003949.

72. Seropian R, Reynolds BM. Wound infections after preoperative depilatory versus razor preparation. Am J Surg 1971;121(3):251–4.

73. Tanner J, Norrie P, Melen K. Preoperative hair removal to reduce surgical site infection. Cochrane Database Syst Rev 2011;(11):CD004122.

74. Braintree Laboratories I. NuLYTELY prescribing information. (MA): Braintree; 2013.

75. Braintree Laboratories I. GoLYTELY prescribing information. (MA): Braintree; 2013.

76. Shieh F, Gnarainam N, Mohamud S, et al. MiraLAX-Gatorade bowel prep versus GoLytely before screening colonoscopy- an endoscopic database study in a community hospital. J Clin Gastroenterol 2012;46:e96–100.

77. Nyberg C, Hendel J, Nielsen OH. The safety of osmotically acting cathartics in colonic cleansing. Nat Rev Gastroenterol Hepatol 2010; 7(10):557–64.

78. Curran M, Plosker G. Oral sodium phosphate solution: a review of its use as a colorectal cleanser. Drugs 2004;64(15):1697–714.

79. Beloosesky Y, Grinblat J, Weiss A, et al. Electrolyte disorders following oral sodium phosphate administration for bowel cleansing in elderly patients. Arch Intern Med 2003;163:803–8.

Update on Antibiotic Prophylaxis for Genitourinary Procedures in Patients with Artificial Joint Replacement and Artificial Heart Valves

CrossMark

Daniel J. Mazur, MD[a],*, Daniel J. Fuchs, MD[b],
Travis O. Abicht, MD[c], Terrance D. Peabody, MD[b]

KEYWORDS

- Antibiotic prophylaxis • Urologic surgical procedures • Bacteremia • Arthroplasty • Endocarditis

KEY POINTS

- Although bacteremia can develop with certain urologic procedures, little evidence exists to support an increased incidence of artificial joint or heart valve infections in patients undergoing genitourinary procedures.
- Antibiotic prophylaxis for patients with artificial joint replacements undergoing genitourinary procedures is recommended for patients at increased risk for joint infection who are having procedures with increased risk for bacteremia. Routine use of antibiotic prophylaxis in all patients with joint replacements remains controversial.
- Routine antibiotic prophylaxis is not recommended for patients undergoing urologic procedures with artificial heart valves solely for the prevention of infectious endocarditis.

INTRODUCTION

Infections are one of the most common and potentially serious complications of operative procedures. Patients with preexisting implanted surgical hardware, such as artificial joints and prosthetic heart valves, are of particular interest because this foreign material may become hematogenously seeded from bacteremia induced during surgical manipulation. These infections are often difficult to eradicate and frequently require surgery to remove the infected material. As a result, the morbidity, mortality, and costs are often high. Consequently, there has been an interest in exploring preventative measures in the perioperative period, mainly through consideration of antibiotic prophylaxis, in an attempt to prevent or reduce bacteremia and seeding of implanted material. Various organizations have released guidelines and statements regarding the use of prophylactic antibiotics for patients undergoing surgical and dental procedures with preexisting surgical implants; however, these

Disclosure statement: The authors have nothing to disclose.
[a] Department of Urology, Feinberg School of Medicine, Northwestern University, 303 East Chicago Avenue, Tarry 16-703, Chicago, IL 60611, USA; [b] Department of Orthopedic Surgery, Feinberg School of Medicine, Northwestern University, 676 North Saint Clair, Suite 1350, Chicago, IL 60611, USA; [c] Department of Surgery-Cardiac Surgery, Feinberg School of Medicine, Northwestern University, 251 East Huron, Galter 3-150, Chicago, IL 60611, USA
* Corresponding author.
E-mail address: d-mazur@md.northwestern.edu

urologic.theclinics.com

recommendations have evolved over time are not without some disagreement. This article specifically focuses on the role of antibiotic prophylaxis in patients undergoing genitourinary procedures with artificial joints and heart valves.

SCOPE AND SIGNIFICANCE OF IMPLANT-ASSOCIATED INFECTION
Artificial Total Joint Replacement Infection

Periprosthetic joint infection (PJI) is a serious complication after total joint arthroplasty. The incidence of PJI is generally low, with contemporary rates ranging from 0.57% to 2.8% for total shoulder arthroplasty, total hip arthroplasty (THA), and total knee arthroplasty (TKA).[1,2] However, arthroplasty is a common surgical procedure with 800,000 or more THA and TKA procedures performed in the United States each year.[3] As a result, the number of PJI cases encountered is significant despite the generally low incidence.

The mainstays of treatment of PJI are antimicrobial therapy and surgery (debridement, implant removal, or amputation).[4] In addition to the morbidity of the infection, extended hospitalization, and further surgery associated with PJI, there is also a significantly greater mortality. Patients undergoing revision arthroplasty for PJI have an increased mortality at 1 year of 10.6% versus 2.0% when compared with revision arthroplasty for aseptic failures.[5]

Cases of PJI following TKA are associated with increased economic costs, with PJI being the most common indication for revision of a TKA.[6] One study showed that PJI had a higher mean annual cost of $116,383 compared with $28,249 in controls.[7] A study of Medicare reimbursements demonstrated a 2.2-fold higher reimbursement for PJIs compared with uninfected controls.[8]

Artificial Heart Valve Infection

Endocarditis is a term used to describe inflammation of the endocardial lining of the heart.[9] Most endocarditis is infectious in nature.[10] The incidence of infectious endocarditis (IE) is low, ranging from 3 to 8 cases per 100,000 persons in industrialized countries.[11,12] Patients with prosthetic valves are at higher risk for endocarditis; however, 50% of IE develops in patients with no known cardiac disease.[9] Prosthetic valve endocarditis (PVE) occurs in 1% to 6% of prosthetic valves with an incidence of 0.3 to 1.2 per patient-year.[13,14]

There is significant morbidity with IE, including the destruction of cardiac tissues and valves, congestive heart failure, embolic events (particularly cerebral complications), the need for extended hospitalization, and the frequent need for surgery for debridement and reconstruction of cardiac structures.[15] Given this, the mortality of PVE is high, with an in-hospital mortality ranging from 14% to 75%.[16,17] Unfortunately, neither the incidence nor the mortality of IE has decreased in the past several decades despite advancements in diagnosis, antimicrobial agents, and surgical techniques.[18]

Given the associated morbidity, mortality, and costs of PJI and PVE-IE, it is no wonder there is an interest in preventing these infections.

PATHOGENESIS OF IMPLANT-ASSOCIATED INFECTION

Implanted devices are at risk for colonization with microorganisms because they serve as artificial sites that create a favorable environment for bacterial growth. Bacteria can bind to the surface, replicate, form a biofilm, and then disperse from the biofilm to allow further spread of the infection. The bacteria in these biofilms can tolerate significantly higher concentrations of antibiotics and may be shielded from the immune system.[19] The presence of a prosthesis alone has also been shown to negatively affect the function of granulocytes.[20] As a result, the presence of implanted material significantly decreases the inoculum of bacteria needed for infection.[21,22]

Most PJI and PVE-IE are caused by gram-positive cocci; however, infection by gram-negative bacteria and fungi also may occur. In both PJI and PVE-IE, the most common microorganisms are staphylococci followed by streptococci and *Enterococcus*.[23,24] The presence of these organisms is not surprising given their ability to form biofilms.[25,26] During the past decade, the percentage of IE caused by staphylococci and *Enterococcus* has increased, whereas that of streptococci has decreased.[24] Of note, the rate of methicillin-resistant *Staphylococcus aureus* (MRSA) seems to be on the increase in PJI.[25]

Bacteremia with hematogenous seeding is the most likely route for introduction of the bacteria to the site of the implanted device after operative and dental procedures. PJI and PVE can also be caused by contamination at the time of implantation. The rates of bacteremia secondary to surgical procedures vary depending on the type of procedure and whether or not periprocedural antibiotics are used. Bacteremia with subsequent prosthesis seeding can occur as long as the prosthesis remains in place; however, the risk of PJI is highest in the early period after total joint implant (TJI). The combined incidence of PJI after TKA and THA in the first 2 years after implantation is 5.9 versus 2.3 per 1000 joint-years compared with postoperative years 3 to 10.[27] Approximately two-thirds of PJI occur within the first year after implanation.[1] It should be noted that these numbers take into account all causes of PJI, not just hematogenous seeding. Additionally, surgical procedures serve as only a minor overall source of bacteremia because exposure can occur from a person's daily activities (see later discussion).

SOURCES OF BACTEREMIA
Urologic Procedures

Because bacteremia is the mechanism by which artificial joints and heart valves are thought to be seeded during later surgical procedures, it is important to understand the incidence of bacteremia with urologic procedures. Interpretation of many studies in this regard is difficult because the rates of sepsis are often reported without associated blood culture data and, therefore, the overall rates of symptomatic and asymptomatic bacteremia are often not known. A meta-analysis examining the use of antibiotics for transurethral procedures (eg, cystoscopy, transurethral resection of prostate, and transurethral resection of bladder tumor) demonstrated bacteremia rates of 6.1% without antibiotics and 2.1% with antibiotic use.[28]

In patients with negative urine and blood cultures undergoing urodynamics without prophylactic antibiotics, 7% demonstrated bacteremia on immediate postprocedure blood cultures.[29] The organisms were *Escherichia coli, Pseudomonas*, and coagulase-negative staphylococci. Two patients had preprocedural positive urine cultures with *E coli* and both had postprocedure *E coli* bacteremia. No patients were symptomatic or needed treatment.

In a randomized study of 50 transrectal prostate biopsies completed without periprocedural antibiotics, bacteremia was found in 28% of subjects not receiving a prebiopsy enema and 4% of those receiving an enema.[30] Blood and urine cultures were taken 15 minutes after the biopsy. The rates of prebiopsy bacteriuria were 44% in the no enema and 52% in the enema group. Both groups had a 44% rate of postbiopsy bacteriuria. Most of the urine cultures had bacterial growth of less than 10,000 colony-forming units (CFU)/mL and none were greater than 50,000 CFU/mL. Only 1 of the 8 subjects with bacteremia (12.5%) was symptomatic necessitating treatment with oral ciprofloxacin. This subject's blood culture grew *E coli*. Other organisms isolated from the blood cultures were one each of *Staphylococcus, Streptococcus*, diphtheroids, *Bacteroides fragilis, Propionibacterium*, and *Gemella morbillorum*, and 2 each of *Enterobacter* and gram-positive rods not otherwise

specified. Only one man had the same organism on prebiopsy urine culture as on blood culture and none had the same organism in postbiopsy urine and blood cultures. In studies using periprocedural antibiotic prophylaxis, the rates of bacteremia with transrectal prostate biopsy are often equal to or less than 1%; however, the rates of fluoroquinolone-resistant bacteria are increasing.[31]

The use of intravesical bacillus Calmette-Guérin (BCG) in patients with prosthetic devices seems to be safe. A phase II trial of BCG plus interferon α-2b therapy for nonmuscle invasive bladder cancer included 13 subjects with artificial heart valves and 43 with orthopedic hardware. It showed that these subjects were no more likely to develop a fever compared with the general population and there were no infectious complications of the prosthetics.[32] Rates of bacteremia posttreatment are not known, however.

A summary of urologic procedures considered by the American Urologic Association (AUA) to be at increased risk for bacteremia is summarized in **Box 1**.

Bacteremia from Other Sources

The risk of bacteremia is not isolated to urologic procedures. Procedures involving the gastrointestinal tract also pose a risk. For example, the rate of bacteremia associated with colonoscopy is 2% to 16%.[33] Dental procedures have potentially high rates of bacteremia. For a tooth extraction or gingivectomy, the median incidence rate of bacteremia is about 65% or higher.[34] Daily activities also can be a source of bacteremia, particularly

---

Box 1
Urologic procedures with increased risk for bacteremia

- Procedures that involve
  1. Stone manipulation
  2. Transmural incision into the urinary tract
  3. Endoscopy of the ureter or renal collecting system
  4. Incision into the bowel
- Transrectal prostate biopsy
- Procedures in patients with higher rates of bacterial colonization (eg, those with indwelling urinary catheters)

Adapted from Wolf JS Jr, Bennett CJ, Dmochowski RR, et al. Best practice policy statement on urologic surgery antimicrobial prophylaxis. J Urol 2008;179: 1384; with permission.

those involving the oral cavity. The median incidence of bacteremia is about 4% for chewing and 18% for toothbrushing.[34] These frequent events may be more significant sources of bacteremia during a person's lifetime compared with occasional surgical procedures.

Given the risk of surgical procedures inducing bacteremia and the potential for hematogenous spread of this bacteria to prosthetic implants, various organizations have developed guidelines to help clinicians with decision making regarding the use of antibiotic prophylaxis in this setting.

ANTIBIOTIC PROPHYLAXIS IN PATIENTS WITH ARTIFICIAL JOINT REPLACEMENTS

Although bacteremia does develop with certain urologic procedures and bacteremia does increase the risk of seeding an artificial joint, there is a lack of evidence to support an increased incidence of TJI in patients undergoing genitourinary procedures. To put it another way, there are no definitive data exists to support a causal link between urologic surgery and PJI. Furthermore, opponents of routine antibiotic prophylaxis cite the risks of anaphylaxis, *Clostridium difficile* infection, and contribution to formation of antibiotic resistant bacteria. To help guide clinicians with their practice, given this uncertainty, in 2003 the AUA and the Academy of Orthopedic Surgeons (AAOS) released an advisory statement regarding antibiotic prophylaxis for patients with total joint replacements undergoing urologic procedures.[35] Antibiotic prophylaxis was not recommended for those with pins, plates, or screws or routinely for those with artificial joint replacements. It was advised that prophylaxis be considered for those with artificial joint replacements who are at increased risk for hematogenous joint infection (**Table 1**) and are undergoing urologic procedures at higher risk for bacteremia (see **Box 1**).

However, subsequent recommendations from each organization have diverged. In 2008, the AUA released a "Best Practice Policy Statement on Urologic Surgery Antimicrobial Prophylaxis."[36] The recommendation was changed to state that prophylaxis is recommended in patients who are both at increased risk of hematogenous total joint infection and undergoing a urologic procedure with increased risk of bacteremia.

The AAOS released an information statement in 2009 recommending that physicians consider antibiotic prophylaxis for all patients with total joint replacements before any invasive procedure that poses a risk of bacteremia.[37] This prophylaxis is considered particularly important for patients at increased risk of hematogenous joint infection (see **Table 1**). This change was made because of consideration given to the morbidity and cost of treating an infected joint prosthesis (see previous discussion) versus the risks of a single dose of antibiotics. The recommendation that prophylaxis be considered for all patients with a prosthesis is in contrast to the AUA's stratified approach of identifying the higher risk patients undergoing higher risk procedures. The AAOS stated that, although the risk for hematogenous seeding of a total joint replacement is highest in the first several years, a risk of seeding remains for the lifetime of the implant and, therefore, antibiotic prophylaxis should be considered throughout the implant's lifetime.

Both the AUA and AAOS are in better agreement about the choice of prophylactic antibiotic if one is to be given. The AUA recommends a single dose of an oral quinolone (ciprofloxacin, 500 mg; levofloxacin, 500 mg; ofloxacin, 400 mg) 1 to 2 hours

---

Table 1
Patients at increased risk for hematogenous prosthetic joint infection according to the American Urologic Association and American Academy of Orthopedic Surgeons

Patients with a Prosthetic Joint Replacement Who	AUA	AAOS
1. Are any patients with a prosthetic joint replacement	No	Yes
2. Are <2 y after joint replacement	Yes	Yes
3. Are immunocompromised	Yes	Yes
4. Have comorbidities (for example malignancy)	Yes	Yes
5. Have had a prior prosthetic joint infection	Yes	Yes
6. Have a megaprosthesis	No comment	Yes

Abbreviations: AAOS, American Academy of Orthopedic Surgeons; AUA, American Urologic Association.
Adapted from Wolf JS Jr, Bennett CJ, Dmochowski RR, et al. Best practice policy statement on urologic surgery antimicrobial prophylaxis. J Urol 2008;179:1384; with permission; and Data from American Academy of Orthopedic Surgeons. Antibiotic prophylaxis for patients after total joint replacement: information statement from the American Academy of Orthopedic Surgeons. Available at: http://orthodoc.aaos.org/davidgrimmmd/Antibiotic%20Prophylaxis%20for%20Patients%20after%20Total%20Joint%20Replacement.pdf. Accessed February 15, 2015.

before the procedure. Intravenous ampicillin 2g (or vancomycin 1g in penicilin allergic patients) plus gentamicin 1.5 mg/kg 30 to 60 minutes before the procedure may be substituted. The AAOS recommends a dose of ciprofloxacin 500 mg orally or 400 mg intravenously 1 hour before the procedure.

Interestingly, in 2012 the AAOS released a guideline with the American Dental Association on the prevention of orthopedic implant infection in patients undergoing dental procedures.[38] The recommendation was that a practitioner might consider discontinuing the routine practice of using prophylactic antibiotics for dental procedures in patients with total joint replacements. This is provocative given that certain dental procedures often carry the highest risk of bacteremia. However, this was given a limited grade of recommendation and it was advised that caution be taken in following this recommendation. The only direct supporting evidence came from one case-control prospective study that did not demonstrate dental procedures to be a risk factor for TJI and that antibiotic prophylaxis before dental procedures did not decrease the risk of TJI.[39] Notably, this statement did not comment specifically on prophylaxis for urologic procedures, did not identify which patients were at particularly high risk of PJI via hematogenous seeding, and did not specify which antibiotic agents were recommended if prophylaxis was used.

Interestingly, practice trends in the medical community do not always follow the recommendations of the national organizations. In 2002, a study was performed in Ireland that polled both orthopedic surgeons and urologists regarding antibiotic prophylaxis for patients with hip and knee arthroplasties.[40] Urologists on average stated that antibiotics were "probably indicated" for routine and lengthy urologic procedures, whereas orthopedic surgeons on average stated that antibiotics were "definitely indicated." A more recent study, published in 2014 after the 2012 AAOS guidelines were released, polled orthopedic surgeons and dentists in Canada.[41] According to survey results, 77% of orthopedic surgeons and 71% of dentists routinely prescribe antibiotic prophylaxis. Although these rates were similar, orthopedic surgeons were more likely than dentists to advocate for lifelong use of antibiotic prophylaxis (63% vs 22%).

ANTIBIOTIC PROPHYLAXIS IN PATIENTS WITH ARTIFICIAL HEART VALVES

Similar to the scenario with artificial joint replacements, there is no strong evidence in humans to support the use of antibiotic prophylaxis to prevent IE in patients undergoing genitourinary

procedures. The American Heart Association (AHA) came out with the first guidelines in 1955 recommending antibiotic prophylaxis against IE for patients with preexisting cardiac conditions before specific dental, gastrointestinal, and genitourinary tract procedures.[42] This was mainly based on observational studies.[43]

However, during the past 2 decades, the pendulum has swung the opposite way to a more restrictive approach toward prophylaxis. This is because, despite the risk of bacteremia associated with some procedures, the risk of developing IE remains exceptionally low. The procedure-related risk of IE for dental procedures in the general population is 1:14,000,000 and decreases only to 1:95,000 for patients with prior IE (a higher risk group).[44,45] This indicates that the number needed to prevent one case of IE in patients undergoing dental procedures is massive. This is further supported in that most patients who develop IE do not have an identifiable proceeding procedure.[46]

The National Institute for Health and Clinical Excellence guidelines issued in 2008 do not recommend antibiotic prophylaxis for patients undergoing genitourinary procedures.[47] The most recent AHA–American College of Cardiology guideline update from 2014 and the European Society of Cardiology guideline statement from 2009 have similar recommendations.[48,49] Neither society recommends antibiotic prophylaxis to prevent IE for patients undergoing genitourinary procedures. These changes are based on questions regarding the efficacy of antimicrobial prophylaxis for IE in most situations. Prophylaxis is considered reasonable for patients at high-risk for adverse outcomes from IE, including patients with prosthetic cardiac valves, who receive dental procedures involving manipulation of gingival tissue or the periapical region of teeth or perforation of the oral mucosa.

There has been one retrospective case-control study published after these guidelines that is the first to show an association between urologic procedures and the development of IE.[50] The study included 384 subjects who were diagnosed with IE during a 10-year period. There was a significant association between the development of enterococcal IE and preceding genitourinary procedures (odds ratio 8.21, 95% confidence interval 3.54–19.05). It should be noted that the exact timing between the events is not reported but up to a 1-year latency period between the procedure and the development of IE was accepted. Antibiotic prophylaxis was routinely given for all urologic procedures, except cystoscopy, in the form of either intravenous gentamicin or amoxicillin-clavulanic acid. It should also be noted that during the study period more than 100,000 urologic procedures were performed at the study institution and there were only 111 cases of enterococcal IE with 24 having a urologic procedure in the preceding year. This highlights the very low incidence of urologic-associated IE despite the statistical significance.

SUMMARY

Although PJI and PVE are uncommon, when they do occur there is a significant increase in morbidity, mortality, and cost. As a result, clinicians have attempted to identify and treat preventable causes of these infections. One consideration has been to use antibiotic prophylaxis before or during surgical procedures to prevent or minimize the effects of procedure-related bacteremia. However, there is currently no strong evidence to correlate urologic procedures with the development of PJI or PVE. As a result, guidelines do not recommend antibiotic prophylaxis for the prevention of endocarditis in patients undergoing urologic procedures. However, guidelines and society statements regarding prophylaxis to prevent infection of an artificial joint in the setting of a genitourinary procedure are more varied. Antibiotic prophylaxis for patients with artificial joint replacements undergoing genitourinary procedures is recommended for patients at increased risk for joint infection who are having procedures with increased risk for bacteremia. The routine use of prophylactic antibiotics in all patients or those undergoing low-risk procedures remains controversial and is not supported by existing evidence.

REFERENCES

1. Phillips JE, Crane TP, Noy M, et al. The incidence of deep prosthetic infections in a specialist orthopaedic prospective study. J Bone Joint Surg Br 2006; 88:943–8.
2. Singh JA, Sperling JW, Schleck C, et al. Periprosthetic infections after total shoulder arthroplasty: a 33-year perspective. J Shoulder Elbow Surg 2012; 21:1534–41.
3. Kurtz SM, Lau E, Schmier J, et al. Infection burden for hip and knee arthroplasty in the United States. J Arthroplasty 2008;23:984–91.
4. Lima AL, Oliveira PR, Carvalho VC, et al. Periprosthetic joint infections. Interdiscip Perspect Infect Dis 2013;2013:1–7.
5. Zmistowski B, Karam JA, Durinka JB, et al. Periprosthetic joint infection increases the risk of one-year mortality. J Bone Joint Surg Am 2013;95:2177–84.
6. Kamath AF, Ong KL, Lau E, et al. Quantifying the burden of revision total joint arthroplasty for periprosthetic infections. J Arthroplasty 2015. [Epub ahead of print].
7. Kapadia BH, McElroy MJ, Issa K, et al. The economic impact of periprosthetic infections following total knee arthroplasty at a specialized tertiary-care center. J Arthroplasty 2014;29:929–32.
8. Yi SH, Baggs J, Culler SD, et al. Medicare reimbursement attributable to periprosthetic joint infection following primary hip and knee arthroplasty. J Arthroplasty 2015;30(6):931–8.e2.
9. Hoen B, Duval X. Infective endocarditis. N Engl J Med 2013;368:1425–33.
10. Thuny F, Grisoli D, Cautela J, et al. Infective endocarditis: prevention, diagnosis, and management. Can J Cardiol 2014;30:1046–57.
11. Federspiel JJ, Stearns SC, Peppercorn AF, et al. Increasing US rates of endocarditis with Staphylococcus aureus: 1999–2008. Arch Intern Med 2012; 172:363–5.
12. Correa de Sa DD, Tleyjeh IM, Anavekar NS, et al. Epidemiological trends of infective endocarditis: a population-based study in Olmsted County, Minnesota. Mayo Clin Proc 2010;85:422–6.
13. Vongpatanasin W, Hillis LD, Lange RA. Prosthetic heart valves. N Engl J Med 1996;335:402–16.
14. Habib G, Thuny F, Avierinos JF. Prosthetic valve endocarditis: current approach and therapeutic options. Prog Cardiovasc Dis 2008;50:274–81.
15. Bedeir K, Reardon M, Ramlawi B. Infective endocarditis: perioperative management and surgical principles. J Thorac Cardiovasc Surg 2014;147:1133–41.
16. Rekik S, Trabelsi I, Znazen A, et al. Prosthetic valve endocarditis: management strategies and prognosis. Neth Heart J 2009;17:56–60.
17. Leport C, Vilde JL, Bricaire F, et al. Late prosthetic valve endocarditis. Bacteriological findings and prognosis in 29 cases. Eur Heart J 1984;5(Suppl C):402–16.
18. Moreillon P, Que YA. Infective endocarditis. Lancet 2004;363:139–49.
19. Arnold WV, Shirtliff ME, Stoodley P. Bacterial biofilms and periprosthetic infections. J Bone Joint Surg Am 2013;95:2223–9.
20. Zimmerli W, Lew PD, Waldvogel FA. Pathogenesis of foreign body infection. Evidence for a local granulocyte defect. J Clin Invest 1984;73:1191–200.
21. Zimmerli W, Waldvogel FA, Vaudaux P, et al. Pathogenesis of foreign body infection: description and characteristics of an animal model. J Infect Dis 1982;146:487–97.
22. Elek SD, Conen PE. The virulence of Staphylococcus pyogenes for man; a study of the problems of wound infection. Br J Exp Pathol 1957;38:573–86.
23. Bjerke-Kroll BT, Christ AB, McLawhorn AS, et al. Periprosthetic joint infections treated with two-stage revision over 14 years: an evolving microbiology profile. J Arthroplasty 2014;29:877–82.

24. Slipczuk L, Codolosa JN, Davila CD, et al. Infective endocarditis epidemiology over five decades: a systematic review. PLoS One 2013;8:e82665.

25. Römling U, Balsalobre C. Biofilm infections, their resilience to therapy and innovative treatment strategies. J Intern Med 2012;272:541–61.

26. Mohamed JA, Huang DB. Biofilm formation by enterococci. J Med Microbiol 2007;56:1581–8.

27. Steckelberg J, Osmon D. Prosthetic joint infection. In: Bisno AL, Waldvogel FA, editors. Infections associated with indwelling medical devices. 3rd edition. Washington, DC: American Society for Microbiology; 2000. p. 173–209.

28. Alsaywid BD, Smith GH. Antibiotic prophylaxis for transurethral urologic surgeries: systematic review. Urol Ann 2013;5:61–74.

29. Onur R, Özden M, Orhan I, et al. Incidence of bacteraemia after urodynamic study. J Hosp Infect 2004;57:241–4.

30. Lindert KA, Kabalin JN. Terris. Bacteremia and bacteriuria after transrectal ultrasound guided prostate biopsy. J Urol 2000;164:76–80.

31. Carignan A, Roussy JF, Lapointe V, et al. Increasing risk of infectious complications after transrectal ultrasound-guided prostate biopsies: time to reassess antimicrobial prophylaxis? Eur Urol 2012;62:453–9.

32. Rosevear HM, Lightfoot AJ, Nepple KG, et al. Safety and efficacy of intravesical bacillus Calmette-Guérin plus interferon α-2b therapy for nonmuscle invasive bladder cancer in patients with prosthetic devices. J Urol 2010;184:1920–4.

33. Cornelius LK, Reddix RN Jr, Carpenter JL. Periprosthetic knee joint infection following colonoscopy. J Bone Joint Surg Am 2003;85:2434–6.

34. Watters W 3rd, Rethman MP, Hanson NB, et al. Prevention of orthopaedic implant infection in patients undergoing dental procedures. J Am Acad Orthop Surg 2013;21:180–9.

35. American Urologic Association, American Academy of Orthopaedic Surgeons. Antimicrobial prophylaxis for urological patients with total joint replacements. J Urol 2003;169:1796–7.

36. Wolf JS Jr, Bennett CJ, Dmochowski RR, et al. Best practice policy statement on urologic surgery antimicrobial prophylaxis. J Urol 2008;179:1379–90.

37. American Academy of Orthopedic Surgeons. Antibiotic prophylaxis for patients after total joint replacement: information statement from the American Academy of Orthopedic Surgeons. 2009. Available at: http://orthodoc.aaos.org/davidgrimmmd/Antibiotic%20Prophylaxis%20for%20Patients%20after%20Total%20Joint%20Replacement.pdf. Accessed February 15, 2015.

38. Rethman MP, Watters W 3rd, Abt E, et al. The American Academy of Orthopedic Surgeons and the American Dental Association clinical practice guideline on the prevention of orthopaedic implant infection in patients undergoing dental procedures. J Bone Joint Surg Am 2013;17:745–7.

39. Berbari EF, Osmon DR, Carr A, et al. Dental procedures as risk factors for prosthetic hip or knee infection: a hospital based prospective case control study. Clin Infect Dis 2010;50:8–16.

40. Kingston R, Kiely P, McElwain JP. Antibiotic prophylaxis for dental or urological procedures following hip or knee replacement. J Infect 2002;45:243–5.

41. Colterjohn T, de Beer J, Petruccelli D, et al. Antibiotic prophylaxis for dental procedures at risk for causing bacteremia among post-total joint arthroplasty patients: a survey of Canadian orthopedic surgeons and dental surgeons. J Arthroplasty 2014;29:1091–7.

42. Jones TD, Baumgartner L, Bellow MT, et al. (Committee on Prevention of Rheumatic Fever and Bacterial Endocarditis, American Heart Association). Prevention of rheumatic fever and bacterial endocarditis through control of streptococcal infections. Circulation 1955;11:317–20.

43. Okell CC, Elliott SD. Bacteraemia and oral sepsis: with special reference to the aetiology of subacute endocarditis. Lancet 1935;226:869–72.

44. Steckelberg JM, Wilson WR. Risk factors for infective endocarditis. Infect Dis Clin North Am 1993;7:9–19.

45. Pallasch TJ. Antibiotic prophylaxis: problems in paradise. Dent Clin North Am 2003;47:665–79.

46. Van der Meer JT, Thompson J, Valkenburg HA, et al. Epidemiology of bacterial endocarditis in the Netherlands. I. Patient characteristics. Arch Intern Med 1992;152:1863–8.

47. National Institute for Health and Clinical Excellence (NICE). Prophylaxis against infective endocarditis. 2008. Available at: https://www.nice.org.uk/guidance/cg64/resources/guidance-prophylaxis-against-infective-endocarditis-pdf. Accessed February 15, 2015.

48. Nishimura RA, Otto CM, Bonow RO, et al, American College of Cardiology/American Heart Association Task Force on Practice Guidelines. 2014 AHA/ACC guideline for the management of patients with valvular heart disease: executive summary: a report of the American College of Cardiology/American Heart Association Task Force on Practice Guidelines. Am Coll Cardiol 2014;63:2438–88.

49. Habib G, Hoen B, Tornos P, et al. Guidelines on the prevention, diagnosis, and treatment of infective endocarditis (new version 2009): the Task Force on the Prevention, Diagnosis, and Treatment of Infective Endocarditis of the European Society of Cardiology (ESC). endorsed by the European Society of Clinical Microbiology and Infectious Diseases (ESCMID) and the International Society of Chemotherapy (ISC) for Infection and Cancer. Eur Heart J 2009;30:2369–413.

50. Mohee AR, West R, Baig W, et al. A case-control study: are urologic procedures risk factors for the development of infective endocarditis? BJU Int 2014;114:118–24.

Preprostate Biopsy Rectal Culture and Postbiopsy Sepsis

Aisha Khalali Taylor, MD[a],*,
Adam Bryant Murphy, MD, MBA, MSCI[b]

KEYWORDS

- Prostate • Biopsy • Urosepsis • Drug resistance • Rectal swab
- Targeted antimicrobial prophylaxis

KEY POINTS

- There has been an increase in bacterial resistance to fluoroquinolones (FQs) in men undergoing transrectal ultrasound-guided prostate biopsy and subsequent urinary tract infections (UTIs) with FQ-resistant uropathogens.
- Prebiopsy rectal swabs have been done to detect the presence of FQ-resistant bacteria, which allows for alteration of the periprocedural antibiotics used for prophylaxis.
- Three main strategies have emerged to address this: (1) the targeted approach whereby the periprocedural prophylaxis is chosen based on the antibiotic susceptibilities of the microbes detected on rectal swab culture, (2) prophylactic rectal cleansing with povidone-iodine, and (3) the augmented approach whereby the prophylaxis regimen includes an FQ and an additional empiric antibiotic or antimicrobial regimen excluding FQs altogether.
- Given concerns about the development of multidrug-resistant bacteria, the authors prefer the targeted approach. Reductions in incidence of postbiopsy UTI, febrile UTI, bacteremia, and hospital admission in comparison with placebo have been demonstrated in the literature, along with the decreased cost of care associated with this approach.
- Urologists face pay-for-performance concerns, and should consider alteration of their biopsy antibiotic prophylaxis regimen to reduce the risk of biopsy-related infectious complications.

INTRODUCTION

Transrectal ultrasound-guided prostate biopsy (TRUSP) has been in use since the early 1980s and is one of the most commonly performed procedures in urology.[1] Approximately 1 million TRUSPs are performed in Europe and the United States annually, and serve as the primary procedure for the histologic diagnosis of prostate cancer.[2–4] Urologists are performing more biopsies per patient and more total biopsies than ever before, which has subsequently led to earlier and more accurate diagnoses of prostate cancer, in addition to significant reductions in death from prostate cancer in a subset of patients at high risk for death from this disease.[5] Since its inception in the 1980s, TRUSP has generally been considered to be a benign, relatively safe outpatient procedure.[6] Occurring in more than 50% of patients, most complications associated with TRUSP historically were minor in nature and included hematuria, urethral bleeding, rectal

[a] Department of Urology, University of Pittsburgh Medical Center, 300 Halket Street, Suite 4710, Pittsburgh, PA 15213, USA; [b] Department of Urology, Northwestern Memorial Hospital, 303 East Chicago Avenue, Tarry Building Room 16-703, Chicago, IL 60611, USA
* Corresponding author.
E-mail addresses: taylora10@upmc.edu; aishakhalalitaylor@gmail.com

Urol Clin N Am 42 (2015) 449–458
http://dx.doi.org/10.1016/j.ucl.2015.06.005

bleeding, and hematospermia.[4,7,8] These complications were typically self-limited and did not require additional treatment.[9] Major complications related to TRUSP during this same period included urinary obstruction (1%–2%), syncope from vasovagal reaction (8%), and bacteremia (0.1%–0.5%), which represented a rare occurrence.[10,11]

Several recent studies exploring hospitalizations after TRUSP, however, have revealed a notable shift in the etiology of complications following TRUSP, with an alarming increase in the occurrence of major infectious complications post-TRUSP including febrile urinary tract infection (UTI), prostatitis, bacteremia, sepsis, septic shock, and in some cases even death.[4,8,12–14] Loeb and colleagues[3] reported a 2.65-fold higher hospitalization admission rate among Medicare patients within 30 days of TRUSP in comparison with the control population using Surveillance Epidemiology and End Results (SEER) data. In addition, this analysis revealed that infectious complications requiring hospitalization among men undergoing TRUSP became more common over time from 1991 to 2007 compared with randomly selected controls.

At present, fluoroquinolones (FQs) are the most commonly used antimicrobial for TRUSP prophylaxis, as they have previously been shown to reduce infectious complications from approximately 25% to 8% compared with placebo.[15,16] Despite prophylaxis with FQs, however, a recent study revealed a 4-fold increase in post-TRUSP infections from 0.52% in 2002 to 2009 to 2.15% in 2011, with 52% of infections caused by FQ-resistant isolates.[13,17] With the increasing rates of drug-resistant post-TRUSP infectious complications, several approaches have been evaluated to reduce the rate of infectious complications in men undergoing TRUSP. These approaches have included 3 main strategies: (1) A targeted approach whereby pre-TRUSP RS culture bacterial identification and antimicrobial sensitivities are used to direct TRUSP antibiotic prophylaxis; (2) prophylactic rectal cleansing with povidone-iodine; and (3) an augmented TRUSP prophylaxis approach whereby standard antimicrobial prophylaxis with an FQ plus the addition of an alternative antimicrobial agent or the use of TRUSP prophylaxis regimens excluding FQs altogether are explored.[8]

Studies to date exploring the effects of povidone-iodine rectal cleansing on post-TRUSP infectious complications have shown similar rates of infectious complications between prophylaxis and control groups. Hwang and colleagues[18] showed a statistically significant difference in rates of bacteremia and sepsis among control versus prophylaxis groups (3.5% vs 0.3%). Other investigators have shown no difference in outcomes.[19]

In 2013, Adibi and colleagues[20] reported on the efficacy of the augmented approach versus the standard approach. Subjects receiving 3 days of ciprofloxacin or sulfamethoxazole/trimethoprim double strength in addition to 1 dose of intramuscular gentamicin before TRUSP between January 2011 and December 2011 were compared with historical controls between January 2010 and December 2010. Urine and blood cultures along with bacterial susceptibilities were obtained at admission and compared between the 2 groups. Cost analysis was done to determine the cost-effectiveness of standard and augmented regimens. The investigators found that the rate of hospitalization attributable to post-TRUSP infections was 3.8% (11 patients among 290 biopsies) in 2010, which decreased to 0.6% (2 patients among 310 biopsies) in 2011 (P<.001). Of the admitted patients who received standard prophylaxis, 73% had fluoroquinolone-resistant *Escherichia coli* urinary infection and/or bacteremia, and only 9% had strains resistant to gentamicin. It was concluded that the augmented regimen resulted in cost savings of $15,700 per 100 patients in comparison with the standard regimen. The investigators did not differentiate which subjects received sulfamethoxazole/trimethoprim versus FQ, making it difficult to establish how many subjects in the intervention arm actually avoided infectious complications secondary to receiving sulfamethoxazole/trimethoprim instead of an FQ in a population with a known high prevalence of FQ-resistant uropathogens. This finding might suggest that a significant number of subjects in the intervention arm were actually overtreated with gentamicin. It is also important that at least 9% of their study subjects were inappropriately treated with gentamicin, ending up with significant infectious complications resistant to this antimicrobial which might otherwise have been avoided altogether had the investigators used the targeted approach.[20] Other investigators have shown similar reductions in infectious complications using the augmented approach.[21,22] Although a seemingly promising approach, the augmented strategy may lead to the accelerated development of multidrug-resistant bacteria, limiting the ability to manage post-TRUSP complications. The authors thus favor the targeted approach, and for the purposes of this review focus on this strategy.

This article provides a review of the following:

- Current TRUSP antimicrobial prophylaxis guidelines (APGs)

- Antimicrobial resistance and its implications on current TRUSP APGs
- The incidence of post-TRUSP infectious complications including urosepsis
- The original data supporting pre-TRUSP rectal swab (RS)
- The RS technique and protocol
- RS and post-TRUSP infectious complications

CURRENT TRANSRECTAL ULTRASOUND-GUIDED PROSTATE BIOPSY ANTIMICROBIAL PROPHYLAXIS GUIDELINES

Historically, the routine administration of antimicrobial prophylaxis for TRUSPs has led to a decline in post-TRUSP complication rates, with UTI rates declining from a range of 8% to 87% down to a range of 3% to 8.6%, and symptomatic bacteremia rates declining from 17.5% to 0.5%.[12,23] Following the publication of several randomized controlled studies demonstrating that antimicrobial prophylaxis with FQs had been shown to significantly decrease the rates of post-biopsy infectious complications in comparison with placebo (8% vs 25%), antimicrobial administration of FQs before TRUSP became standard practice.[23–28] A large randomized controlled trial (RCT) involving 537 patients receiving oral ciprofloxacin or placebo before TRUSP revealed the incidence of bacteriuria to be significantly lower in the group receiving antimicrobial prophylaxis.[27] In a 3-armed RCT including 231 patients comparing placebo, a single dose of ciprofloxacin and tinidazole, and the same combination twice a day for 3 days, the incidence of all infectious complications, specifically UTI, was significantly lower in both antimicrobial groups. Furthermore, the single dose was as effective as the 3-day dosing regimen.[15,29–31]

The optimal course for antimicrobial prophylaxis before TRUSP is still unclear. Several RCTs have confirmed the equivalence of single-dose or 1-day regimens compared with 3-day regimens, but despite this there is significant variation among practicing urologists regarding length of antimicrobial prophylaxis for TRUSPs (ranging from a single dose to 7 days).[2,32–34] FQs are still recommended by the American Urologic Association and European Association of Urology as the agents of choice for antimicrobial prophylaxis because of their broad-spectrum coverage for E coli, the etiologic agent for most infections after prostate biopsy. FQs have favorable pharmacokinetics, reaching high and long-lasting concentrations in the urine and prostatic tissue, and offer the ease of oral administration.[28,33–36]

It is important, however, that the benefit of empiric antimicrobial prophylaxis with FQs and the recommendations for its use were based on studies predating the twenty-first century, which had a lower prevalence of antibiotic-resistant uropathogens.[5]

ANTIMICROBIAL RESISTANCE AND ITS IMPLICATIONS ON CURRENT TRANSRECTAL ULTRASOUND-GUIDED PROSTATE BIOPSY ANTIMICROBIAL PROPHYLAXIS GUIDELINES

There has since been a significant upsurge in antimicrobial resistance, particularly to FQs, since the development of the original APGs for TRUSP. It has been suggested that this increase in antimicrobial resistance is in part due to the increased use of antimicrobials not only to treat infectious disease but also for the prevention of disease and enhancement/growth in livestock and poultry.[5] FQ-resistant E coli have been shown to be highly prevalent in animal food sources given feed containing FQs. Given the widespread use of FQs in both humans and animals, it is probable that FQ-resistant E coli are increasingly likely to be present in the colonic flora of men undergoing TRUSP.[37]

The widespread use of FQs as prophylactic agents for TRUSP has led to the emergence of FQ-resistant post-TRUSP genitourinary infections.[1,38] In a study involving single-dose prophylaxis with ciprofloxacin in urologic procedures, FQ-resistant E coli were isolated from 3% of patients before prophylaxis, with this rate increasing to 12% just 7 days after FQ prophylaxis.[39] Qi and colleagues[17] recently published prevalence rates of FQ resistance in men undergoing evaluation for TRUSP, and found that 17% of 991 men carried FQ-resistant E coli. Detailed analysis of resistance mechanisms and plasmid analysis further revealed that along with bacterial strain typing, this population harbored organisms with heterogeneous phenotypic susceptibility. Taken together, these data suggest that universal prophylaxis with FQs would not provide optimal coverage for patients undergoing TRUSPs and that the current APGs for TRUSP should be updated.

INCIDENCE OF POST–TRANSRECTAL ULTRASOUND-GUIDED PROSTATE BIOPSY INFECTIOUS COMPLICATIONS, INCLUDING UROSEPSIS

Infectious complications of TRUSPs ranging from bacteriuria to urosepsis have previously been shown to occur in 1% to 4% of patients.[25,40] Carignan and colleagues[13] reported an alarming trend of increasing infectious complications among 5798 TRUSPs performed in Canadian men between 2002 and 2011 (**Fig. 1**). During the study period, 48 cases of urosepsis (20 with documented bacteremia) were noted. The total incidence of post-TRUSP infectious complications increased from 0.52 infections per 100 biopsies in 2002 to 2009, to 2.15 infections per 100 biopsies in 2010 to 2011 (P<.001). E coli was the predominant pathogen (in 75% of cases).

Despite a recent upward trend in the rate of infectious complications post-TRUSP, particularly secondary to FQ-resistant organisms, the actual incidence of post-TRUSP urosepsis is surprisingly low. Lange and colleagues[39] revealed that between 2001 and 2006 there was a 0.5% incidence of urosepsis following 4749 TRUSPs. Of the 24 patients with post-TRUSP urosepsis, 94% had blood isolates of E coli that were 100% resistant to FQs. In 2007, 240 TRUSPs performed at Long Beach Veterans Affairs Medical Center yielded an estimated 0.8% incidence of sepsis.[40] Most recently, Pinkhasov and colleagues[41] published the largest incidence rate of post-TRUSP urosepsis, reporting a 1.2% rate among a 1000-patient cohort undergoing TRUSP between September 2001 and August 2010.

Although the incidence and absolute numbers of post-TRUSP urosepsis hospitalizations are small, the costs of these events can be exorbitant, including admissions to intensive care units. The authors previously reported that the total cost of managing 9 patients with post-TRUSP infectious complications with FQ-resistant organisms treated according to the TRUSP APGs was $13,219. Duplessis and colleagues[23] estimated a

cost exceeding $15,000 to treat infectious complications in 3 patients receiving FQ prophylaxis based on the APGs. As health care gradually morphs into a system designed to reward physicians for keeping patients healthy and minimizing the cost of care, reducing these complications and subsequent hospitalizations can yield significant cost savings for both private and public health care payers. This policy should drive urologists to update our current prophylaxis approach to reduce the morbidity associated with our primary prostate cancer detection strategy.[5,42]

ORIGINAL DATA SUPPORTING PRE–TRANSRECTAL ULTRASOUND-GUIDED PROSTATE BIOPSY RECTAL SWAB

The rationale for a targeted approach to antimicrobial prophylaxis for TRUSP using RS was initially described in 2010. Batura and colleagues[43] determined the prevalence of antimicrobial resistance in the intestinal flora of patients undergoing prostate biopsy in London (United Kingdom) between January 2007 and December 2008. Of 592 patients who underwent TRUSP, 445 (75.1%) had an RS before TRUSP, which revealed a 10.6% prevalence of FQ-resistant organisms. Post-TRUSP, UTIs developed in 6 patients and bacteremia in 2. All infections were caused by E coli that were resistant to ciprofloxacin except for 1 UTI that was caused by ciprofloxacin-sensitive Pseudomonas aeruginosa. As there was a strong correlation between the antimicrobial sensitivity of organisms causing infections after biopsy and those isolated from the recent swabs, the study suggested that RS cultures before biopsy could

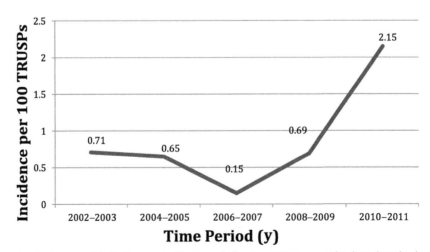

Fig. 1. Increasing incidence of infectious complications following TRUSP over the last decade. (*Adapted from* Carignan A, Roussy JF, Lapointe V, et al. Increasing risk of infectious complications after transrectal ultrasound-guided prostate biopsies: time to reassess antimicrobial prophylaxis? Eur Urol 2012;62:453; with permission.)

provide guidance for selecting appropriate antimicrobial prophylaxis and treatment of TRUSP-associated infection.[5,43]

Rectal Swab Technique and Protocol

RSs are collected in the clinic when TRUSP is advised, preferably at least 5 to 7 days before TRUSP to allow adequate time for results and subsequent response. To ensure relative stability of the rectal flora, the authors collect specimens no more than 14 days before the biopsy. Swabs are cultured on blood agar plates containing 1 μg/mL ciprofloxacin; these plates are incubated at 35° to 37°C in a CO_2 incubator and assessed for growth at 36 to 48 hours. The blood agar plate is used as a quality control indicator for specimen adequacy. As such, RS from blood agar plates without growth are considered to represent inadequate specimen collection. Specimens with growth on blood agar but no growth on MacConkey with ciprofloxacin agar at 48 hours are considered to contain organisms sensitive to FQs. Specimens with growth of gram-negative bacteria on blood and MacConkey with ciprofloxacin agar undergo organism identification and antimicrobial susceptibility testing using an automated microbial system (Vitek R2).

Patients with FQ-sensitive coliforms isolated by RS receive FQ prophylaxis based on the standard APG protocol while those with FQ-resistant organisms receive targeted antimicrobial prophylaxis based on RS data with or without FQs (**Fig. 2**).[44]

RECTAL SWAB AND POST–TRANSRECTAL ULTRASOUND-GUIDED PROSTATE BIOPSY INFECTIOUS COMPLICATIONS

Although some have advocated for the use of multiple antimicrobials to enhance prophylaxis, it has been well established that antimicrobial resistance in fact increases in severity and frequency with the increased exposure to antimicrobials over time.[12] Even prior remote exposure to FQs has been shown to be a risk factor for FQ resistance and infectious complications among patients undergoing TRUSP.[44,45] Furthermore, resistance persists for months and even years after antimicrobial exposure.[15] Thus, even if antimicrobial prophylaxis might be transiently effective in newly biopsied patients, it will inevitably lead to more infectious complications among men requiring subsequent biopsies.[4]

It should follow that the targeted approach to antimicrobial prophylaxis for TRUSP may represent a more optimal strategy. Within the last few years, several studies with varying patient populations undergoing TRUSP have evaluated the efficacy of the targeted approach to antimicrobial prophylaxis. These studies are reviewed here; the reader is referred to **Table 1** for a summary of their results.

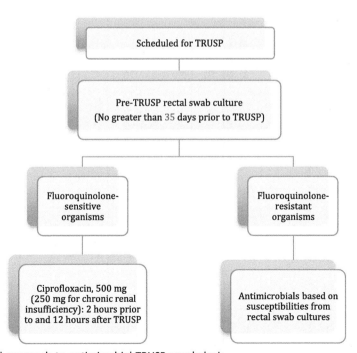

Fig. 2. The targeted approach to antimicrobial TRUSP prophylaxis.

Table 1
Targeted antimicrobial prophylaxis for TRUSP and impact on infectious complications; visual summary of most current literature

Authors,[Ref.] Year	Dates of Analysis	Study Design	Total No. of Patients	No. of Patients Undergoing Empiric Approach	No. of Patients Undergoing Targeted Approach	Post-TRUSP Infectious Complications, Empiric Arm (%)	Post-TRUSP Infectious Complications, Targeted Arm (%)	Prevalence of Resistant Organisms Isolated by RS (%)
Taylor et al,[44] 2012	Jul 2010–Mar 2011	Prospective	457	345	112	2.6	0	19.6
Duplessis et al,[22] 2012	May 2010–Mar 2011	Prospective with historical controls	338	103	235	2.9	0	14
Liss et al,[45] 2015	May 2013–Apr 2014	Retrospective	5355	3553	1802	0.44	0.56	25
Dai et al,[46] 2015	Feb 2013–Feb 2014	Retrospective	487	173	314	2.9	1.9	12.1
Summers et al,[8] 2015	Jun 2013–Jun 2014	Prospective with historical controls	2926	2759	167	2.8	0.6	14

The authors' group[44] evaluated targeted pre-TRUSP prophylaxis between July 2010 and March 2011. Rates of post-TRUSP infectious complications among 112 men undergoing the targeted approach using RS were compared with those among 345 men who received empiric therapy based on the current TRUSP APG protocol at Northwestern Memorial Hospital in Chicago, Illinois. The prevalence of FQ-resistant organisms was 19.6% among men who underwent RS. There were no infectious complications in the 112 men who received targeted antimicrobial prophylaxis, while there were 9 cases (including 1 case of sepsis) among the 345 men who received empiric therapy (P = .12). FQ-resistant organisms caused 7 of these infections. This study suggested that the infection rate was low when appropriate prophylaxis was provided. Conversely, when prophylaxis was empiric the post-TRUSP infectious complications were ~3%, with a 0.28% rate of urosepsis.[44]

In addition to poor infectious outcomes, it was shown that the cost of care could be dramatically increased by ineffective prophylaxis. In this study the total cost of managing infectious complications for patients in the empiric group was $13,219. The calculated cost of targeted versus empiric prophylaxis per 100 men undergoing TRUSP was $1346 versus $5,598, respectively. Cost-effectiveness analysis revealed that targeted prophylaxis yielded cost savings of $4499 per post-TRUSP infectious complication averted. Per estimation, 38 men would need to undergo RS before TRUSP to prevent 1 infectious complication.[44]

Duplessis and colleagues[22] evaluated the benefit of the targeted approach among 235 patients in their hospital population in San Diego between June 1, 2013, and June 1, 2014, and compared the rates of infectious complications within 30 days of TRUSP with those of 2759 historical controls from Jan 1, 2006 to May 31, 2013. Patients with FQ-susceptible organisms received FQ. A 14% prevalence of FQ resistance was noted among patients undergoing RS. Moreover, the investigators found that the average annual infectious complication rate within 30 days of TRUSP was reduced from 2.8% to 0.6% before and after implementation of the targeted approach, although this difference was not statistically significant (P = .13).[22]

Dai and colleagues[46] also examined the effect of RS culture-directed prophylaxis on the prevalence of post-TRUSP associated infections through a retrospective analysis evaluating 487 patients undergoing TRUSP between February 2013 and February 2014. Of 487 patients, 314 received pre-TRUSP RS while 173 did not. The investigators noted an FQ-resistant organism prevalence rate of 12.1% among patients who underwent RS. In addition, the RS group had fewer infectious complications (1.9% vs 2.9%; P = .5) than those patients who underwent the empiric approach. On multivariate analysis, a decreased odds of infection was associated with the targeted approach (odds ratio, 0.70; 95% confidence interval, 0.20–2.50; P = .6). However, these findings were not statistically significant, as their study was underpowered.[46]

The largest study conducted to date examining the effect of targeted prophylaxis on post-TRUSP sepsis was a nonrandomized multicenter retrospective analysis of 5355 patients in 13 Kaiser Permanente urology departments undergoing TRUSP.[47] Between May 1, 2013 and April 30, 2014, 3553 patients underwent the standard empiric approach while 1802 underwent the targeted approach. The investigators noted a prevalence rate of 25% of FQ-resistant organisms among men undergoing RS. Surprisingly there was no statistical difference in post-TRUSP sepsis between the empiric and targeted antimicrobial groups (incidence 0.44% vs 0.56%). Of importance, patients in the empiric arm of this study actually underwent an augmented approach (FQ + an additional antimicrobial). As previous studies have shown that the augmented approach can reduce the incidence of sepsis, this factor could have significantly lowered the infectious complication rates among those patients in the empiric group of this study.[47]

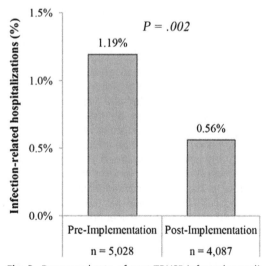

Fig. 3. Decreased rate of post-TRUSP infected complications with updated TRUSP prophylaxis protocol. (*From* Womble PR, Linsell SM, Gao Y, et al, Michigan Urological Surgery Improvement Collaborative. A statewide intervention to reduce hospitalizations after prostate biopsy. J Urol 2015. [Epub ahead of print]; with permission.)

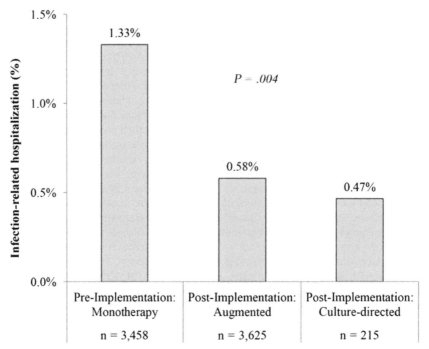

Fig. 4. Decreased rate of post-TRUSP infected complications with updated TRUSP prophylaxis protocol. Standard prophylaxis versus Augmented versus Targeted. (*From* Womble PR, Linsell SM, Gao Y, et al, Michigan Urological Surgery Improvement Collaborative. A statewide intervention to reduce hospitalizations after prostate biopsy. J Urol 2015. [Epub ahead of print]; with permission.)

Womble and colleagues[42] not only demonstrated the high efficacy of the targeted approach to TRUSP prophylaxis to reduce post-TRUSP infectious complications, but in addition demonstrated the remarkable feasibility by which the targeted approach could be utilized on a large scale. Data on patient demographics, comorbidities, prophylactic antibiotics, and post-TRUSP complications were prospectively entered into an electronic registry by trained abstractors in 30 practices participating in a Michigan statewide registry from March 2012 through May 2014. During this period each practice implemented one or both of the interventions aimed at addressing FQ resistance; the targeted and/or the augmented approach. The investigators identified all patients with post-TRUSP infection–related hospitalization within 30 days after the procedure and compared the frequency of these occurrences before (5028 TRUSP) and after (4087 TRUSP) implementation of the quality improvement interventions. There was a statistically significant 53% decrease in the overall proportion of patients with post-TRUSP–related hospitalizations from before versus after (1.19% vs 0.56%, P = .002) implementation of the quality improvement interventions (**Fig. 3**).[42]

Although the investigators demonstrated decreased post-TRUSP infectious complications in both targeted (0.47%) and augmented (0.57%) prophylaxis arms (**Fig. 4**), they favored the targeted approach secondary to the inherent risk of increasing antimicrobial resistance known to be associated with the augmented approach.[42]

SUMMARY

TRUSP remains the standard procedure for the accurate histologic diagnosis of prostate cancer. The American Urologic Association and European Association of Urology both recommend FQs as the agents of choice for antimicrobial prophylaxis for TRUSP despite the alarming increasing incidence of FQ-resistant organisms noted among men undergoing TRUSP. Two approaches have been proposed to reduce post-TRUSP infectious complications: the targeted approach whereby pre-TRUSP RS culture data are used to direct TRUSP prophylaxis, and the augmented approach whereby standard antimicrobial prophylaxis with an FQ plus the addition of an alternative antimicrobial agent or the use of TRUSP prophylaxis regimens excluding FQs altogether have been suggested. Augmented empiric antimicrobial prophylaxis, in light of the rising rates of FQ-resistant and extended spectrum β-lactamase–producing organisms, encourages overtreatment in approximately 86% of men undergoing TRUSP because their flora are sensitive to FQs, and promotes poor antibiotic stewardship.[5,42] Antimicrobial prophylaxis using RS culture has been used since 2010 and offers a promising approach toward reducing post-TRUSP infectious complications, as it is a microbiologically sound strategy that has been shown to be efficacious, cost-effective, and feasible on a large scale.[8,23,42,45–47] Additional RCTs are needed to further evaluate the efficacy and efficiency of this approach. Although severe post-TRUSP infection related hospitalizations are rare, these events are expensive (potentially including admissions to intensive care units), and reducing these admissions can yield significant cost savings for both private and public payers. Moving forward, it is the authors' belief that the current APGs for TRUSP prophylaxis should be revised to reduce the morbidity associated with the principal diagnostic test for prostate cancer.[5]

REFERENCES

1. Gottesman T, Yossepowich O, Harari-Schwartz O, et al. The value of rectal cultures in treatment of sepsis following post-transrectal ultrasound-guided prostate biopsy. Urol Int 2015. [Epub ahead of print].
2. Center MM, Jemal A, Lortet-Tieulent J, et al. International variation in prostate cancer incidence and mortality rates. Eur Urol 2012;61:1079.
3. Loeb S, Carter HB, Berndt S, et al. Complications after prostate biopsy data from SEER-Medicare. J Urol 2011;186:1830.
4. Loeb S, Vellekoop A, Ahmed HU, et al. Systematic review of complications of prostate biopsy. Eur Urol 2013;64:876.
5. Schaeffer AJ. The impact of collateral damage on urological care. J Urol 2012;187(5):1527–8.
6. Djavan B, Margreiter M. Biopsy standards for detection of prostate cancer. World J Urol 2007;11:7.
7. Norberg M, Holmberg L, Haggman M, et al. Determinants of complications after multiple transrectal core biopsies of the prostate. Eur Radiol 1996;6:457.
8. Summers SJ, Patel DP, Hamilton BD, et al. An antimicrobial prophylaxis protocol using rectal swab cultures for transrectal prostate biopsy. World J Urol 2015. [Epub ahead of print].
9. Enlund AL, Varenhorst E. Morbidity of ultrasound-guided transrectal core biopsy of the prostate without prophylactic antibiotic therapy: a prospective study in 415 cases. Br J Urol 1997;79:777.
10. Djavan B, Waldert M, Zlotfa A, et al. Safety and morbidity of first and repeat transrectal ultrasound-guided prostate needle biopsies: results of a prospective European prostate cancer detection study. J Urol 2001;166:856–60.
11. Raaijmakers R, Kirkels WJ, Roobol MJ, et al. Complication rates and risk factors of 5802 transrectal ultrasound-guided sextant biopsies of the prostate within a population-based screening program. Urology 2002;60:826–30.
12. Liss MA. Infection: prostate biopsy-infection and prior fluoroquinolone exposure. Nat Rev Urol 2011;8:592.
13. Carignan A, Roussy JF, Lapointe V, et al. Increasing risk of infectious complications after transrectal ultrasound-guided prostate biopsies: time to reassess antimicrobial prophylaxis? Eur Urol 2012;62:453.
14. Carlson WH, Bell DG, Lawen JG, et al. Multi-drug resistant *E. coli* urosepsis in physicians following transrectal ultrasound guided prostate biopsies—3 cases including one death. Can J Urol 2010; 17:5135.
15. Aron M, Rajeev TP, Gupta NP. Antimicrobial prophylaxis for transrectal needle biopsy of the prostate: a randomized controlled study. BJU Int 2000; 35:682.
16. Rodriguez LV, Terris MK. Risks and complications of transrectal ultrasound guided prostate needle biopsy: a prospective study and review of the literature. J Urol 1998;160:2115.
17. Qi C, Malczynski M, Schaeffer AJ, et al. Characterization of ciprofloxacin resistant *Escherichia coli* isolates among men undergoing evaluation for transrectal ultrasound guided prostate biopsy. J Urol 2013;190:2026–32.
18. Hwang EC, Jung SI, Seo YH, et al. Risk factors for and prophylactic effect of povidone-iodine rectal cleansing on infectious complications after prostate biopsy: a retrospective cohort study. Int Urol Nephrol 2015;4:595–601.
19. Abughoshs Z, Margolick J, Goldberg SL, et al. A prospective randomized trial of povidone-iodine prophylactic cleansing of the rectum before transrectal ultrasound guided prostate biopsy. J Urol 2013;189:1326.
20. Adibi M, Hornberger D, Bhat, et al. Reduction in hospital rates due to post-prostate biopsy infections after augmenting standard antibiotic prophylaxis. J Urol 2013;189:535.
21. Kehinde EO, Al-Maghrebi M, Sheikh M, et al. Combined ciprofloxacin and amikacin prophylaxis in the prevention of septicemia after transrectal ultrasound guided biopsy of the prostate. J Urol 2013; 189:911.
22. Duplessis CA, Bavaro M, Simons MP, et al. Rectal cultures before transrectal ultrasound-guided prostate biopsy reduce post-prostatic biopsy infection rates. Urology 2012;79:556.

23. Shandera KC, Thibault GP, Deshon GE Jr. Efficacy of one dose fluoroquinolone before prostate biopsy. Urology 1998;52:641.

24. Sieber PR, Rommel FM, Agusta VE, et al. Antibiotic prophylaxis in ultrasound guided transrectal prostate biopsy. J Urol 1997;157:2199.

25. Taylor HM, Bingham JB. Antimicrobial prophylaxis for transrectal prostate biopsy. J Antimicrob Chemother 1997;39:115.

26. Kapoor DA, Klimberg IW, Malek GH, et al. Single dose oral ciprofloxacin versus placebo for prophylaxis during transrectal prostate biopsy. Urology 1998;52:552.

27. Zani EL, Clark OA, Rodrigues Netto N Jr. Antibiotic prophylaxis for transrectal prostate biopsy. Cochrane Database Syst Rev 2011;(5):CD006576.

28. Remynse LC, Sweeney PJ, Brewton KA, et al. Intravenous piperacillin/tazobactam plus fluoroquinolone prophylaxis prior to prostate ultrasound biopsy reduces serious infectious complications and is cost effective. J Urol 2011;3:139.

29. Tal R, Livine PM, Lask DM, et al. Empirical management of urinary tract infections complicating transrectal ultrasound guided prostate biopsy. J Urol 2003;169:1762.

30. Sabbagh R, McCormack M, Peloquin F, et al. A prospective randomized trial of 1-day versus 3-day antimicrobial prophylaxis for transrectal ultrasound guided prostate biopsy. Can J Urol 2004;11:2216.

31. Shigemura K, Tnaka K, Yasuda M, et al. Efficacy of 1-day prop medication with fluoroquinolone for prostate biopsy. World J Urol 2005;23:356.

32. Wolf JS, Bennett CJ, Dmochowski RR, et al. Best practice policy statement on urologic surgery antimicrobial prophylaxis. J Urol 2008;179:1379.

33. Drusano GL, Preston SL, Van Guilder M, et al. A population pharmacokinetic analysis of the penetration of the prostate by levofloxacin. Antimicrob Agents Chemother 2000;44:2046.

34. Yu X, Susa M, Weile J, et al. Rapid and sensitive detection of fluoroquinolone-resistant Escherichia coli from urine samples using a genotyping DNS microarray. Int J Med Microbiol 2007;297:417.

35. Naber KG. Use of quinolones in urinary tract infections and prostatitis. Rev Infect Dis 1989;52:552.

36. Saenz Y, Zarazaga M, Brinas L, et al. Antibiotic resistance in Escherichia coli isolates obtained from animals, foods and humans in Spain. Int J Antimicrob Agent 2001;67:353–8.

37. Otrock Z, Oghlakian G, Salamoun M, et al. Incidence of urinary tract infection following transrectal ultrasound guided prostate biopsy at a tertiary-care medical center in Lebanon. Infect Control Hosp Epidemiol 2004;25:873.

38. Wagenlehner F, Stower-Hoffman J, Schneider-Brachert W, et al. Influence of a prophylactic single dose of ciprofloxacin on the level of resistance of Escherichia coli to fluoroquinolones in urology. Int J Antimicrob Agent 2000;15:207.

39. Lange D, Zappavigna C, Hamidizadeh R, et al. Bacterial sepsis after prostate biopsy—a new perspective. J Urol 2009;74:1200–5.

40. Young JL, Liss MA, Szabo RJ. Sepsis due to fluoroquinolone-resistant Escherichia coli after transrectal ultrasound-guided prostate needle biopsy. Urology 2009;74:332.

41. Pinkhasov GI, Lin YK, Palmerola R, et al. Complications following prostate needle biopsy requiring hospital admission or emergency department visits—experience from 1000 consecutive cases. BJU Inter 2012;110:369–74.

42. Womble PR, Linsell SM, Gao Y, et al, Michigan Urological Surgery Improvement Collaborative. A statewide intervention to reduce hospitalizations after prostate biopsy. J Urol 2015. [Epub ahead of print].

43. Batura D, Rao GG, Nielsen PB. Prevalence of antimicrobial resistance in intestinal flora of patients undergoing prostatic biopsy: implications for prophylaxis and treatment of infections after biopsy. BJU Int 2010;106:1017–20.

44. Taylor AK, Zembower TR, Nadler RB, et al. Targeted antimicrobrial prophylaxis using rectal swab cultures in men undergoing transrectal ultrasound guided prostate biopsy is associated with reduced incidence of post-operative infectious complications and cost of care. J Urol 2012;187:1275–9.

45. Liss MA, William K, Moskowitz D, et al. Comparative effectiveness of targeted vs. empiric antibiotic prophylaxis to prevent sepsis from transrectal prostate biopsy: a retrospective analysis. J Urol 2015;15:5347.

46. Dai J, Leone A, Mermel L, et al. Rectal swab culture-directed antimicrobial prophylaxis for prostate biopsy and risk of postprocedure infection, 2015. Rectal swab culture-directed antimicrobial prophylaxis for prostate biopsy and risk of postprocedure infection: a cohort study. Urology 2015;85:8–14.

47. Akduman B, Akduman D, Hunsu T, et al. Long-term fluoroquinolone use before the prostate biopsy may increase the risk of sepsis caused by resistant microorganisms. Urol 2011;78:250–6.

Treatment of the Infected Stone

Tracy Marien, MD, Nicole L. Miller, MD*

KEYWORDS

- Struvite • Calcium carbonate apatite • Staghorn • Obstructive pyelonephritis • Kidney stones
- Urinary tract infection

KEY POINTS

- Infection stones result from urease-producing bacteria and are struvite and/or calcium carbonate apatite in composition.
- Optimal management of infection stones is complete stone removal, and failure to achieve complete stone clearance results in a high recurrence rate.
- Obstructive pyelonephritis is a urologic emergency and can result in urosepsis and death.
- Emergent decompression with retrograde ureteral stent placement or percutaneous nephrostomy tube (PCNT) placement and broad-spectrum antibiotics are imperative to treating patients with obstructive pyelonephritis.

INTRODUCTION

An infected kidney stone can refer to stones that form because of urinary tract infections (UTIs) with urease-producing bacteria, secondarily infected stones of any composition, or stones obstructing the urinary tract leading to pyelonephritis. Most commonly, kidney stones that form secondary to urease-producing bacteria are composed of struvite or calcium carbonate apatite, and presentation is frequently incidental and generally nonemergent. Secondarily infected metabolic stones have also been described. These stones are frequently colonized with non–urease-producing bacteria and often have discordant culture results compared with the lower urinary tract. Obstructive pyelonephritis secondary to urinary tract calculi is considered a urologic emergency, and immediate treatment is indicated to avoid serious complications, including urosepsis and death. Given the difference in pathophysiology and treatment approach, these entities are discussed separately.

Infection Stones

Infection stones are most commonly composed of magnesium ammonium phosphate (ie, struvite) and/or calcium carbonate apatite. These stones result from chronic infections with urease-producing bacterial pathogens and frequently form large branched stones known as staghorn calculi. The incidence of infection stones has overall decreased during the last 30 years, likely due to improved medical care. They are more common in women (10%–11% vs 4% in men) and elderly patients.[1,2] The pathogenesis of struvite and calcium carbonate apatite stone formation is presented in **Fig. 1**.[3,4] Urease from bacteria splits urea into ammonia and carbon dioxide. Ammonia reacts with water to become ammonium and hydroxide ions, which creates an alkaline milieu. In this alkaline environment, the ammonium combines with magnesium, phosphate, and water to create magnesium ammonium phosphate stones. The carbon dioxide eventually breaks down to carbonate, which combines with calcium and phosphate to

Department of Urologic Surgery, Administrative Office, A-1302 Medical Center North, Vanderbilt University Medical Center, Nashville, TN 37232-2765, USA
* Corresponding author. Department of Urologic Surgery, Administrative Office, A-1302 Medical Center North, Vanderbilt University Medical Center, Nashville, TN 37232-2765.
E-mail address: nicole.miller@vanderbilt.edu

Urol Clin N Am 42 (2015) 459–472
http://dx.doi.org/10.1016/j.ucl.2015.05.009

urologic.theclinics.com

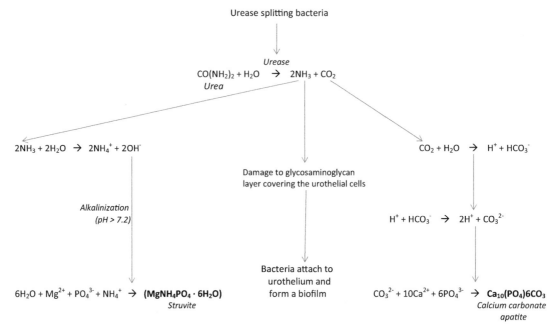

Fig. 1. Pathogenesis of infection stones. Urease from bacteria splits urea (ie, carbamide) into ammonia and carbon dioxide. The ammonia combines with water to produce ammonium and hydroxide. Hydroxide results in an alkalosis of the urine leading to the formation of magnesium ammonium phosphate (ie, struvite). The ammonia also damages the glycosaminoglycan layer causing urothelial damage, allowing the bacteria to attach to the urothelium and form a biofilm. Carbon dioxide complexes with water to form bicarbonate and then carbonate. Carbonate combines with calcium and phosphate forming calcium carbonate apatite.

form calcium carbonate apatite stones. The most common urease-producing bacterial pathogens are *Proteus* spp, *Klebsiella* spp, *Providencia* spp, *Morganella morganni*, and *Staphylococcus aureus*.[5,6] Infection stones are commonly asymptomatic or present with UTIs, flank or abdominal pain, fevers, gross hematuria, or less commonly with sepsis or renal insufficiency.[7] Patients with indwelling catheters, neurogenic bladder, and urinary diversion have the highest risk of developing infection stones due to chronic bacterial colonization. The natural history of these stones is associated with progressive morbidity and mortality, with the 10-year mortality rate reported at 28% with nonsurgical management versus 7% with surgical treatment.[8]

Secondarily infected stones, which are nonstruvite and non–calcium carbonate apatite stones associated with infection, have been described.[9] In a series of 125 patients undergoing percutaneous nephrolithotomy (PCNL), de Cógáin and colleagues[9] found that 24 (23%) of 106 patients with nonstruvite stones had positive stone cultures. A history of neurogenic bladder was associated with positive stone culture in both patients with infected nonstruvite and struvite stones in this series. Non–urease-producing bacteria, including *Escherichia coli* and *Enterococcus* spp, are the predominant

organisms colonizing these metabolic stones.[9,10] Whether these stones form and become secondarily infected or whether these stones result from a nidus of infection that propagates stone formation is unclear. Theories for how bacteria could be a nidus for nonstruvite and non–calcium carbonate apatite stones include kidney cell injury and inflammation potentiating crystal retention, alteration of the microenvironment by bacterial metabolic activity, or biofilm that acts as a matrix for stone growth.[9] In general, sending a sample for stone culture should be considered for all patients undergoing PCNL to help target antibiotic therapy in the event of a postoperative infection. Patients should make appropriate dietary modifications and receive specific medical therapy based on metabolic studies to prevent recurrent urolithiasis. Further studies are necessary to elucidate the exact role and clinical significance of bacteria in these stones.

Obstructive Pyelonephritis

Pyelonephritis is an infection of the kidney with typical presentation including but not limited to fever, flank pain, and irritative lower urinary tract symptoms. Obstructive pyelonephritis is a complicated UTI and considered a urologic emergency because of the significant risk of morbidity and mortality.[11–13] Borofsky and colleagues[12] identified 1712 patients from the Nationwide Inpatient Sample between 2007 and 2009 who had ureteral calculi and sepsis and found a 19% rate of mortality if decompression was not performed versus 9% for those who underwent surgical decompression. Ureteral stones are responsible for approximately two-thirds of the occurrences of obstructive pyelonephritis.[14]

PATIENT EVALUATION OVERVIEW
Infection Stones

Patients with infection stones typically do not present with acute colic and instead are found incidentally or due to complaints of vague abdominal or back pain, recurrent UTIs, and/or gross hematuria.[7] **Box 1** provides a summary of the initial evaluation of these patients. A focused history and physical examination should be performed.

A urinalysis (UA) may show an alkaline pH (>7.0) and evidence of an infection, including leukocyte esterase, white blood cells (WBCs), nitrite, and blood. Magnesium ammonium phosphate crystals (which are coffin shaped) may also be noted on the UA of a patient with infection stones. Urine culture should be done, and is likely to grow a urease-producing bacteria. A basic metabolic panel is used to assess kidney function, as infectious staghorn calculi have a high risk of causing renal insufficiency.[8] Hematocrit, platelet count, and coagulation panel values are necessary for surgical planning.

Box 1
Initial evaluation of patients with suspicion for infection stones

History

- Symptoms
  - Flank pain, abdominal pain, fevers, chills, gross hematuria
  - LUTS: dysuria, hematuria, urgency, frequency
- Urologic history
  - UTI, pyelonephritis
  - Urolithiasis
  - Urinary diversion and/or neurogenic bladder
  - Anatomic abnormalities (UPJO, strictures)
  - Chronic indwelling catheters, SPT or CIC
  - Urethral strictures
  - Prior urologic surgeries
- Anticoagulation or antiplatelet therapy (and if these can be held)

Physical examination

- Fever/hypothermia, vital signs
- CVAT, abdominal/suprapubic tenderness
- Musculoskeletal deformities

Laboratory tests

- UA and urine culture
- BMP, CBC, coagulation panel
- ± Blood cultures (if presenting acutely with fever/concern for sepsis)

Radiology

- Noncontrast CT scan (gold standard)
- KUB and/or renal US (best used for follow-up)
- ± Renogram

Abbreviations: BMP, basic metabolic panel; CBC, complete blood count; CIC, clean intermittent catheterization; CT, computed tomography; CVAT, costovertebral angle tenderness; KUB, kidney ureter bladder radiography; LUTS, lower urinary tract symptoms; SPT, suprapubic tube; UA, urinalysis; UPJO, ureteropelvic junction obstruction; US, ultrasonography; UTI, urinary tract infection.

Imaging with noncontrast computerized tomography (CT) is the gold standard for both diagnosis and surgical planning. Kidney, ureter, and bladder radiography and/or renal ultrasonography (US) may be used for follow-up. A renogram should be performed if poor function is suspected in the affected kidney.

Obstructive Pyelonephritis

Initial evaluation of patients presenting with obstructive pyelonephritis most frequently begins in the emergency room (ER). **Box 2** provides a summary of the initial evaluation of these patients. A focused history and physical examination should be performed, with careful attention paid to vital signs and hemodynamic stability. Findings of poor performance status and a history of paralysis in patients with obstructive pyelonephritis should alert the medical practitioner to an increased risk for sepsis.[13] The use of anticoagulation or antiplatelet therapy must be assessed. For patients with paralysis and contractures, physical examination should also assess mobility of the patient's lower body and the ability to place them in lithotomy position for cystoscopy. Patients with severe lower extremity contractures that prohibit cystoscopic access may require PCNTs for decompression.

UA may show signs of infection, with positivity for leukocyte esterase, WBCs, blood, and nitrite; however, a negative UA result does not rule out infection. The urine proximal to an obstructing stone may be infected, whereas the voided urine

---

Box 2
Initial evaluation of patients with obstructive pyelonephritis

History
- Symptoms
  - Flank pain, abdominal pain, nausea, vomiting, fevers, chills
  - LUTS: dysuria, hematuria, urgency, frequency
- Urologic history
  - UTI, pyelonephritis
  - Urolithiasis
  - Anatomic abnormalities (UPJO, strictures)
  - Urologic surgeries
- Past history of malignancy, irradiation, abdominal surgeries (risks for ureteral obstruction)
- Risk factors for infection (DM, HIV/AIDS, performance status, paralysis, other immunocompromised states)
- Anticoagulation or antiplatelet therapy

Physical examination
- Fever/hypothermia, hemodynamic stability
- CVAT, abdominal pain/suprapubic pain

Laboratory tests
- UA, CBC, BMP, ± albumin, ± CRP
- Voided urine culture and blood culture at presentation
- Urine culture from the kidney(s) at the time of decompression

Radiology
- Noncontrast CT abdomen and pelvis
- Ultrasonography (can consider as first line if patient is stable and there is low suspicion for stone) ± KUB

Abbreviations: AIDS, acquired immune deficiency syndrome; BMP, basic metabolic panel; CBC, complete blood count; CRP, c-reactive protein; CVAT, costovertebral angle tenderness; DM, diabetes mellitus; HIV, human immunodeficiency virus; KUB, kidney ureter bladder radiography; LUTS, lower urinary tract symptoms; UPJO, ureteropelvic junction obstruction.

distal to this may be sterile. Glucosuria should alert the clinician to poorly controlled or undiagnosed diabetes mellitus. The practitioner should be aware that patients with thrombocytopenia[13,15,16] and low serum albumin levels[13,15] are at an increased risk of developing septic shock and should be monitored appropriately. Urine and blood cultures should be sent on presentation, and a urine culture from the kidney(s) should be obtained at the time of decompression. Although some series have found C-reactive protein (CRP) levels helpful in distinguishing between infected and sterile hydronephrosis[17] as well as for identifying those patients who will develop urosepsis,[13] the utility of CRP in the management of obstructive pyelonephritis is unclear.

Imaging is required to differentiate nonobstructive from obstructive pyelonephritis. Although US can detect hydronephrosis and has the advantage of avoiding ionizing radiation, it is user dependent, limited by body habitus, and frequently suboptimal in identifying the specific source of ureteral obstruction. Some advocate for bedside US in the ER to screen for hydronephrosis before CT scan to avoid radiation and unnecessary costs.[18] US performed in the ER has a reported sensitivity of 80% and specificity of 83%.[19] A bedside US by the ER physician may be reasonable as an initial evaluation for ureteral obstruction in a stable patient. Ultimately, however, a CT scan should be obtained to confirm the diagnosis and clearly characterize the cause of obstruction, which affects the choice of decompression procedure as well as guides future definitive surgical therapy.

PHARMACOLOGIC TREATMENT OPTIONS
Infection Stones

Infection stones are optimally managed surgically with the goal of complete stone clearance. After surgery, pharmacologic preventative measures can be considered, including acidification of the urine, inhibition of urease, chemolysis via topical application, and suppressive antibiotic therapy. Medical therapy alone can also be considered for those unable to undergo surgery. Crystallization of infection stones occurs at a pH greater than 7.0 to 7.2. Acidification of the urine to less than pH 6.5 can greatly increase the solubility of this type of infection stone. Urinary acidification with ascorbic acid, ammonium chloride, ammonium sulfate, ammonium nitrite, and L-methionine has been reported.[6,20] L-Methionine is an oral medication that is metabolized to sulfate and hydrogen ions.[21] In vitro studies using L-methionine have shown excellent ability to dissolve infection stones,[22] and older in vivo series have shown

favorable urinary acidification.[23] Contemporary in vivo studies are needed to assess for safety and efficacy. Urinary acidification is rarely implemented today.

Acetohydroxamic acid (AHA) is an oral agent that acts as a urease inhibitor. AHA was initially described in the 1960s and is the only US Food and Drug Administration (FDA)-approved urease inhibitor.[24] Hydroxyurea was also investigated as an oral urease inhibitor but was found to be inferior to AHA.[25] AHA works well because it achieves high levels in the urine and can penetrate bacterial cell walls. Randomized and placebo-controlled studies have proved AHA's ability to significantly reduce stone growth; however, it does not decrease existing stone burden.[26–28] Griffith and colleagues[26] in a randomized, double-blind, placebo-controlled trial of AHA in 210 patients with spinal cord injury reported a significant decrease in stone growth for those receiving AHA versus placebo (33% and 60%, respectively). However, many patients experience psychoneurologic, hematologic, and gastrointestinal side effects, with 22% unable to tolerate AHA.[27,29] The presence of renal insufficiency increases the risk of toxicity and results in decreased efficacy. Thus, AHA is contraindicated for patients with a creatinine level greater than 2.5 mg/dL[2]. It is also contraindicated in pregnant women and women of childbearing age who are not using birth control. The American Urological Association (AUA) guidelines state that AHA may be offered only after surgical options have been exhausted for patients with residual or recurrent struvite stones.[30] They also encourage the use of AHA in patients with abnormal lower urinary tracts (ie, neurogenic bladder or urinary diversion) and struvite and/or calcium carbonate apatite stones because of the high risk for recurrent stone formation.[31]

Topical chemolysis and dissolution with Renacidin irrigant (10% hemiacidrin) or Suby G solution (3.2% citric acid) into the collecting system has also been described.[32–34] In the 1960s, 6 patients died after treatment with Renacidin, which led to the ban of this irrigant by the FDA. Further investigation found that these deaths were related to administration of the irrigant under high pressure resulting in pyelovenous back flow, systemic absorption, urosepsis, and subsequent death.[35] Dissolution therapy for infection stones via PCNTs, ureteral stents, and/or access sheaths is now considered safe and effective as long as it is performed in the setting of sterile urine, with prophylactic antibiotics and at low renal pelvic pressures.[34] Postoperative application is limited for multiple reasons including the need to know the stone composition before administration, difficulty maintaining a low-pressure system, need for constant nursing care, need for replacement/ exchange of ureteral stents and nephrostomy tubes when they become obstructed, and need for prolonged hospitalization. For those patients with infection stones who are not cured with surgical stone removal, dissolution therapy can be considered and is currently approved by the FDA for use in this setting.

In theory, the eradication of urease-producing bacteria in the urinary tract with antibiotics should halt the formation of infection stones, and older series have even reported that infection stones may dissolve in sterile urine[36,37]; however, antibiotics do not penetrate infection stones. Ultimately, surgical removal is required to achieve sterility. There are anecdotal reports of decreased recurrence of infection stones by placing patients on suppressive antibiotic therapy for several months after surgical stone removal, but there are no series in the literature studying this approach. With increasing rates of antimicrobial resistance, evidence is needed to justify the use of prolonged antimicrobial therapy in this patient population. Another suggested approach is to check a urine culture every month for 3 months after surgical removal of infection stones and treat as needed.[38] Further studies are necessary to clearly state the role of suppressive antibiotics after surgical removal of infection stones.

Obstructive Pyelonephritis

Obstructive pyelonephritis requires dual therapy with broad-spectrum antibiotics and emergent decompression. Selection of empiric antibiotic therapy can be complicated because of the increasing antimicrobial resistance both nationally and worldwide.[39–42] Choice of empiric antibiotic therapy can be guided by reviewing prior urine culture data, urine culture gram-staining result,[43] the hospital's antibiogram, and antimicrobial stewardship's recommendations.[44] In general, the patient should be administered broad-spectrum antibiotics to cover for common gram-negative pathogens with or without antibiotics to cover gram-positive pathogens. One series reported on their experience with obstructive pyelonephritis and found that 79% of bacterial pathogens were gram-negative rods, with E coli being the most common (66%) and Enterococcus spp making up two-thirds of the gram-positive pathogens.[44] Of the 65 patients in this series, 2 had candida in their urine specimens. Coverage for gram-positive pathogens should be initiated if the patient presents with sepsis, if gram-positive bacteria are noted on gram staining, and if the patient has a history of prior UTIs with gram-positive pathogens. Once the organisms in the urine and blood cultures are determined, the patient should be switched to a 1- to 2-week course of culture-specific antibiotics.[45]

NONPHARMACOLOGIC TREATMENT OPTIONS
Infection Stones

Dietary modifications to prevent infection stones have generally focused on reducing urinary phosphorous and magnesium levels by avoiding dietary foods and vitamin supplements high in these elements. Shorr and Carter[46] proposed a regimen in the 1940s of a low-phosphate, low-calcium diet with oral estrogens (to decrease calcium excretion) and an aluminum hydroxide gel to bind phosphate in the gut. Although studies found significant stone dissolution and reduced stone growth[46] as well as decreased stone recurrence following PCNL[47] on this regimen, the Shorr diet has been shown to result in significant metabolic abnormalities related to the aluminum hydroxide, including constipation, anorexia, lethargy, bone pain, and hypercalciuria.[48] The Shorr diet with aluminum hydroxide is not currently recommended.

Obstructive Pyelonephritis

There is no role for nonpharmacologic treatment of obstructive pyelonephritis in the acute setting. Long-term efforts to decrease recurrent nephrolithiasis and UTIs through dietary measures are indicated.

SURGICAL TREATMENT OPTIONS
Infection Stones

Surgical management with the goal of complete stone clearance is the standard of care for patients with infection stones. **Table 1** provides a summary of surgical treatment options for infection stones as recommended by AUA guidelines and reported in the literature.

For those well enough to undergo surgical intervention, the current AUA guidelines recommend PCNL monotherapy as the treatment of choice for staghorn calculi.[31] PCNL in combination with flexible ureteroscopy results in less access tracts and decreased blood loss.[59] PCNL and ureteroscopy may be performed simultaneously in the prone position with a split leg bed, avoiding time needed to reposition from dorsal lithotomy to prone.[60,61] Combination therapy for the treatment of infection stones refers to the use of PCNL with shockwave lithotripsy (SWL). Segura and colleagues[62] reported a disappointing stone free rate of 23% in their series of 16 consecutive

Table 1
Surgical approaches for infection stones

Surgery	Indication	Evidence
PCNL (± URS, ± flexible nephroscopy)	First line per AUA guidelines	Preminger et al,[31] 2005
PCNL + SWL	When calyces cannot be accessed with nephroscopy or additional access tracts	Preminger et al,[31] 2005; Merhej et al,[49] 1998
SWL monotherapy (+stent or PCNT)	Stone burden <500 mm² with no/minimal dilation of the collecting system	Preminger et al,[31] 2005; Lam et al,[50] 1992
URS monotherapy	May consider for partial staghorn stones in patients unable to undergo PCNL	Healy & Ogan,[51] 2007
ANL (open or lap/RAL)	PCNL failure, extremely large stones, aberrant collecting system anatomy (ie, calyceal diverticulum, infundibular stenosis), unfavorable body habitus for PCNL (ie, morbid obesity, skeletal deformities), pelvic or transplant kidneys	Preminger et al,[31] 2005; Bove et al,[52] 2012; Assimos,[53] 2001; King et al,[54] 2014; Ghani et al,[55] 2013; Giedelman et al,[56] 2012; Simforoosh et al,[57] 2008; Elbahnasy et al,[58] 2011

Abbreviations: ANL, anatrophic lithotripsy; lap, laparoscopic; RAL, robotic-assisted laparoscopic; SWL, shockwave lithotripsy; URS, ureteroscopy.

patients undergoing PCNL followed by SWL. Based on this study, the current AUA guidelines state that if SWL is to be performed with PCNL, PCNL should be the first modality used to treat these patients as well as the last because clearance of all fragments after SWL is unlikely.[31] SWL may be used in cases in which residual stones cannot be treated with flexible nephroscopy or via another access tract. However, in general, flexible nephroscopy and ureteroscopy obviates SWL for inaccessible calyces.[31] Although older series have found SWL monotherapy with stent or PCNT acceptable treatment of smaller stone burden (<500 mm²) with no or minimal dilation of the renal collecting system, most urologists who treat complex stone disease still perform PCNL in this cohort.[50] Open surgery with anatrophic nephrolithotomy (ANL) is not appropriate for most patients with infection or staghorn stones per the AUA guidelines, although it may be considered for cases in which the stone is not expected to be removed by a reasonable number of less invasive procedures. Although open stone removal results in stone free rates similar to those of PCNL, this approach is associated with increased morbidity, convalescence period, hospital stay, narcotic requirement, and complications.[63] A minimally invasive alternative to open ANL is laparoscopic and robotic ANL, which have recently been described.[54–57]

In preparation for surgery, a noncontrast CT scan is obtained to delineate the anatomy and guide the surgical approach. A renogram should be obtained if there is concern for a poorly functioning renal unit, and nephrectomy considered if poor function is confirmed and the contralateral kidney is normal.

Patients with suspected infection stones are at increased risk for infectious complications after PCNL. Preplacement of PCNT allows for drainage, aspiration, and culture of stagnant and infected urine. By administering a course of antibiotics based on this pelvic urine culture, some have shown a decreased rate of postoperative bacteremia, systemic inflammatory response syndrome (SIRS), and sepsis,[64,65] which is likely because stone culture results correlates more closely with renal pelvic than bladder culture results.[66] In a retrospective review of 219 patients, Benson and colleagues[64] reported a 6% rate of SIRS/sepsis at the time of PCNL in those undergoing concurrent PCNT placement versus none in those undergoing preplaced PCNT.

If bladder urine culture results are positive, patients undergoing stone treatment without preplaced PCNT should be treated with a course of preoperative antibiotics with the goal of sterilizing the urine. For those patients without positive results on preoperative urine culture, current AUA guidelines recommend limiting perioperative antibiotics to less than 24 hours except for those patients with external urinary catheters present before surgery, with risk factors (ie, advanced age, anatomic abnormalities of the urinary tract, poor nutritional status, tobacco use, chronic corticosteroid use, immunodeficiency, or prolonged hospitalization), or with bacteriuria.[67] However, several series have shown significant reduction in postoperative sepsis by administering all patients undergoing PCNL a prophylactic course of antibiotics.[68,69] Mariappan and colleagues[69] found that 52 patients who had dilated collecting systems, stone burden greater than 2 cm, and no confounding factors predisposing to UTIs who received a 1-week course of ciprofloxacin before PCNL had a 3-fold lower risk of postoperative UTI and SIRS than 46 patients who received standard perioperative antibiotics on the day of surgery. Bag and colleagues[68] prospectively randomized 101 patients with greater than 2.5-cm kidney stones and/or hydronephrosis with sterile preoperative urine cultures to a 7-day course of nitrofurantoin versus no antibiotics before PCNL and found a statistically significant lower rate of postoperative SIRS (19% vs 49%), endotoxemia (18% vs 42%), positive result on kidney urine culture (0% vs 10%), and positive result on stone culture (8% vs 30%) in the arm receiving nitrofurantoin. Although these 2 small series support a week of preoperative antibiotics before PCNL, larger, prospective, randomized studies are underway to better elucidate the risks and benefits of empiric antibiotics used in this setting.

Given the known discordance between results of bladder urine culture and stone culture, strong consideration should be given to sending a sample for stone culture to help target antibiotic therapy if the patient develops a postoperative infection. Multiple series have examined the relationship between results of preoperative urine culture from the bladder and kidney stone culture and found poor correlation between the two.[70,71] One series by Eswara and colleagues[70] reported on 328 consecutive patients who underwent stone surgery and found for those 11 patients who developed sepsis, readmission urine culture result correlated with stone culture result in 64% of cases and with preoperative urine culture result in only 9% of cases ($P = .02$). A stone culture at the time of surgery may be helpful to guide antibiotic therapy in the setting of postoperative UTI and/or urosepsis.

Obstructive Pyelonephritis

Although older series may support withholding emergency decompression in patients with fever and obstructing urolithiasis,[72] it is clear that decompression with retrograde ureteral stent placement or PCNT is imperative to decrease morbidity and mortality.[12] Some have theorized that ureteral stent placement is inferior to PCNT because of the risk of exacerbating infection via stone manipulation and by providing suboptimal drainage compared with a larger-caliber nephrostomy tube. Pearle and colleagues[73] randomized 42 consecutive patients with obstructing ureteral stones and clinical evidence of infection to drainage with PCNT or retrograde ureteral stent placement and found that neither modality was superior in promoting rapid recovery after drainage, although ureteral stent placement was found to be more than twice as costly as PCNT ($1137 vs $2401). The only benefit of PCNT versus ureteral stent placement in this setting was found as a secondary end point from a series out of Syria, which reported that patients who underwent decompression with PCNT required shorter antibiotic courses than those managed with stents.[74]

Although ureteral stent placement and PCNT have both been shown to be effective methods of decompression, in some circumstances one method is indicated over the other (**Table 2**). The presence of hemodynamic instability may limit

---

Table 2
Mode of decompression considerations for obstructive pyelonephritis

Favoring Ureteral Stent	Favoring PCNT
• Interventional radiologist unavailable • Failed PCNT attempt • Uncorrected coagulopathy • Minimal hydronephrosis • Unfavorable anatomy for percutaneous access	• Urologist unavailable • Failed ureteral stent attempt • Difficult retrograde access (ie, urinary diversion, renal transplant) • Inability to access the bladder (ie, urethral stricture, lower extremity contractures) • Steinstrasse and/or large stone burden • Concern for impacted ureteral stone • Inability to tolerate general anesthesia

the use of general anesthesia. Although most urologists place ureteral stents under general anesthesia, several series have shown that retrograde ureteral stent placement under local anesthesia is safe and effective, with less than 10% rate of failure.[75–77] A retrospective review of 119 primary ureteral stent placements reported by Sivalingam and colleagues[75] compared 46 cases undergoing stent placement with local anesthesia with 73 cases with general anesthesia and found no statistical difference in placement failure (1.3% for those under general anesthesia vs 8.7% for those under local anesthesia, $P = .07$) and no complications in either group. However, the cost was 4-fold greater in the group undergoing stent placement with general anesthesia ($30,060 vs $7700).

When attempting ureteral stent placement under local anesthesia, the authors recommend the use of lidocaine jelly and a flexible cystoscope for improved patient tolerance. Patient consent should be obtained for both procedures before being sedated or undergoing anesthesia in the event that the first attempt at decompression fails. This method prevents delay in implementing a secondary procedure that may be time sensitive and life saving.

At the time of decompression, a kidney urine culture should be done. Given the risk of urosepsis after decompression, patients should be observed in a monitored setting such as an intensive care unit. A Foley catheter is also recommended for maximum decompression of the urinary collecting system. After a 1- to 2-week course of culture-specific antibiotics, the patient can be scheduled for definitive stone treatment.[45]

TREATMENT RESISTANCE/COMPLICATIONS
Infection Stones

Patients with infection stones undergoing surgical stone removal are at increased risk of adverse events compared with those undergoing surgery for metabolic stones. Higher rates of infectious and bleeding complications are likely related to bacterial colonization of the stones and chronic inflammation related to persistent infection. Thus, although one would expect similar rates of urinary extravasation (7%), renal pelvis perforation (3%), colonic injury (0.2%–0.8%), and pleural injury (0%–3%) for all patients undergoing PCNL, those with infection stones are likely to experience higher rates of infectious and bleeding complications than the following rates that are typically reported: bleeding (8%), blood transfusion (6%–17%), fever (11%–32%), and sepsis (0.3%–5%).[78,79]

Similarly, although complications for all comers undergoing SWL includes bacteriuria (8%–24%),

bacteremia (14%), sepsis (<1–3%), steinstrasse (3%), perinephric hematomas (20%–25%), symptomatic perinephric hematoma (<1%), and gastrointestinal tract injury (2%), patients undergoing SWL for infection stones have even higher risks of these postoperative infectious adverse events.[80–83] Some have even shown that performing SWL in the setting of a staghorn stone with a positive urine culture result and urinary obstruction increases the risk of postoperative sepsis.[83] Similarly, if an infection stone is treated ureteroscopically either because a more invasive approach could not be safely performed or because there was low suspicion for infection stone at the time of surgical planning, these patients are at higher risk for postoperative infectious complications and especially sepsis related to increased intrarenal pressures secondary to irrigation. Use of a ureteral access sheath at the time of ureteroscopy may decrease intrarenal pressures and risks of postoperative systemic infection. Otherwise these patients are at similar risks to other patients undergoing ureteroscopy for urolithiasis, including risks of bleeding (0.3%–2%), stricture (0.5%–3%), ureteral perforation (0%–15%), extravasation (<1%), ureteral avulsion (<0.5%), and steinstrasse (rare).[84] Open ANL is now rarely performed given the development and success of minimally invasive techniques and the morbidity related to this procedure, including the risk of serious complications such as pneumothorax, pulmonary embolism, wound infection, acute tubular necrosis, rhabdomyolysis, hemorrhage, vascular injuries, and urinoma.[53] Of the small series publishing their outcomes of robotic and laparoscopic ANL, reported complications include gross hematuria requiring continuous bladder irrigation, blood transfusion, splenic injury necessitating splenectomy, and vascular fistula.[54,56,85]

Obstructive Pyelonephritis

Patients with obstructive pyelonephritis are at risk to develop urosepsis and its sequelae, including acute kidney injury and death. Mortality rates for patients with obstructive pyelonephritis and sepsis are reported at 9% for those undergoing surgical decompression and 19% for those without decompression.[12] Potential complications related to nephrostomy tube placement include bleeding, although severe bleeding requiring transfusion is rare (1%–3%); liver, splenic, or pleural injury (0.1%–0.3%); and rarely colonic or small-bowel injury.[86,87] Ureteral stent placement can be complicated by ureteral perforation and malposition requiring another procedure for decompression. In addition, ureteral stents can cause significant bother specifically related to urinary symptoms. Quality of life has been shown to be superior for patients with ureteral stones managed with PCNTs than for those with ureteral stents.[74,88]

EVALUATION OF OUTCOMES AND LONG-TERM RECOMMENDATIONS
Infection Stones

PCNL monotherapy stone free rates range from 82% to 93%.[50,89] Lower stone free rates have been reported with SWL and PCNL combination therapy ranging from 67% to 78% even when PCNL is last.[49,50] Lam and colleagues[50] report a stone free rate of 92% for renal stones less than 500 mm^2 that were in a nondilated collecting system treated with SWL monotherapy in a series of 12 patients. Stone free rates after open ANL are reported to be high, ranging from 80% to 100%.[90,91] Stone free rates after pure laparoscopic ANL are reported at 80% to 88%,[85,92] whereas early experience with the robotic-assisted laparoscopic approach reports fairly low stone free rates at 29% to 33%.[54,55]

The presence of residual stone fragments in patients with infection stones composed of struvite and/or calcium carbonate apatite significantly increases the risk of stone recurrence, with a 0% to 10% recurrence rate for those who are stone free postoperatively versus 40% to 85% in the setting of residual stone fragments.[20,29] Patients who are rendered stone free have a lower rate of postoperative UTI (38%) versus those with residual fragments (64%).[29]

After surgery, preventative measures may be helpful including dietary modifications as previously described in the nonpharmacologic section and urinary acidification and urease inhibitors as described in the pharmacologic section of this article. Sterilization of the urine with antibiotics may help decrease stone recurrence, as persistent infection is known to increase the risk of stone recurrence. However, there is not much more than anecdotal evidence of this approach in the literature, and the best regimen in terms of antibiotic selection, duration, and dosing is unknown. Antibiotic use in this setting can be even more complicated when stone and/or renal pelvic urine cultures resistance patterns show no oral options. For those patients with secondarily infected metabolic stones, a full metabolic workup with a 24-hour urine study should be performed. Metabolic evaluation may also be beneficial in patients with infection stones given the findings of a recent series comparing postoperative stone events in patients with struvite stones with and without metabolic evaluation and directed medical therapy. In this series, 39 patients with pure and mixed struvite stones who underwent metabolic evaluation and directed treatment had significantly less stone events postoperatively compared with 17 patients with pure struvite stones and no metabolic workup or management.[93]

Obstructive Pyelonephritis

Vahlensieck and colleagues[14] reported on their experience with 57 patients treated for obstructive pyelonephritis during a 5-year period and found that 32% go on to have recurrent UTIs and 11% experience recurrent obstructive pyelonephritis over a 5-year follow-up period. For those patients with recurrent UTIs and no obvious cause that can be definitively treated (ie, incomplete bladder emptying secondary to benign prostatic hypertrophy), prophylactic antibiotics may be beneficial. Metabolic evaluation is recommended even in patients with first-time stone formation who have a history of obstructive pyelonephritis given the potential risk of sepsis with future stone events.

SUMMARY/DISCUSSION
Infection Stones

Infection stones are struvite and/or calcium carbonate apatite in composition and occur as a result of UTI with urease-producing bacteria. Surgery with the aim of complete stone removal is the mainstay of treatment. PCNL is the treatment of choice for most patients with large infection stones per AUA guidelines. In certain circumstances, other surgical approaches including combination therapy for SWL with PCNL, SWL monotherapy, ureteroscopy, and open and laparoscopic/robotic approaches may be appropriate. A course of preoperative antibiotics has been shown to decrease the rate of SIRS/sepsis after PCNL. Nonsurgical approaches with dietary measures, urease inhibitors, and dissolution therapy may be useful adjuncts to surgical intervention or as a primary treatment of those who are medically unfit to undergo a surgical procedure.

Obstructive Pyelonephritis

Obstructing ureteral stones with concurrent UTI is a urologic emergency and requires immediate decompression, broad-spectrum antibiotics, and close monitoring for urosepsis. Obstructive pyelonephritis with sepsis without decompression has a 19% mortality rate. PCNT and retrograde ureteral stenting are both adequate for decompression. Long-term interventions to prevent recurrent infections and stones is useful given the high rate of recurrent UTIs and 10% risk of recurrent obstructive pyelonephritis in these patients.

REFERENCES

1. Knoll T, Schubert AB, Fahlenkamp D, et al. Urolithiasis through the ages: data on more than 200,000 urinary stone analyses. J Urol 2011;185(4):1304–11.

2. Daudon M, Dore JC, Jungers P, et al. Changes in stone composition according to age and gender of patients: a multivariate epidemiological approach. Urol Res 2004;32(3):241–7.

3. Choong S, Whitfield H. Biofilms and their role in infections in urology. BJU Int 2000;86(8):935–41.

4. Rahman NU, Meng MV, Stoller ML. Infections and urinary stone disease. Curr Pharm Des 2003;9(12): 975–81.

5. Hedelin H. Uropathogens and urinary tract concretion formation and catheter encrustations. Int J Antimicrob Agents 2002;19(6):484–7.

6. Bichler KH, Eipper E, Naber K, et al. Urinary infection stones. Int J Antimicrob Agents 2002;19(6):488–98.

7. Schwartz BF, Stoller ML. Nonsurgical management of infection-related renal calculi. Urol Clin North Am 1999;26(4):765–78, viii.

8. Koga S, Arakaki Y, Matsuoka M, et al. Staghorn calculi – long-term results of management. Br J Urol 1991;68(2):122–4.

9. de Cógáin MR, Lieske JC, Vrtiska TJ, et al. Secondarily infected nonstruvite urolithiasis: a prospective evaluation. Urology 2014;84(6):1295–300.

10. Tavichakorntrakool R, Prasongwattana V, Sungkeeree S, et al. Extensive characterizations of bacteria isolated from catheterized urine and stone matrices in patients with nephrolithiasis. Nephrol Dial Transplant 2012;27(11):4125–30.

11. Yoshimura K, Utsunomiya N, Ichioka K, et al. Emergency drainage for urosepsis associated with upper urinary tract calculi. J Urol 2005;173(2):458–62.

12. Borofsky MS, Walter D, Shah O, et al. Surgical decompression is associated with decreased mortality in patients with sepsis and ureteral calculi. J Urol 2013;189(3):946–51.

13. Yamamoto Y, Fujita K, Nakazawa S, et al. Clinical characteristics and risk factors for septic shock in patients receiving emergency drainage for acute pyelonephritis with upper urinary tract calculi. BMC Urol 2012;12:4.

14. Vahlensieck W, Friess D, Fabry W, et al. Long-term results after acute therapy of obstructive pyelonephritis. Urol Int 2015;94(4):436–41.

15. Tambo M, Okegawa T, Shishido T, et al. Predictors of septic shock in obstructive acute pyelonephritis. World J Urol 2014;32(3):803–11.

16. Kamei J, Nishimatsu H, Nakagawa T, et al. Risk factors for septic shock in acute obstructive pyelonephritis requiring emergency drainage of the upper urinary tract. Int Urol Nephrol 2014;46(3):493–7.

17. Angulo JC, Gaspar MJ, Rodriguez N, et al. The value of C-reactive protein determination in patients with renal colic to decide urgent urinary diversion. Urology 2010;76(2):301–6.

18. Carnell J, Fischer J, Nagdev A. Ultrasound detection of obstructive pyelonephritis due to urolithiasis in the ED. Am J Emerg Med 2011;29(7):843.e1–3.

19. Watkins S, Bowra J, Sharma P, et al. Validation of emergency physician ultrasound in diagnosing hydronephrosis in ureteric colic. Emerg Med Australas 2007;19(3):188–95.

20. Flannigan R, Choy WH, Chew B, et al. Renal struvite stones-pathogenesis, microbiology, and management strategies. Nat Rev Urol 2014;11(6):333–41.

21. Hesse A, Heimbach D. Causes of phosphate stone formation and the importance of metaphylaxis by urinary acidification: a review. World J Urol 1999; 17(5):308–15.

22. Jacobs D, Heimbach D, Hesse A. Chemolysis of struvite stones by acidification of artificial urine – an in vitro study. Scand J Urol Nephrol 2001;35(5): 345–9.

23. Jarrar K, Boedeker RH, Weidner W. Struvite stones: long-term follow up under metaphylaxis. Ann Urol 1996;30(3):112–7.

24. Bernardo NO, Smith AD. Chemolysis of urinary calculi. Urol Clin North Am 2000;27(2):355–65.

25. Martelli A, Buli P, Cortecchia V. Urease inhibitor therapy in infected renal stones. Eur Urol 1981; 7(5):291–3.

26. Griffith DP, Khonsari F, Skurnick JH, et al. A randomized trial of acetohydroxamic acid for the treatment and prevention of infection-induced urinary stones in spinal cord injury patients. J Urol 1988;140(2):318–24.

27. Griffith DP, Gleeson MJ, Lee H, et al. Randomized, double-blind trial of Lithostat (acetohydroxamic acid) in the palliative treatment of infection-induced urinary calculi. Eur Urol 1991;20(3):243–7.

28. Williams JJ, Rodman JS, Peterson CM. A randomized double-blind study of acetohydroxamic acid in struvite nephrolithiasis. N Engl J Med 1984;311(12):760–4.

29. Iqbal MW, Youssef R, Neisius A, et al. Contemporary management of struvite stones using combined endourological and medical treatment: predictors of unfavorable clinical outcome. J Endourol 2013. [Epub ahead of print].

30. Pearle MS, Goldfarb DS, Assimos DG, et al. Medical management of kidney stones: AUA guideline. J Urol 2014;192(2):316–24.

31. Preminger GM, Assimos DG, Lingeman JE, et al. Chapter 1: AUA guideline on management of staghorn calculi: diagnosis and treatment recommendations. J Urol 2005;173(6):1991–2000.

32. Kachrilas S, Papatsoris A, Bach C, et al. The current role of percutaneous chemolysis in the management of urolithiasis: review and results. Urolithiasis 2013; 41(4):323–6.

33. Angermeier K, Streem SB, Yost A. Simplified infusion method for 10% hemiacidrin irrigation of renal pelvis. Urology 1993;41(3):243–6.

34. Gonzalez RD, Whiting BM, Canales BK. The history of kidney stone dissolution therapy: 50 years of optimism and frustration with Renacidin. J Endourol 2012;26(2):110–8.

35. Mulvaney WP, Henning DC. Solvent treatment of urinary calculi: refinements in technique. J Urol 1962; 88:145–9.

36. Griffith DP, Bragin S, Musher DM. Dissolution of struvite urinary stones. Experimental studies in vitro. Invest Urol 1976;13(5):351–3.

37. Griffith DP, Moskowitz PA, Carlton CE Jr. Adjunctive chemotherapy of infection-induced staghorn calculi. J Urol 1979;121(6):711–5.

38. Bichler KH, Eipper E, Naber K. Infection-induced urinary stones. Urologe A 2003;42(1):47–55 [in German].

39. Goettsch W, van Pelt W, Nagelkerke N, et al. Increasing resistance to fluoroquinolones in Escherichia coli from urinary tract infections in the Netherlands. J Antimicrob Chemother 2000;46(2):223–8.

40. Cullen IM, Manecksha RP, McCullagh E, et al. An 11-year analysis of the prevalent uropathogens and the changing pattern of Escherichia coli antibiotic resistance in 38,530 community urinary tract infections, Dublin 1999–2009. Ir J Med Sci 2013;182(1):81–9.

41. Cullen IM, Manecksha RP, McCullagh E, et al. The changing pattern of antimicrobial resistance within 42,033 Escherichia coli isolates from nosocomial, community and urology patient-specific urinary tract infections, Dublin, 1999–2009. BJU Int 2012;109(8): 1198–206.

42. Karlowsky JA, Kelly LJ, Thornsberry C, et al. Trends in antimicrobial resistance among urinary tract infection isolates of Escherichia coli from female outpatients in the United States. Antimicrob Agents Chemother 2002;46(8):2540–5.

43. MacFadden DR, Ridgway JP, Robicsek A, et al. Predictive utility of prior positive urine cultures. Clin Infect Dis 2014;59(9):1265–71.

44. Marien T, Mass AY, Shah O. Antimicrobial resistance patterns in cases of obstructive pyelonephritis secondary to stones. Urology 2015;85(1):64–8.

45. Nicolle LE. A practical guide to the management of complicated urinary tract infection. Drugs 1997; 53(4):583–92.

46. Shorr E, Carter AC. Aluminum gels in the management of renal phosphatic calculi. J Am Med Assoc 1950;144(18):1549–56.

47. Lavengood RW Jr, Marshall VF. The prevention of renal phosphatic calculi in the presence of infection by the Shorr regimen. J Urol 1972;108(3):368–71.

48. Lotz M, Zisman E, Bartter FC. Evidence for a phosphorus-depletion syndrome in man. N Engl J Med 1968;278(8):409–15.

49. Merhej S, Jabbour M, Samaha E, et al. Treatment of staghorn calculi by percutaneous nephrolithotomy and SWL: the Hotel Dieu de France experience. J Endourol 1998;12(1):5–8.

50. Lam HS, Lingeman JE, Barron M, et al. Staghorn calculi - analysis of treatment results between initial percutaneous nephrostolithotomy and extracorporeal shock-wave lithotripsy monotherapy with reference to surface-area. J Urol 1992;147(5):1219–25.

51. Healy KA, Ogan K. Pathophysiology and management of infectious staghorn calculi. Urol Clin North Am 2007;34(3):363.

52. Bove AM, Altobelli E, Buscarini M. Indication to open anatrophic nephrolithotomy in the twenty-first century: a case report. Case Rep Urol 2012;2012: 851020.

53. Assimos DG. Anatrophic nephrolithotomy. Urology 2001;57(1):161–5.

54. King SA, Klaassen Z, Madi R. Robot-assisted anatrophic nephrolithotomy: Description of technique and early results. J Endourol 2014;28(3):325–9.

55. Ghani KR, Rogers CG, Sood A, et al. Robot-assisted anatrophic nephrolithotomy with renal hypothermia for managing staghorn calculi. J Endourol 2013; 27(11):1393–8.

56. Giedelman C, Arriaga J, Carmona O, et al. Laparoscopic anatrophic nephrolithotomy: developments of the technique in the era of minimally invasive surgery. J Endourol 2012;26(5):444–50.

57. Simforoosh N, Aminsharifi A, Tabibi A, et al. Laparoscopic anatrophic nephrolithotomy for managing large staghorn calculi. BJU Int 2008;101(10):1293–6.

58. Elbahnasy AM, Elbendary MA, Radwan MA, et al. Laparoscopic pyelolithotomy in selected patients with ectopic pelvic kidney: a feasible minimally invasive treatment option. J Endourol 2011;25(6):985–9.

59. Marguet CG, Springhart WP, Tan YH, et al. Simultaneous combined use of flexible ureteroscopy and percutaneous nephrolithotomy to reduce the number of access tracts in the management of complex renal calculi. BJU Int 2005;96(7):1097–100.

60. Landman J, Venkatesh R, Lee DI, et al. Combined percutaneous and retrograde approach to staghorn calculi with application of the ureteral access sheath to facilitate percutaneous nephrolithotomy. J Urol 2003;169(1):64–7.

61. Hamamoto S, Yasui T, Koiwa S, et al. Successful results of endoscopic combined intrarenal surgery against large calculi; simultaneous use of flexible ureteroscopy and mini-percutaneous nephrolithotomy overcame the drawbacks of the monotherapy of percutaneous nephrolithotomy. J Urol 2013; 189(4):E626–7.

62. Segura JW, Patterson DE, Leroy AJ. Combined percutaneous ultrasonic lithotripsy and extracorporeal shock-wave lithotripsy for struvite staghorn calculi. World J Urol 1987;5(4):245–7.

63. Rodrigues Netto N Jr, Lemos GC, Palma PC, et al. Staghorn calculi: percutaneous versus anatrophic nephrolithotomy. Eur Urol 1988;15(1–2):9–12.

64. Benson AD, Juliano TM, Miller NL. Infectious outcomes of nephrostomy drainage before percutaneous nephrolithotomy compared to concurrent access. J Urol 2014;192(3):770–4.

65. Eswara JR, Lee H, Dretler SP, et al. The effect of delayed percutaneous nephrolithotomy on the risk of bacteremia and sepsis in patients with neuromuscular disorders. World J Urol 2013;31(6):1611–5.

66. Mariappan P, Smith G, Bariol SV, et al. Stone and pelvic urine culture and sensitivity are better than bladder urine as predictors of urosepsis following percutaneous nephrolithotomy: A prospective clinical study. J Urol 2005;173(5):1610–4.

67. Wolf JS, Bennett CJ, Dmochowski RR, et al. Best practice policy statement on urologic surgery antimicrobial prophylaxis. J Urol 2008;179(4):1379–90.

68. Bag S, Kumar S, Taneja N, et al. One week of nitrofurantoin before percutaneous nephrolithotomy significantly reduces upper tract infection and urosepsis: a prospective controlled study. Urology 2011;77(1):45–9.

69. Mariappan P, Smith G, Moussa SA, et al. One week of ciprofloxacin before percutaneous nephrolithotomy significantly reduces upper tract infection and urosepsis: a prospective controlled study. BJU Int 2006;98(5):1075–9.

70. Eswara JR, Sharif-Tabrizi A, Sacco D. Positive stone culture is associated with a higher rate of sepsis after endourological procedures. Urolithiasis 2013; 41(5):411–4.

71. Margel D, Ehrlich Y, Brown N, et al. Clinical implication of routine stone culture in percutaneous nephrolithotomy - a prospective study. Urology 2006;67(1): 26–9.

72. Klein LA, Koyle M, Berg S. The emergency management of patients with ureteral calculi and fever. J Urol 1983;129(5):938–40.

73. Pearle MS, Pierce HL, Miller GL, et al. Optimal method of urgent decompression of the collecting system for obstruction and infection due to ureteral calculi. J Urol 1998;160(4):1260–4.

74. Mokhmalji H, Braun PM, Martinez Portillo FJ, et al. Percutaneous nephrostomy versus ureteral stents for diversion of hydronephrosis caused by stones: a prospective, randomized clinical trial. J Urol 2001;165(4):1088–92.

75. Sivalingam S, Tamm-Daniels I, Nakada SY. Office-based ureteral stent placement under local anesthesia for obstructing stones is safe and efficacious. Urology 2013;81(3):498–502.

76. McFarlane JP, Cowan C, Holt SJ, et al. Outpatient ureteric procedures: a new method for retrograde ureteropyelography and ureteric stent placement. BJU Int 2001;87(3):172–6.

77. Adeyoju AB, Collins GN, Brooman P, et al. Outpatient flexible cystoscope-assisted insertion of ureteric catheters and ureteric stents. BJU Int 1999;83(7):748–50.

78. Michel MS, Trojan L, Rassweiler JJ. Complications in percutaneous nephrolithotomy. Eur Urol 2007;51(4): 899–906.

79. de la Rosette J, Assimos D, Desai M, et al. The clinical research office of the endourological society percutaneous nephrolithotomy global study: indications, complications, and outcomes in 5803 patients. J Endourol 2011;25(1):11–7.

80. D'Addessi A, Vittori M, Racioppi M, et al. Complications of extracorporeal shock wave lithotripsy for urinary stones: to know and to manage them – a review. ScientificWorldJournal 2012;2012:619820.

81. Wazir BG, Iftikhar ul Haq M, Faheem ul H, et al. Experience of extracorporeal shockwave lithotripsy for kidney and upper ureteric stones by electromagnetic lithotriptor. J Ayub Med Coll Abbottabad 2010; 22(2):20–2.

82. Razvi H, Fuller A, Nott L, et al. Risk factors for perinephric hematoma formation after shockwave lithotripsy: a matched case-control analysis. J Endourol 2012;26(11):1478–82.

83. Skolarikos A, Alivizatos G, de la Rosette J. Extracorporeal shock wave lithotripsy 25 years later: complications and their prevention. Eur Urol 2006;50(5): 981–90.

84. D'Addessi A, Bassi P. Ureterorenoscopy: avoiding and managing the complications. Urol Int 2011; 87(3):251–9.

85. Aminsharifi A, Hadian P, Boveiri K. Laparoscopic anatrophic nephrolithotomy for management of complete staghorn renal stone: clinical efficacy and intermediate-term functional outcome. J Endourol 2013;27(5):573–8.

86. Uppot RN. Emergent nephrostomy tube placement for acute urinary obstruction. Tech Vasc Interv Radiol 2009;12(2):154–61.

87. Winer AG, Hyams ES, Shah O. Small bowel injury during percutaneous nephrostomy tube placement causing small bowel obstruction. Can J Urol 2009; 16(6):4950–2.

88. Joshi HB, Okeke A, Newns N, et al. Characterization of urinary symptoms in patients with ureteral stents. Urology 2002;59(4):511–6.

89. Desai M, Jain P, Ganpule A, et al. Developments in technique and technology: the effect on the results of percutaneous nephrolithotomy for staghorn calculi. BJU Int 2009;104(4):542–8.

90. Assimos DG, Wrenn JJ, Harrison LH, et al. A comparison of anatrophic nephrolithotomy and percutaneous nephrolithotomy with and without extracorporeal shock wave lithotripsy for management of patients with staghorn calculi. J Urol 1991; 145(4):710–4.

91. Morey AF, Nitahara KS, McAninch JW. Modified anatrophic nephrolithotomy for management of staghorn calculi: is renal function preserved? J Urol 1999;162(3 Pt 1):670–3.

92. Simforoosh N, Radfar MH, Nouralizadeh A, et al. Laparoscopic anatrophic nephrolithotomy for management of staghorn renal calculi. J Laparoendosc Adv Surg Tech A 2013;23(4): 306–10.

93. Kaplan A, Shin R, Iqbal M, et al. Patients with struvite stones. SESAUA presentation. Savannah (GA), March 19, 2015.

Treatment of Fungal Urinary Tract Infection

Lewis Thomas, MD, Chad R. Tracy, MD*

KEYWORDS

- Funguria • Candiduria • Fungus ball • Candidemia • Fluconazole • Flucytosine • Amphotericin B

KEY POINTS

- Candiduria is a common condition particularly in patients with diabetes, urinary catheters, or recent antibiotics or steroids, or in those who were recently hospitalized.
- Asymptomatic candiduria does not typically necessitate antifungal treatment, although workup and modification of candiduria risk factors are important.
- For symptomatic patients, fluconazole is the mainstay of therapy because it readily accumulates in high levels in the urine. Almost all cases of *Candida* cystitis can be treated with fluconazole.
- Care must be taken in treating patients with candiduria with nephrolithiasis or fungal bezoars, because urinary tract manipulation or failure to drain obstructed systems can lead to *Candida* pyelonephritis or candidemia.
- Noncandidal funguria is very rare and mostly occurs in patients who are severely immunocompromised.

INTRODUCTION

Fungal colonization or infection of the urinary system is common, particularly in patients with severe illness. Among funguria cases, *Candida* sp make up the majority of pathogens, representing greater than 95% of positive result of urine cultures.[1] Candiduria is rare in healthy individuals (<2% of urine cultures) but common among hospitalized individuals and in those with significant comorbidities (up to 40%). In addition, candiduria is increasing in prevalence, representing 22% of nosocomial urinary tract infections (UTIs) in 1986 to 1989 and 40% in 1992 to 1997.[1,2] Fortunately, candiduria is often asymptomatic and follows a benign clinical course, with a minimal number of candiduria cases leading to candidemia.[3] However, invasive candidal infection (cystitis, pyelonephritis, prostatitis, epididymo-orchitis, and fungemia) can prove difficult to treat, and in cases of pyelonephritis or fungemia, can carry significant morbidity and mortality. Urologists, in particular, must take care in treating patients with candiduria, because urologic manipulation can easily transform benign asymptomatic candiduria into a morbid and invasive infection.

CANDIDURIA
Patient Evaluation

The workup of candiduria hinges on determining if the candiduria represents contamination, colonization, or infection. In addition, the patient's clinical status governs how quickly the workup must take place and the appropriateness of starting empirical therapy. Predisposing factors are present in 90% of patients with candiduria and include the following[3]:

- Diabetes mellitus
- Recent antibiotic usage
- Urinary tract instrumentation and indwelling catheters
- Recent surgical procedures

Disclosure Statement: The authors have nothing to disclose.
Department of Urology, University of Iowa Hospitals and Clinics, 200 Hawkins Drive, Iowa City, IA 52242, USA
* Corresponding author.
E-mail address: Chad-Tracy@uiowa.edu

urologic.theclinics.com

- Urinary tract disease (including neurogenic bladder, urolithiasis, bladder outlet obstruction, ureteropelvic junction obstruction)
- Bedridden status
- Pregnancy
- Other factors such as presence of malignancy, immunosuppressive medication usage, and renal transplantation; however, studies in intensive care unit (ICU) populations have not shown these to be risk factors, suggesting that high acuity of care may be the overarching risk factor[3–5]
- Nonmodifiable risk factors for candiduria such as extremes of age and female gender[1] (Table 1)

Initial Evaluation

A full history and physical examination including comprehensive genitourinary examination for both men and women is recommended. Initial laboratory evaluation includes urinary dipstick, microscopy, and urine culture. Concern for funguria should be informed to the microbiology laboratory because some Candida sp grow slowly on routine culture. Urine markers to differentiate infection from colonization have been proposed (including leukocyte esterase, urine culture colony count, presence of candidal casts, and presence of pseudohyphae) but are limited by poor accuracy, particularly in the presence of

indwelling catheters or concomitant urologic disease.[6]

Further Evaluation

In 2011, Fisher and colleagues[7] proposed a workup for patients with candiduria based on symptoms, presence of predisposing factors, and clinical status. An overview of their workup for asymptomatic patients is presented in **Fig. 1**. Repeating a urinalysis and culture is the first step in therapy for all asymptomatic patients. The authors recommend use of clean catheters for collection in order to decrease the risk of contamination. In patients with an indwelling catheter, the catheter should be exchanged before repeat collection. In asymptomatic healthy outpatients, contamination of the urine (either poor collection technique or postcollection contamination) is thought to cause most candiduria cases.[1] Persistent candiduria requires workup for predisposing factors, including postvoid residual (PVR) to rule out urinary retention; renal and bladder ultrasonography (US) to look for hydronephrosis, urolithiasis, fungus balls, and renal abscesses; and hemoglobin A_{1c} for diagnosis of diabetes mellitus. If no predisposing factors are identified and no symptoms develop, then observation with repeat culture is appropriate (1–3 months). Asymptomatic outpatients with identifiable predisposing factors should be treated by first addressing the

Table 1
Frequency of concomitant conditions among patients diagnosed with candiduria/funguria in different populations

	Inpatient (%)	Outpatient (%)	ICUs (%)
Strong Risk Factors			
Diabetes mellitus	39	29	22 (insulin dependent)
Indwelling catheter use	83	15	98
Recent antibiotic use	85	46	98
Urinary tract disease	38	36–59[a]	N/A
Possible Risk Factors			
Pregnancy	2	23	NA
Malignancy	22	10	13
Immunosuppression	4.3 (neutropenia)	3	6 (25% with steroid use)
Recent surgery	52	NA	42
Renal transplant	4	NA	1
Gender and Age			
Gender (female)	60	82	49[b]
Age (mean)	64.5	46	61.2

Abbreviation: N/A, not assessed.
[a] Incompletely assessed and reported as individual conditions.
[b] Women represented just 34% of the ICU cohort.
Data from Refs.[3–5]

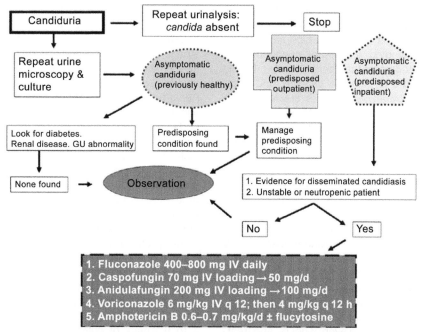

Fig. 1. Algorithm for the management of asymptomatic candiduria. IV, intravenous. (*From* Fisher JF, Sobel JD, Kauffman CA, et al. *Candida* urinary tract infections–treatment. Clin Infect Dis 2011;52(Suppl 6):S458; with permission.)

predisposing condition and then repeating the urine culture (usually 1–2 weeks later).

For asymptomatic inpatients (particularly in the ICU), candidemia leading to hematogenous renal seeding and subsequent candiduria is possible, and all inpatients with candiduria should undergo an assessment of candidemia risk. Risk factors include central venous catheters, total parenteral nutrition, antibiotic use, high severity of disease (high Acute Physiology and Chronic Health Evaluation score), recent surgery (particularly abdominal surgery), acute renal failure, gastric acid suppression, and nasogastric tube use.[8,9] For patients at risk of candidemia, workup should include blood cultures and a skin and ophthalmologic examination to investigate for characteristic pustular lesions and chorioretinitis. Empirical therapy should also be considered in the population with high candidemia risk. In patients with a significant urologic history, imaging should be performed to rule out urinary tract obstruction.

Candiduria rarely results in symptoms, and alternative diagnoses should be considered in patients thought to have a symptomatic fungal UTI. Immediate repeat culture to rule out bacterial UTI and to confirm the candiduria is recommended, as well as a workup for predisposing factors (including renal US and PVR).[6] *Candida* prostatitis and epididymo-orchitis are rare entities, but if they are suspected clinically, additional imaging

(transrectal US for prostatitis and scrotal US for epididymo-orchitis, or computed tomography [CT] for prostatitis) is recommended to rule out abscess formation.[6]

Antimicrobial Treatment

In 2000, Sobel and colleagues[10] randomized patients with asymptomatic candiduria to either placebo or 14 days of fluconazole, 200 mg (Diflucan). Although more fluconazole-treated patients were candida free at the end of the treatment course, by 2 weeks posttherapy candida-free rates were similar between the 2 groups (68% vs 65%). Of note, no patient in either group developed pyelonephritis or candidemia, highlighting that spontaneous clearance of candiduria occurs commonly and that treatment may not benefit asymptomatic patients. A subanalysis looking at clearance by 1 week versus 2 weeks of fluconazole did show improvement in candida-free rates with 2 weeks of therapy. This finding has been extrapolated to treatment of symptomatic patients. Importantly, patients at high risk of candidemia (neutropenic patients, neonates) and patients undergoing urologic procedures should be considered for treatment regardless of symptoms.

Patients with symptomatic cystitis should be treated with antifungal agents. The mainstay of treatment for uncomplicated cystitis is oral fluconazole. Fluconazole is an azole antifungal that inhibits synthesis of fungal membrane elements (ergosterol)[11] and is excreted in high amounts by the kidneys, leading to urinary concentrations often 10 times greater than serum levels.[7] Nearly all urine isolates of Candida albicans and most isolates of Candida glabrata are susceptible to fluconazole because of the high urinary concentrations (see Treatment Resistance/Complications section).[12] The recommended dosage for symptomatic cystitis is 200 mg daily for 14 days. Other azoles are not readily excreted in the urine (including itraconazole, voriconazole, and posaconazole) making these agents ineffective for the treatment of candiduria.[7]

In patients with resistant strains, flucytosine (Ancobon) may be used. Flucytosine is taken up by susceptible fungi and converted into 5-fluorouracil, which inhibits protein and DNA synthesis, leading to fungal toxicity.[13] Most isolates of C glabrata are sensitive to flucytosine, whereas approximately 30% to 40% of C albicans isolates display resistance. Dosing is 25 mg/kg every 6 hours, and treatment is typically for 7 to 10 days. Prolonged courses of flucytosine should be avoided because development of resistance or toxicity is common.[7,14]

Nearly all urinary isolates of Candida are susceptible to amphotericin B deoxycholate (AmB). AmB is a polyene antifungal and works by binding fungal membrane ergosterol resulting in membrane disorganization and micropore formation.[15] Unfortunately, because of its significant toxicity (see section on Toxicities), it should not be used as a primary treatment unless otherwise necessary. When delivered intravenously, the nonlipid form should be used because the lipid form does not readily accumulate in the urine. Recommended dosing for amphotericin B is 0.3 to 0.6 mg/kg daily for 1 to 7 days, although some studies have shown reasonable efficacy with one-time dosing (0.3 mg/kg).[7]

For patients with resistant bacteria or those with contraindications to systemic antifungal therapy, AmB can also be administered intravesically. AmB bladder irrigation dose is typically 50 mg in 1 L of sterile water instilled continuously over 24 hours using a 3-way Foley catheter (42 mL/h). In a trial comparing continuous bladder irrigation with AmB to fluconazole (200 mg × 7 days), 94.4% of patients on AmB had negative result of urine cultures 24 h after conclusion of therapy, with 78% remaining candiduria free at 5 to 9 days after therapy. However, there was no significant difference in these rates compared with those of oral fluconazole, underscoring the limited use of AmB bladder irrigation especially in patients without catheters.[16]

In cases of pyelonephritis, it is essential to obtain speciation and antifungal sensitivities because inappropriate treatment of resistant strains may increase the risk of candidemia or treatment failure. Fluconazole is the first-line therapy for pyelonephritis (400 mg/d for 14 days). Renal tissue concentration of fluconazole is less substantial than urinary concentration, and secondary antibiotics such as flucytosine (25 mg/kg every 6 hours × 14 days) or AmB (0.5–0.7 mg/kg daily × 14 days) should be used if the minimum inhibitory concentration (MIC) of fluconazole is greater than 16 µg/mL. Although flucytosine and AmB may be used together to decrease flucytosine resistance, combination therapy is limited by bone marrow toxicity.[14] Caspofungin has shown some promise in patients with pyelonephritis (including 3 with ascending infection) but is not considered a standard therapy because of poor urinary concentrations (Table 2).[7,17]

Patients with intrarenal or perirenal abscesses should be treated with abscess drainage and 4 to 6 weeks of culture-appropriate antifungals (fluconazole or amphotericin B at pyelonephritis dosing). Microabscesses do not typically require drainage, but imaging should be done to ensure resolution after therapy. Patients with a compromised renal unit, persistent infection, or evidence of emphysematous pyelonephritis should be considered for nephrectomy.[18–21]

Candida may also cause prostatitis or epididymo-orchitis. Both disorders should be treated with fluconazole, 400 mg/d for 2 to 4 weeks, or amphotericin B, 0.5 to 0.7 mg/kg daily for 4 weeks.[7,22,23] Testicular or prostatic abscesses may develop and require urgent drainage. Patients with prostatic abscesses should undergo suprapubic tube placement (when obstructed) followed by transurethral resection (unroofing) or percutaneous/transrectal drainage.[24–27] The authors typically perform needle drainage in peripheral abscesses or in critically ill patients and transurethral resection in patients with large, multifocal, or periurethral lesions. Surgical management of epididymo-orchitis is necessary when epididymal or testicular abscess is noted. Abscesses are common, and orchiectomy is frequently necessary. Aggressive surgical management of abscesses, even if bilateral, is warranted, because a high rate of associated candidemia has been reported.[28]

Many of the above-mentioned disease states are caused by or accompanied by candidemia. In cases of candidemia with candiduria, guidelines for treatment of candidemia should be followed.

Table 2
Commonly used medications for treatment of genitourinary fungal infections

Drug	Route	Dose	Dose in Renal Impairment	Side Effects	Cost	Monitoring
Fluconazole	Oral	200 mg q day × 14 d (cystitis) 400 mg q day × 14 d (pyelonephritis or resistant cystitis) 400 mg q day × 2–4 wk (prostatitis)	See section titled Treatment in Cases of Renal Failure Normal dose once following dialysis	Hepatotoxicity (major) Headache (minor) Nausea (minor) Abdominal pain (minor)	Low	Liver function tests at start of therapy and weekly
Flucytosine	Oral	25 mg/kg q 6 h × 7–10 d (cystitis) 25 mg/kg q 6 h × 14 d (pyelonephritis)	12.5 mg/kg q 6 h for CrCl 20–40 mL/min 6.125 mg/kg q 6 h for CrCl 10–20 mL/min Normal dose once following dialysis	Bone marrow suppression (major) Rash (minor) Diarrhea (minor) Hepatotoxicity (minor)	Very high	Creatinine levels q 2–3 d to ensure appropriate dosing Flucytosine blood levels after 3–5 d of therapy Drawn 2 h postdose. Target is 30–80 µg/mL If unable to measure blood levels: frequent monitoring (q 3–5 d) for white blood cell and platelet counts
Amphotericin B	IV	0.3–0.6 mg/kg/d × 1–7 d (cystitis) 0.5–0.7 mg/kg/d × 14 d (pyelonephritis) 0.5–0.7 mg/kg/d × 2–4 wk (prostatitis) 0.3–0.7 mg/kg/d × 4–6 wk (epididymo-orchitis)	No dose adjustment necessary	Renal dysfunction (major) Acute infusion reactions (major) Anemia/pancytopenia (moderate)	Moderate	Creatinine daily Electrolytes every 2–3 d Acute infusion (4–6 h postinfusion) Blood cell count every 3–7 d

Abbreviations: CrCl, creatinine clearance; IV, intravenous.

Nonantimicrobial Treatment

Conservative management of funguria relies on alleviating predisposing factors, including the removal of indwelling urologic devices, improving urinary tract drainage, stopping systemic antibiotics, and treating underlying medical problems such as diabetes and immunosuppression. Patients should have indwelling urethral catheters removed as soon as possible because this alone results in clearance of funguria in 75% of patients within 2 weeks.[10] For patients who are catheter dependent, changing the catheter can result in resolution of funguria in 20% of cases. When possible, all efforts should be made to change from an indwelling catheter to clean intermittent catheterization (CIC) because patients with an indwelling catheter are 10 times more likely to develop candiduria than those who practice CIC.[10,29]

For patients with urinary retention/stasis (PVR >100 mL) management should include attempts at improving drainage. For men, the most common cause of obstruction is benign prostatic hyperplasia (BPH), whereas for women the causes are more varied. Patients with long-standing diabetes or other neurologic problems may have a hypotonic bladder. Urodynamics can help elucidate bladder functionality and guide therapy in such cases.

As previously mentioned, recurrent UTIs may increase the risk of funguria because of the frequent use of antibiotics. Nonantimicrobial management strategies to reduce UTI risk (increased fluids, improved hygiene, use of vaginal estrogen, use of cranberry supplementation, etc) can lead to reduction in funguria.

Special Situations

Patients with funguria and an obstructing stone should undergo prompt decompression with either a nephrostomy tube or ureteral stent. Before definitive stone procedure, 7 to14 days of culture-directed antifungal therapy should be administered given the high risk of sepsis in this at-risk population.[30]

As with other types of infected stones, the goal should be complete stone removal. For ureteroscopic procedures, the authors use a ureteral access sheath and small flexible scope to keep intrarenal pressures low and allow for basket removal of fragments. For larger stones, percutaneous removal is preferred because of the superior stone-free rate.[31] For both percutaneous nephrostolithotomy (PCNL) and ureteroscopic removal, additional antifungals (7–14 days) should be given after the procedure with removal of any urologic devices (eg, stent) completed while the patient is on therapy.

Fungus balls (bezoars) are conglomerations of fungal cells and sloughed renal epithelial and urothelial cells, which can cause upper tract or bladder outlet obstruction and occur most commonly in neonates in the ICU (high candidemia and candiduria risk). On renal US, fungus balls appear as echogenic nonshadowing intracollecting system masses (**Fig. 2**), whereas on excretory imaging using CT, they are typically identified as a filling defect in the collecting system.[32]

Initial management of fungus balls involves placement of a percutaneous nephrostomy (PCN) tube, which allows for relief of high collecting system pressures, reduction in candidal burden, appropriate microbiological diagnosis, and restoration of renal function.[33,34] Although percutaneous drainage and systemic antifungal therapy may clear the fungus ball, some patients require additional interventions. Renal pelvis irrigation with antifungal agents may clear remaining debris (**Table 3**), but similar to percutaneous stone dissolution, irrigation can cause increased intrarenal pressure and sepsis, making irrigation contraindicated in patients with distal obstruction.[33,35–37]

Adult patients who fail conservative measures should be considered for percutaneous removal. Use of a large-caliber working channel allows for easy fragmentation/removal/suctioning of the entire fungus ball and copious irrigation of the collecting system. After the procedure, the authors recommend a short period of continued PCN drainage in order to facilitate clearance of any remaining organisms. Although efficacious, percutaneous removal does carry potential morbidity that may limit its use in the critically ill.[38] For patients who are unable to tolerate traditional percutaneous removal, some investigators

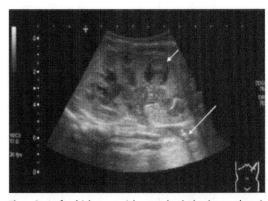

Fig. 2. Left kidney with marked hydronephrosis with a fungus ball in the collecting system (*short white arrow*) and in the upper ureter (*long white arrow*). (*From* Bisht V, Voort JV. Clinical practice: obstructive renal candidiasis in infancy. Eur J Pediatr 2011;170(10):1229; with permission.)

Table 3
Upper tract irrigation regimens for treatment of renal fungus balls

Drug	Dose	Rate
Adult Dosing		
Fluconazole	300 mg in 500 mL D5W	40 mL/h continuous
Amphotericin B	50 mg/L sterile water 200 µg/mL	40 mL/h continuous 5 mL q 6 h × 9 d Catheter clamped for 1 h postadministration
Pediatric/Neonatal Dosing		
Fluconazole	0.04–2 mg/mL in normal saline	25mL in 1hr twice daily
Amphotericin B	0.05 mg/mL in 5% dextrose	5–45 mL/h twice daily
Streptokinase	3000 U/mL	5 mL twice daily × 3 d. Catheter clamped for 1 h postadministration

Abbreviation: D5W, 5% dextrose in water.
Data from Refs.[33,35,37]

have described removal with an atherectomy device, fragmentation with guidewire, or instillation of streptokinase.[35,36] A treatment algorithm for neonatal renal candidiasis is shown in Fig. 3, although a similar algorithm would be appropriate for adult patients, with the exception that streptokinase use in adults is not well described.

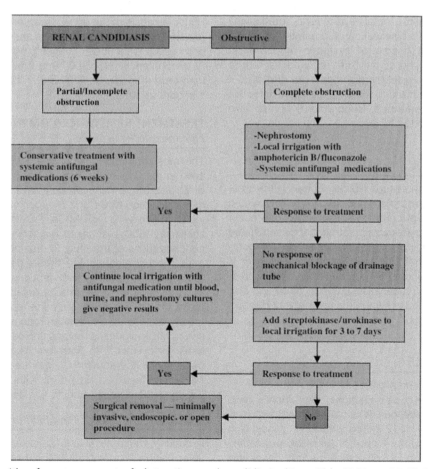

Fig. 3. Algorithm for management of obstructive renal candidiasis. (*From* Bisht V, Voort JV. Clinical practice: obstructive renal candidiasis in infancy. Eur J Pediatr 2011;170(10):1230; with permission.)

NON-*CANDIDA* FUNGAL URINARY TRACT DISEASE

Similar to candiduria, non-*Candida* funguria presents in comorbid (particularly immunocompromised) patients with either systemic fungal disease or significant lower urinary tract dysfunction; however, asymptomatic colonization is not widely reported. In asymptomatic patients, contamination of samples should be considered because many fungi are widely distributed and common in hospital environments. As human immunodeficiency virus (HIV)/AIDS is a common predisposing factor, the authors recommend HIV testing for any patient diagnosed with a noncandidal genitourinary (GU) fungal infection. Principles of management are similar to those for *Candida* infections, namely, extended courses of antifungals, removal of macroscopic foci of infection, and reduction of predisposing risk factors.

Aspergillosis

Reported genitourinary infections include renal fungal bezoars, renal abscesses (particularly with systemic disease), and prostatic infection. A prolonged course of systemic amphotericin B (0.5–1 mg/kg/d) may be required for up to 3 months. Surgical management with drainage of abscesses similar to that for candidal infection should be performed. Nephrectomy should also be considered.[27,39]

Cryptococcus

Cryptococcal infection typically occurs in the presence of disseminated disease. However, isolated residual foci of cryptococcal infection can occur in the prostate following treatment of disseminated disease and are thought to be reservoirs for recurrent infection.[40] The most common treatment is high-dose fluconazole (up to 600 mg/d). Suppressive doses of fluconazole (200 mg daily) can also be used to reduce symptoms and prevent disseminated infection.[41,42]

Blastomycosis

Epididymitis and prostatitis are the most common GU blastomycosis infections. Treatments have included intravenous (IV) amphotericin B with total dosage of 1 to 2 g (disseminated cases with GU involvement). A case of localized prostatitis/epididymitis in an otherwise healthy man was treated with ketoconazole, 400 mg, for 1 year and initial partial epididymectomy.[43]

Mucormycosis

Mucormycosis may present as an isolated renal infection or as a component of systemic infection. Both localized and systemic infections carry a high mortality rate. For localized unilateral disease, nephrectomy and systemic amphotericin B therapy (>1 g total dose) is a common treatment regimen. Bilateral disease has mostly proved to be fatal. Reversal of immunosuppression (cessation of corticosteroids, immune stimulation with granulocyte-macrophage colony-stimulating factor) has been used successfully in some patients.[39,44,45]

Coccidiomycosis

Reported sites of coccidia infection include epididymis, testis, prostate, and kidney. GU coccidiomycosis typically presents as part of systemic disease. IV amphotericin B is the usual therapy (total dose of 500–2500 mg). Long-term systemic azole agents have also been used. Serologic antibody testing can be used to monitor clinical course.[39]

Histoplasmosis

Histoplasmosis of the urinary system is typically a result of disseminated disease in an immunocompromised patient (mostly patients with HIV/AIDS). IV amphotericin B (>2000 mg total dose) and long-term itraconazole (200 mg × 12 weeks) is a standard treatment.[39]

TREATMENT RESISTANCE/COMPLICATIONS
Fluconazole Resistance

The most common fluconazole-resistant fungus seen in the urinary system is *C glabrata*. Studies of *C glabrata* urinary isolates have shown both higher average MICs and a larger percentage of isolates with very high MICs.[12] Determination of sensitivity (MICs) is based on achievable serum concentrations of the drug. In prostatitis, epididymitis, and pyelonephritis, tissue concentrations are closer to serum concentrations and serum MICs should be appropriate for determining resistance. However, because urine concentrations greatly exceed serum concentrations, the role of serum MICs in guiding therapy choice is less applicable for cystitis.[46–48] Therefore, fluconazole can be a useful therapy for *C glabrata* cystitis with MIC values less than 128 μg/mL, although a higher dosage (400 mg daily) should be used.

Treatment in Cases of Renal Failure

In patients with renal failure/compromise, fluconazole dosing is typically reduced. However, reduced dosing combined with reduced excretion results in lower urinary concentrations and possible therapeutic failure. Fisher and colleagues[49] argue that given patient tolerance of high fluconazole doses (1600 mg/d in other fungal infections), 400 mg/d of fluconazole is a safe and effective dose for patients with urinary infection and renal failure,[7] although frequent hepatic monitoring is recommended. Flucytosine, on the other hand, carries significant toxicity associated with serum drug accumulation and must be adjusted in renal failure/compromise. Amphotericin B does not require renal dose adjustment, but abnormal renal function is a risk factor for AmB-related nephrotoxicity.

Toxicities

The main toxicities of amphotericin B include renal toxicity, acute infusion reactions, and anemia. Renal toxicity, which can occur in up to 80% of patients, can include oliguria, azotemia, electrolyte disturbances, and diabetes insipidus. Most changes in renal function are reversible with discontinuation of therapy. In order to reduce toxicity, other nephrotoxic drugs should be eliminated and patients may be given salt loading (1 L saline before drug administration). Acute infusion reactions occur in approximately 50% of patients and include local irritation/thrombophlebitis (reduced with central line infusion) or systemic symptoms (fever, nausea/vomiting, headache, chills). Systemic reactions can be palliated with a combination of acetaminophen/nonsteroidal anti-inflammatory drugs, diphenhydramine, and antiemetics. Preemptive use of these medications in patients with previous reactions is recommended. Anemia and pancytopenia may occur with AmB therapy and usually occur after treatment and resolve without therapy. Patients receiving AmB require acute infusion monitoring, daily creatinine measurements, and frequent electrolyte monitoring for the first 1 to 2 weeks of treatment (may be spaced after that).[50]

The main flucytosine-related toxicity is dose-dependent bone marrow suppression. Monitoring with blood counts and flucytosine serum concentration should be done every 3 to 5 days. Renal function should be checked frequently (2–3 days) to ensure appropriate dosing.[51,52]

Fluconazole is a well-tolerated medication. The notable side effect of hepatotoxicity is rare (0.98/100 patient-days therapy) and typically resolves even with continuation of therapy.[53] The authors check transaminase levels with initiation of therapy and then weekly.[54] Mild transaminase level elevation does not warrant discontinuation of therapy, but doubling or quadrupling of levels should prompt consideration of discontinuation of therapy.

EVALUATION OF OUTCOME AND LONG-TERM RECOMMENDATIONS
Evaluation of Outcomes

Evaluation of treatment outcomes in patients with funguria should include 3 different assessments. The first assessment is for clearance of the organism. For asymptomatic patients with persistent candiduria, the authors typically repeat cultures at 1 to 2 weeks after risk factor reduction (such as catheter removal or completion of antibiotic course). For patients with persistent candiduria with no remaining modifiable risk factors, they repeat cultures every 1 to 3 months until candiduria resolves. For those with resolved candiduria, the authors typically carry out follow-up at 3 months and then as appropriate based on their urologic condition. Repeat cultures are not performed at visits past 3 months unless clinically indicated. For uncomplicated infections (cystitis), the authors typically follow-up for symptom and culture assessment 1 to 2 weeks after treatment completion. For complex infections, they typically treat until culture negativity (often × 2); cultures are not repeated unless symptoms return.

The second assessment is for resolution of macroscopic infection. For patients with a fungal bezoar and a nephrostomy tube, antegrade pyelography can be done every 2 to 3 days during therapy. For those managed with percutaneous treatment, CT with antegrade pyelography on postoperative day 1 is useful for determining the next steps in care. For perinephric abscesses or prostatic collections, CT or US imaging may be used to detect persistent disease.

The third assessment is for risk factor reduction and prevention of further infection. The basic principles for prevention are the same as those outlined for nonmedical treatment, and assessment depends on the specific risk factor. Other strategies to prevent repeat infections including use of prophylactic antifungals have not been widely used.

Summary/Discussion

Funguria is commonly encountered by practicing urologists. Most candiduria is benign and should be treated with risk factor reduction and surveillance. However, complex invasive infections including pyelonephritis, fungal bezoars, infected nephrolithiasis, prostatitis, abscesses, and disseminated candidiasis can occur. Management of invasive infections follows principles similar to treatment of bacterial infections, namely, treatment with culture-appropriate antimicrobials, relief of urinary obstruction, removal of foreign bodies, and drainage of abscesses. Fluconazole is the mainstay of drug treatment, despite an increasing prevalence of non-albicans species that often are fluconazole resistant. Amphotericin B and flucytosine are common therapies for resistant infections. Other strategies, such as local irrigation (bladder or collecting), have a role in managing complex funguria cases. Noncandidal funguria is a rare entity, typically noted in severely ill and immunocompromised patients. Treatment standards for noncandidal funguria are lacking, but principles remain the same.

REFERENCES

1. Sobel JD, Fisher JF, Kauffman CA, et al. *Candida* urinary tract infections—epidemiology. Clin Infect Dis 2011;52(suppl 6):S433–6.
2. Richards MJ, Edwards JR, Culver DH, et al. Nosocomial infections in combined medical-surgical intensive care units in the United States. Infect Control Hosp Epidemiol 2000;21(8):510–5.
3. Kauffman CA, Vazquez JA, Sobel JD, et al. Prospective multicenter surveillance study of funguria in hospitalized patients. Clin Infect Dis 2000;30(1):14–8.
4. Álvarez-Lerma F, Nolla-Salas J, León C, et al. Candiduria in critically ill patients admitted to intensive care medical units. Intensive Care Med 2003;29(7):1069–76.
5. Colodner R, Nuri Y, Chazan B, et al. Community-acquired and hospital-acquired candiduria: comparison of prevalence and clinical characteristics. Eur J Clin Microbiol Infect Dis 2008;27(4):301–5.
6. Kauffman CA. Diagnosis and management of fungal urinary tract infection. Infect Dis Clin North Am 2014;28(1):61–74.
7. Fisher JF, Sobel JD, Kauffman CA, et al. *Candida* urinary tract infections—treatment. Clin Infect Dis 2011;52(suppl 6):S457–66.
8. Blumberg HM, Jarvis WR, Soucie JM, et al. Risk factors for candidal bloodstream infections in surgical intensive care unit patients: the NEMIS prospective multicenter study. Clin Infect Dis 2001;33(2):177–86.
9. Puzniak LP, Teutsch S, Powderly W, et al. Has the epidemiology of nosocomial candidemia changed? Infect Control Hosp Epidemiol 2004;25(8):628–33.
10. Sobel JD, Kauffman CA, McKinsey D, et al. candiduria: a randomized, double-blind study of treatment with fluconazole and placebo. Clin Infect Dis 2000;30(1):19–24.
11. Ghannoum MA, Rice LB. Antifungal agents: mode of action, mechanisms of resistance, and correlation of these mechanisms with bacterial resistance. Clin Microbiol Rev 1999;12(4):501–17.
12. Pfaller MA, Diekema DJ, Sheehan DJ. Interpretive breakpoints for fluconazole and *Candida* revisited: a blueprint for the future of antifungal susceptibility testing. Clin Microbiol Rev 2006;19(2):435–47.
13. Vermes A, Guchelaar H-J, Dankert J. Flucytosine: a review of its pharmacology, clinical indications, pharmacokinetics, toxicity and drug interactions. J Antimicrob Chemother 2000;46(2):171–9.
14. White TC, Marr KA, Bowden RA. Clinical, cellular, and molecular factors that contribute to antifungal drug resistance. Clin Microbiol Rev 1998;11(2):382–402.
15. Adler-Moore J, Proffitt RT. AmBisome: liposomal formulation, structure, mechanism of action and pre-clinical experience. J Antimicrob Chemother 2002;49(suppl 1):21–30.
16. Fan-Havard P, O'Donovan C, Smith SM, et al. Oral fluconazole versus amphotericin B bladder irrigation for treatment of candidal funguria. Clin Infect Dis 1995;21(4):960–5.
17. Sobel JD, Bradshaw SK, Lipka CJ, et al. Caspofungin in the treatment of symptomatic candiduria. Clin Infect Dis 2007;44(5):e46–9.
18. Clerckx C, Wilmes D, Aydin S, et al. *Candida glabrata* renal abscesses in a peritoneal dialysis patient. Perit Dial Int 2012;32(1):114–5.
19. High KP, Quagliarello VJ. Yeast perinephric abscess: report of a case and review. Clin Infect Dis 1992;15(1):128–33.
20. Li WY, Wu VC, Lin WC, et al. Renal *Candida tropicalis* abscesses in a patient with acute lymphoblastic leukemia. Kidney Int 2007;72(3):382.
21. Harrabi H, Marrakchi C, Daoud E, et al. Bilateral emphysematous pyelonephritis caused by *Candida glabrata*: an exceptional entity. Nephrol Ther 2010;6(6):541–3 [in French].
22. Kauffman CA, Fisher JF, Sobel JD, et al. *Candida* urinary tract infections—diagnosis. Clin Infect Dis 2011;52(suppl 6):S452–6.
23. Wise GJ, Shteynshlyuger A. How to diagnose and treat fungal infections in chronic prostatitis. Curr Urol Rep 2006;7(4):320–8.
24. Arrabal-Polo MA, Jimenez-Pacheco A, Arrabal-Martin M. Percutaneous drainage of prostatic abscess: case report and literature review. Urol Int 2012;88(1):118–20.
25. Bastide C, Carcenac A, Arroua F, et al. Prostatic abscess due to *Candida tropicalis*. Prostate Cancer Prostatic Dis 2005;8(3):296–7.
26. Elert A, von Knobloch R, Nusser R, et al. Isolated candidal prostatitis. J Urol 2000;163(1):244.
27. Kaplan-Pavlovcic S, Masera A, Ovcak Z, et al. Prostatic aspergillosis in a renal transplant recipient. Nephrol Dial Transplant 1999;14(7):1778–80.
28. Jenkin GA, Choo M, Hosking P, et al. Candidal epididymo-orchitis: case report and review. Clin Infect Dis 1998;26(4):942–5.
29. Goetz LL, Howard M, Cipher D, et al. Occurrence of candiduria in a population of chronically catheterized patients with spinal cord injury. Spinal Cord 2009;48(1):51–4.

30. Kumar S, Bag S, Ganesamoni R, et al. Risk factors for urosepsis following percutaneous nephrolithotomy: role of 1 week of nitrofurantoin in reducing the risk of urosepsis. Urol Res 2012;40(1):79–86.

31. Akman T, Binbay M, Ozgor F, et al. Comparison of percutaneous nephrolithotomy and retrograde flexible nephrolithotripsy for the management of 2–4 cm stones: a matched-pair analysis. BJU Int 2012; 109(9):1384–9.

32. Atlani M, Sharma RK. Intermittent renal graft obstruction by fungal ball—case report. NDT Plus 2011;4:279–80.

33. Bell DA, Rose SC, Starr NK, et al. Percutaneous nephrostomy for nonoperative management of fungal urinary tract infections. J Vasc Interv Radiol 1993;4(2):311–5.

34. Watson RA, Esposito M, Richter F, et al. Percutaneous nephrostomy as adjunct management in advanced upper urinary tract infection. Urology 1999;54(2):234–9.

35. Bisht V, Voort JV. Clinical practice: obstructive renal candidiasis in infancy. Eur J Pediatr 2011;170(10): 1227–35.

36. Irby PB, Stoller ML, McAninch JW. Fungal bezoars of the upper urinary tract. J Urol 1990;143(3):447–51.

37. Chung BH, Chang SY, Kim SI, et al. Successfully treated renal fungal ball with continuous irrigation of fluconazole. J Urol 2001;166(5):1835–6.

38. Chitale SV, Shaida N, Burtt G, et al. Endoscopic management of renal candidiasis. J Endourol 2004;18(9):865–6.

39. Wise GJ. Genitourinary fungal infections: a therapeutic conundrum. Expert Opin Pharmacother 2001;2(8):1211–26.

40. Ndimbie OK, Dekker A, Martinez AJ, et al. Prostatic sequestration of Cryptococcus neoformans in immunocompromised persons treated for cryptococcal meningoencephalitis. Histol Histopathol 1994;9(4): 643–8.

41. Bozzette SA, Larsen RA, Chiu J, et al. Fluconazole treatment of persistent Cryptococcus neoformans prostatic infection in AIDS. Ann Intern Med 1991; 115(4):285–6.

42. Yip SK, Cheng C, Wong MY, et al. Cryptococcal prostatic abscess in an immunocompromised patient: a case report and review of the literature. Ann Acad Med Singap 1998;27(6):873–6.

43. Seo R, Oyasu R, Schaeffer A. Blastomycosis of the epididymis and prostate. Urology 1997;50(6):980–2.

44. Weng DE, Wilson WH, Little RF, et al. Successful medical management of isolated renal zygomycosis: case report and review. Clin Infect Dis 1998; 26(3):601–5.

45. Gonzalez CE, Couriel DR, Walsh TJ. Disseminated zygomycosis in a neutropenic patient: successful treatment with amphotericin B lipid complex and granulocyte colony-stimulating factor. Clin Infect Dis 1997;24(2):192–6.

46. Latimer FG, Colitz CM, Campbell NB, et al. Pharmacokinetics of fluconazole following intravenous and oral administration and body fluid concentrations of fluconazole following repeated oral dosing in horses. Am J Vet Res 2001;62(10):1606–11.

47. Walsh TJ, Foulds G, Pizzo PA. Pharmacokinetics and tissue penetration of fluconazole in rabbits. Antimicrobial Agents Chemother 1989;33(4):467–9.

48. Finley RW, Cleary JD, Goolsby J, et al. Fluconazole penetration into the human prostate. Antimicrobial Agents Chemother 1995;39(2):553–5.

49. Fisher MA, Talbot GH, Maislin G, et al. Risk factors for amphotericin B-associated nephrotoxicity. Am J Med 1989;87(5):547–52.

50. Gallis HA, Drew RH, Pickard WW. Amphotericin B: 30 years of clinical experience. Rev Infect Dis 1990;12(2):308–29.

51. Vermes A, van Der Sijs H, Guchelaar HJ. Flucytosine: correlation between toxicity and pharmacokinetic parameters. Chemotherapy 2000;46(2):86–94.

52. Perfect JR, Dismukes WE, Dromer F, et al. Clinical practice guidelines for the management of cryptococcal disease: 2010 update by the Infectious Diseases Society of America. Clin Infect Dis 2010; 50(3):291–322.

53. Fischer MA, Winkelmayer WC, Rubin RH, et al. The hepatotoxicity of antifungal medications in bone marrow transplant recipients. Clin Infect Dis 2005; 41(3):301–7.

54. Como JA, Dismukes WE. Oral azole drugs as systemic antifungal therapy. N Engl J Med 1994; 330(4):263–72.

Current Concepts in Infections Associated with Penile Prostheses and Artificial Sphincters

Matthias D. Hofer, MD, Chris M. Gonzalez, MD*

KEYWORDS

- Penile prosthesis • Artificial urinary sphincter • Infection

KEY POINTS

- Improved design and understanding of infections has lowered infection rates associated with penile prostheses (PPs) and artificial sphincters.
- Treatment of infection consists of immediate removal and antimicrobial therapy.

INTRODUCTION

Implantation of PPs and artificial urinary sphincters (AUSs) have gained widespread acceptance for the treatment of refractory erectile dysfunction (ED) and incontinence, respectively. In the past 3 decades, improved device design and an increased understanding of the pathophysiology of device infections have contributed to a decrease in infection rates. However, understanding the concepts related to infection prevention and management remains critical. In this article, the authors review and discuss these concepts and provide outlines for the practicing urologists for both infection prevention and treatment.

INFECTIONS OF PENILE PROSTHESES

In the United States, ED affects about 25% of men older than 40 years.[1] First-line therapy for ED includes oral phosphodiesterase type 5 inhibitors, intraurethral prostaglandin suppositories, or vacuum erection device. If these treatments fail, intracavernous injections of vasoactive agents have been shown to be effective.[2] If conservative medical therapy fails or the patient is apprehensive to self-injections, placement of a PP can be considered. The first PP implantation was reported by Scott and colleagues[3] in 1973. In the early years, mechanical failure of the implant was the most frequent complication.[4] Reliability and durability of prostheses have improved over the past 4 decades with failure rates decreasing to 15% at 5 and 30% at 10 years.[5] Device infection now poses the most significant risk for patients. However, in the past decade, the understanding of the mechanisms and causes of infection has increased, which has led to markedly decreased infection rates.[6] At present, the most commonly implanted device for ED treatment is the inflatable PP, a 3-piece device consisting of 2 corporal cylinders, a pump, and a separate reservoir.[4] An alternative for patients is the semirigid (malleable) prosthesis or a 2-piece PP.

Superficial Skin Infections Versus Prosthesis Infections

Superficial surgical site infections at the suture line need to be distinguished from actual infection at

Department of Urology, Feinberg School of Medicine, Northwestern University, 675 North St Clair Street, Galter 20-150, Chicago, IL 60611, USA
* Corresponding author.
E-mail address: cgonzalez@nmff.org

Urol Clin N Am 42 (2015) 485–492
http://dx.doi.org/10.1016/j.ucl.2015.05.008
0094-0143/15/$ – see front matter © 2015 Elsevier Inc. All rights reserved.

the implanted device site. These superficial skin infections are limited to the skin around the suture line without bacterial contamination of device components and present rapidly after implantation similar to other postsurgical incision infections. These infections can successfully be treated with antibiotics. In contrast, actual device-associated infections usually occur months to years after implantation and require surgical therapy. However, they can also develop within days after the implantation and it can be difficult to differentiate them from superficial skin infections. Skin erythema at the suture line is present in both, and there may be some fluctance surrounding the newly implanted components from postoperative edema. Similarly, in both instances, the patient reports pain or tenderness, which may be postoperative pain due to the space-occupying pump. In the absence of clear evidence of PP infection (eg, purulent drainage, significant and increasing edema), a trial of oral antimicrobials such as bactrim or ciprofloxacin can be attempted.[6] This trial may also be diagnostic, because the symptoms persistently improve in cases of superficial skin infection, whereas the recurrence of symptoms after stopping the antibiotics is consistent with an actual PP infection requiring explantation.

Acute and Chronic Penile Implant Infections

Infections that involve the implanted device can present as acute or chronic infections. In acute infections, patients present within days or weeks after surgery and are often very ill because of systemic effects of the infection. Hallmarks of the physical examination are fever with or without chills, erythema of the scrotum and/or penile shaft, fluctance around the pump or cylinders, purulent drainage from the incision site, and a pump that may be fixed to the scrotal wall.[6] Imaging such as a computed tomographic (CT) scan or preferably an MRI[7] may aid in the diagnosis and should be considered for evaluating the location and also involvement of the intra-abdominal reservoir. One advantage of the MRI is that it allows assessment of penile anatomy in 3 orthogonal planes and can be used to differentiate PP-associated infections from some of the other conditions associated with similar symptoms. For example, in a patient complaining of shaft pain, the MRI can differentiate a buckling cylinder that is too large for the patient from a soft tissue infection.[7] If the implantation has been recent, however, it may be difficult to discern postoperative edema from infection, particularly on a CT scan.

Chronic infections associated with prostheses present months after surgery with the classic findings of a patient with persistent scrotal or penile pain, whereas systemic symptoms are absent and the patient has a normal white blood cell count. Chronic device infection may ultimately lead to extrusion of the prosthesis.[8] Imaging to confirm the diagnosis is not necessary but may facilitate surgical planning, such as identification of rear-tip extenders that must be removed during explantation.

Microorganisms involved in the device-related infection are usually acquired during the initial surgery and therefore come from the surgical team or the patient himself and usually originate from a cutaneous source.[6] In up to 80% of infected PP, Staphylococcus epidermidis is isolated, and in the remaining 20%, gram-negative bacteria including Proteus mirabilis, Pseudomonas aeruginosa, Escherichia coli, and Serratia marcescens are found.[9] Device contamination during surgery can lead to the generation of biofilm, which is produced by bacteria and results in a glycocalyx-containing slimelike coating of the device. Biofilm protects the contained bacteria from the patient's immune system as well as from antibiotics at concentrations up to 1500 times higher than those required to affect the same bacteria not protected by biofilm.[10] Furthermore, bacteria in biofilm can exchange plasmids coding for antibiotic resistance.[11] Up to 80% of PP explanted for mechanical failure contain bacteria in the absence of a clinically apparent infection, and a critical threshold of biofilm may exist before an infection becomes apparent.[10] Biofilms persist after device explantation, and thus a thorough washout procedure is critical for salvage reimplantations of PPs.

Risk factors for PP infections are concomitant infections of the urinary tract or other body sites with subsequent hematogenous spread[12] as well as extended operative time, which occurs when the implantation is combined with other reconstructive surgery[13] or when implantation is performed by inexperienced surgeons.[14] There is conflicting evidence regarding whether diabetes mellitus or quadriplegia is a risk factor for implant infection.[13,14]

Treatment of Infections Associated with Prostheses

Unlike superficial surgical site infections that are amenable to antimicrobial therapy, an infection involving the PP requires removal of the implant. Explantation should also ensue upon suspicion of a device infection to prevent further patient deterioration. During explantation it is crucial that all components of the PP be removed. Although partial removal of infected parts with salvage reimplantation while leaving uninfected parts in place has been described,[15] the eventual outcome can be considered poor. Bacteria migrate along the tubing, and reinfection of any of the components can occur.[6] In addition, implantation of new parts of a device may lead to transition of bacteria contained in biofilm to their planktonic (activated) state. Explantation of an infected prosthesis should occur promptly because the infection progresses and results in tissue edema followed by necrosis of the penile shaft and glans and may culminate in life-threatening sepsis. Systemic antibiotics alone are unable to clear the infection owing to poor tissue penetration because the implant components are encapsulated by dense fibrous tissue with poor vascularization. In addition, the appropriate concentration of antibiotics required to destroy bacteria contained in the biofilm cannot be reached.

In the past 3 decades, immediate salvage procedure algorithms replacing the infected implant with a new prosthesis have become the most commonly performed approach for the treatment of an infection associated with PP. There are 2 important aspects specific to PP explantation. First, the cavity in the corpora cavernosa that is left behind by an explanted cylinder should be filled, for example, with a new PP, because otherwise, in addition to penile shrinkage, the corporal scar makes a later reimplantation attempt very difficult.[6] One alternative to avoid replacement of an infected PP with a new one is to temporarily implant a malleable prosthesis.[16] However, this again requires implantation of a synthetic device that can act as a substrate for the (re-)development of biofilm. The second aspect is that salvage is associated with a reinfection rate of up to 13%.[13] Explantation followed by a prolonged course of antibiotics to further clear remaining organisms has therefore been propagated.

A novel approach combining antibiotic delivery while preserving corporal spaces has recently been described by Swords and colleagues.[17] The investigators describe filling the corpora cavernosa with a cast made of high-purity calcium sulfate that had been mixed with tobramycin and vancomycin and acts as a spacer before reimplantation of an inflatable PP several weeks later. This technique, however, is still in the experimental phase.

Salvage Reimplantation

Salvage reimplantation that combines the explantation of a PP with immediate replacement has become the most popular approach. This procedure is indicated for patients who are not immunosuppressed, who do not have significant comorbidities limiting operative time, and who continue to have an indication for a PP. During explantation, all nonabsorbable sutures that may have been used during the initial implant should be removed because they may harbor microorganisms. A second abdominal incision to remove the reservoir may be necessary. Once the device is removed, cultures are sampled and all areas of prior implant components are irrigated with antiseptic and antibiotic solutions. In the first description of this washout in 1996,[18] the use of vancomycin-gentamicin solution in water followed by half-strength hydrogen peroxide and half-strength povidone-iodine was recommended. Hydrogen peroxide eradicates anaerobic bacteria efficiently, and povidone-iodine is 99% bactericidal. These solutions are injected into the corpora using a 60-mL syringe or through a red rubber catheter to ensure that all areas of the prior implant are reached. Similarly, antibiotic and iodine solution can be injected into the tract of the reservoir; however, hydrogen peroxide should not be used because it may leak into the peritoneal cavity. Mulcahy[6] as well as Brant and colleagues[18] advocate for the use of a water pick to irrigate the cavities mechanically with antibiotic solution to break up and remove the biofilm[6,18]; however, the use of a large syringe should also generate sufficient pressure. Finally, all cavities are irrigated with the same solutions in reverse order so that the foamy hydrogen peroxide and the povidone-iodine are cleared by the antibiotic solution. Brant and colleagues[18] recommend changing of gowns and gloves and redraping of the field at this point before implantation of the new PP.[18] The sterile packaging of the new implant should not be opened until this stage to avoid accidental contamination. Once the new device has been implanted and the wound is closed, the patient is administered an antibiotic with good tissue penetration such as trimethoprim-sulfamethoxazole for 30 days.[6] The rationale for this extended course is based on reports by Henry and colleagues[19] who found that the pump scar tissue grew bacteria in 25% of patients after the antiseptic washout, which is putatively eliminated by the oral antibiotic regimen. Overall, the success rates of this salvage procedure are over 80%.[20] Failed salvage procedures have been attributed to short incubation time of washout solutions used, organisms with increased virulence, and also the presence of excessive cellulitis.[21] Excessive cellulitis should be treated with a 3-day course of intravenous antibiotics before salvage reimplantation.[21] Relative contraindications to a salvage procedure are a patient who is too ill to undergo the procedure and an infection that is unlikely to be cleared by the procedure. Examples of these situations are immunocompromised patients, patients with tissue necrosis at the implant sites, and bilateral erosion of cylinders into the fossa navicularis.[21] Of note, unilateral erosion of a cylinder is not a contraindication because the other cylinder may be replaced followed by implantation of the second cylinder at a later time.[21] In certain circumstances, delayed salvage can be considered, which entails explantation of the components of the device and washout with multiple Jackson-Pratt drains placed into the pump, reservoir, and corporal cavities before the wound is closed.[22] Antibiotic solution is instilled through the drains for 72 hours before a new implant is placed. Success rates using this technique are similar to those for immediate salvage.[22]

The Effect of Antibacterial Coatings

One improvement in the design of newer-generation PP was the development of antimicrobial coatings. Rifampin/minocycline coatings help in the prevention of bacterial adherence during and after the procedure, although serum levels of both antibiotics used for impregnation remain very low. Another variation is hydrophilic surface coatings that allow the uptake of antibiotic during soaking before implantation. This variation has the advantage of tailoring the antibiotic to the surgeon's discretion and the site's susceptibility profile. In vitro studies have suggested that the hydrophilic coating may have an improved antibacterial effect over rifampin/minocycline coating,[23] yet both coatings seem to be equally effective clinically. A recent report by Serefoglu and colleagues[24] analyzed over 36,000 primary PPs with hydrophilic coating and found that the infection rate of coated devices decreased to 1.4% compared to 4.6% for uncoated models at 11 years follow-up. Similarly, Carson and colleagues[25] analyzed over 35,000 PPs coated with rifampin/minocycline with up to 7.7 years of follow-up and found a 1.1% infection rate compared with 2.5% infection rate of nonimpregnated implants. Although infection rates in diabetic patients were significantly higher at 1.9%, the overall rate remains relatively low.[26] There are concerns in the continuing effectiveness of the antibacterial coatings used mainly in regard to the development of bacterial resistance. However, it seems that the risk of emergence of bacteria resistant to rifampin and minocycline is rather low, as a randomized prospective study on intravenous central line catheters has shown.[27] Overall, the antibacterial modification of PP seems to have significantly reduced the risk of device infection.

Preventing Penile-Prosthesis-Associated Infection

Colonization during implantation is the single most important factor for PP infection. Therefore, prevention of contamination by the surgical team, the patient, and the operating room environment are critical and are summarized in **Table 1**. In 2013, a

---

Table 1
Measures for infection prevention for penile implants and artificial sphincters

Topic	Recommendation
Intraoperative systemic antibiotics	Intravenous vancomycin and gentamicin for 24 h; vancomycin should be infused 1 h before incision
Postoperative antibiotics	Oral antibiotics for 1–2 wk, use of bactrim if MRSA is prevalent in the hospital or the community
Patient optimization	Optimized blood sugar control (HbA$_{1c}$<10%), negative result of urine culture
Preoperative showering of patient	Recommended if the patient has poor skin conditions
Antiseptic cleansing of operative site	Chlorhexidine preparation, which is allowed to dry for 3 min before incision
Surgeon's hand preparation	Scrubbing if it is the first surgery of the day or the hands are grossly contaminated, alcohol-based rubbing for the following procedures
Device use	Use of surface-modified devices recommended (except sphincters)
Intraoperative measures	Soaking of the implant in rifampin/gentamicin solution, irrigating the wound before implantation with rifampin/gentamicin solution, handling of the device predominantly by the surgeon, multilayered wound closure

Abbreviations: HbA$_{1c}$, hemoglobin A$_{1c}$; MRSA, methicillin-resistant *Staphylococcus aureus*.

panel of experts defined clinical guidelines to decrease the rates of penile infections[28] and provided the basis for the following recommendations.

Preoperative antibiotics

Although the American Urological Association has published a best practice statement in 2008[29] recommending the use of a first- or second-generation cephalosporin in combination with an aminoglycoside for 24 hours (aztreonam when renal insufficiency is present), the rising prevalence of methicillin-resistant bacteria advocates for the use of vancomycin instead of cephalosporin in conjunction with an aminoglycoside such as gentamicin to achieve both gram-positive and gram-negative coverage.[28] Care should be taken to infuse vancomycin with sufficient lead time before skin incision to allow for maximum blood concentration of this antibiotic (typically 1 hour). There has traditionally been a great variety in postoperative antibiotic management after prosthesis implantation,[30] and based on the expert opinion in the guideline, a 5- to 14-day course of oral antibiotics with trimethoprim-sulfamethoxazole (or doxycycline if the patient has a sulfa allergy) has been recommended.[28]

Patient preparation

Katz and colleagues[31] have shown that optimized blood sugar control (hemoglobin A_{1c} <10%) and a negative result of preoperative urine culture can reduce the risk of PP infection. A randomized controlled trial has shown a decreased incidence of surgical site infections by Staphylococcus aureus among patients who are nasal carriers with preoperative showering with chlorhexidine soap and the application of nasal mupirocin.[32] This regimen may be beneficial for patients with poor skin conditions.[28] Preparation of the surgical site should include cleansing using a chlorhexidine-alcohol-based solution because it has been found to be superior over traditional povidone-iodine solutions in reducing bacterial skin flora and surgical site infections[33,34] while not increasing irritation of the genital skin or urethral meatus.[34] The chlorhexidine-alcohol-based solution should be allowed to dry for 3 minutes before incision.[28] There is lack of evidence regarding whether the surgical team should scrub their hands with soap and brush or rub their hands with alcohol-based solution. It seems that performing a scrub for the first surgery of the day, or when the hands of the team members become grossly dirty, is appropriate followed by rubbing the hand with alcohol-based solutions for subsequent procedures.[28]

Intraoperative measures to decrease penile-prosthesis-associated infections

Soaking of the implant in rifampin/gentamicin solution, irrigating the wound before implantation with the same solution, handling of the device predominantly by the surgeon, and multilayered wound closure have been shown to contribute to the prevention of PP-associated infection.[31] It remains unclear whether the use of tissue glue to seal the wound is beneficial, and thus it cannot be recommended.[28] There is lack of evidence whether limiting traffic through the operating room during the procedure or leaving drains in place postoperatively has an impact on PP-associated infection risk.[28]

ARTIFICIAL URINARY SPHINCTERS

AUSs have become the gold standard for the treatment of severe urinary incontinence with over 90% of patients reporting satisfaction with the device.[35,36] AUSs are predominantly implanted for the treatment of postprostatectomy incontinence. The most commonly implanted AMS 800 model (American Medical Systems, Minnetonka, MN, USA) was first introduced in 1983, and despite some minor modifications in cuff sizes, tubing, and connectors, the basic design has been unchanged.[37]

Infections and Erosions Due to Artificial Urinary Sphincters

About 20% of AUSs require explantation, half due to infection and erosion and the other half due to mechanical failure or urethral atrophy.[38] AUS infections occur predominantly in connection with cuff erosion, and vice versa, which makes it difficult if not impossible to separate these events reliably because one may dictate the other. In turn, cuff erosions lead to subsequent infection of the cuff and the remaining parts of the AUS. In both instances, the entire AUS and its components must be explanted. The overall AUS explantation rate has been reported to be 8.3% to 10%, with the rate of explantation specifically due to infection being 2% to 2.5%, with the remaining explantations being due to cuff erosion.[38,39] In contrast to PPs, coating of the AUS with rifampin/minocycline has not been found to decrease infection rates.[40]

A recent multicenter prospective study analyzed the risk factors of AUS erosion and found that prior radiation therapy, prior implantation of a UroLume stent (American Medical Systems, Minnetonka, MN, USA), and a cuff size of 3.5 cm (smallest available cuff) were significantly associated with cuff erosion and/or infection.[41] Another risk factor for erosion is a previous history of cuff erosion, with an explantation rate approaching 20%.[38] Based on the time that has elapsed between surgery and erosion, the cause of erosion may be determined. Early erosions (weeks after implantation) are usually due to urethral injury during the implantation. Late erosions (several months to years) are caused by urethral atrophy such as that encountered after radiation therapy, small AUS cuff, and urethral catheter placement without prior deactivation of the AUS.[37]

A special consideration for AUS placement is the combination with bladder augmentation with small bowel. Catto and colleagues[42] reported on 86 patients who underwent bladder augmentation and AUS placement, of whom in 56 (65%) patients the AUS was placed simultaneously. The increased overall risk of infection of the AUS in patients with bladder augmentation compared with that in patients who received only an AUS was similar, although infections occurred earlier in patients with bladder augmentation (within 3 years after the procedure).

A final consideration is combined implantation of a PP and AUS where there seems to be no increased risk of infection or complication for either device.[43]

Microorganisms Involved in Infections Associated with Artificial Urinary Sphincters

The causative organisms associated with AUS infections and erosions are predominantly skin flora. Cultures isolated from infected AUS devices showed growth of gram-positive cocci in two-thirds of cases (S aureus in approximately 50% and S epidermidis in nearly 30%) and gram-negative cocci in the remaining third (P aeruginosa, E coli, and P mirabilis).[39] A considerably high rate of methicillin-resistant organisms, 50% in cultures isolated that grew gram-positive organisms, must be taken into account in surgical planning.

The Approach to a Sphincter-Associated Infection or Erosion

Management of an AUS-associated infection involves explantation of all components of the device while covering the patient for systemic infectious complications with antibiotics. This procedure resembles closely the management of an infected PP. However, although successful salvage AUS implantation at the time of removal for infection has been described[44] an immediate salvage AUS reimplantation should be approached with caution. Concomitant involvement of the urethra in the infectious process predisposes it to early urethral erosion. In the case of a cuff erosion, the urethra is compromised and neither urethral regeneration nor reliable reinfection prevention can be achieved.

After AUS explantation, a prolonged course of antibiotics and urethral and periurethral tissue recovery is recommended. Reimplantation can be attempted after approximately 3 months while diverting the urine with a suprapubic or urethral catheter for the initial 6 weeks.[38] Before AUS reimplantation, a cystoscopy is necessary to assess the viability of the urethra and potential development of a urethral stricture at the prior cuff site.[38] The success rate of AUS reimplantation is 60% to 70% in cases with prior infection or erosion,[38,45] although it has been suggested that the rates may be lower in less-experienced centers because of the challenging periurethral dissection secondary to scar, altered tissue planes, and poor vascularization.[38] Extensive mobilization of the urethra during reimplantation should be avoided to preserve blood supply.[38] Determination of an appropriate site for the new cuff depends on tissue viability via cystoscopy and intraoperative findings.[38] If the urethra is atrophic, or the patient has risk factors for erosion, transcorporal cuff placement should be considered. This approach may also be chosen to avoid posterior urethral injury when the dissection is particularly difficult.[38] For transcorporal placement, the cuff is placed through the interposing corporal tissue surrounding the dorsal aspect of the urethra. This technique provides 2 distinct advantages. First, the urethra does not have to be mobilized off the corpora cavernosa at the implantation site avoiding compromise of blood supply, and second, the interposed tissue acts as bolster to allow sufficient closing pressure of the cuff while dispersing the pressure exerted by the cuff. Success rates of transcorporal sphincter implantations have been reported as high as 76%, and it is important to note that erectile function remained intact in men who were potent preoperatively.[46] Alternative approaches to avoid cuff erosion in high-risk men include wrapping the urethra with xenograft tissue such as porcine small intestine submucosa.[47] Success rates of nearly 40% in a high-risk population of patients with multiple previous AUS were achieved; however, this approach should be considered experimental until more data are available.[47]

Guide to Artificial Urinary Sphincter Implantation

The concepts described for PP to prevent infection also apply to AUS. Perioperative antibiotic treatment and meticulous sterile technique is the mainstay of infection prevention. One study has recommended a 5-day preoperative course of chlorhexidine scrub of the abdomen and perineum because this has decreased bacterial colonization[39]; however, actual infection rates of the implanted AUSs were not reported. As described above, salvage implantation of an AUS is not recommended and the use of an antibacterial-coated device seems to be of little or no additional benefit.

OVERALL SUMMARY

PPs and AUSs are commonly implanted urologic devices with overall low infection rates. Improved device design with antibacterial coating has contributed to lowering infection rates in PP. Similarly, improved understanding of the pathophysiology of device infections has enabled perioperative strategies to minimize the risk of device infections.

Treatment of a PP- or AUS-associated infection consists of immediate removal of the device in conjunction with systemic antibiotic coverage. Thorough washout of the implantation site is required to remove remnants of bacterial biofilm. Salvage reimplantation of PP has become the standard approach in most patients, whereas tissue regeneration is required before an AUS-associated infection site can be reimplanted.

REFERENCES

1. Foster SA, Annunziata K, Shortridge EF, et al. Erectile dysfunction with or without coexisting benign prostatic hyperplasia in the general US population: analysis of US National Health and Wellness Survey. Curr Med Res Opin 2013;29:1709–17.
2. Hatzimouratidis K, Amar E, Eardley I, et al. Guidelines on male sexual dysfunction: erectile dysfunction and premature ejaculation. Eur Urol 2010;57: 804–14.
3. Scott FB, Bradley WE, Timm GW. Management of erectile impotence. Use of implantable inflatable prosthesis. Urology 1973;2:80–2.
4. Muench PJ. Infections versus penile implants: the war on bugs. J Urol 2013;189:1631–7.
5. Carson CC, Mulcahy JJ, Govier FE. Efficacy, safety and patient satisfaction outcomes of the AMS 700CX inflatable penile prosthesis: results of a long-term multicenter study. AMS 700CX Study Group. J Urol 2000;164:376–80.
6. Mulcahy JJ. Current approach to the treatment of penile implant infections. Ther Adv Urol 2010;2:69–75.
7. Moncada I, Jara J, Cabello R, et al. Radiological assessment of penile prosthesis: the role of magnetic resonance imaging. World J Urol 2004;22: 371–7.
8. Montague DK. Periprosthetic infections. J Urol 1987; 138:68–9.
9. Carson CC. Infections in genitourinary prostheses. Urol Clin North Am 1989;16:139–47.
10. Silverstein AD, Henry GD, Evans B, et al. Biofilm formation on clinically noninfected penile prostheses. J Urol 2006;176:1008–11.
11. Donlan RM. Biofilms: microbial life on surfaces. Emerg Infect Dis 2002;8:881–90.
12. Carson CC, Robertson CN. Late hematogenous infection of penile prostheses. J Urol 1988;139:50–2.
13. Jarow JP. Risk factors for penile prosthetic infection. J Urol 1996;156:402–4.
14. Cakan M, Demirel F, Karabacak O, et al. Risk factors for penile prosthetic infection. Int Urol Nephrol 2003; 35:209–13.
15. Furlow WL, Goldwasser B. Salvage of the eroded inflatable penile prosthesis: a new concept. J Urol 1987;138:312–4.
16. Kohler TS, Modder JK, Dupree JM, et al. Malleable implant substitution for the management of penile prosthesis pump erosion: a pilot study. J Sex Med 2009;6:1474–8.
17. Swords K, Martinez DR, Lockhart JL, et al. A preliminary report on the usage of an intracorporal antibiotic cast with synthetic high purity CaSO4 for the treatment of infected penile implant. J Sex Med 2013;10:1162–9.
18. Brant MD, Ludlow JK, Mulcahy JJ. The prosthesis salvage operation: immediate replacement of the infected penile prosthesis. J Urol 1996;155:155–7.
19. Henry GD, Carson CC, Wilson SK, et al. Revision washout decreases implant capsule tissue culture positivity: a multicenter study. J Urol 2008;179: 186–90 [discussion: 90].
20. Carson CC. Penile prosthesis implantation and infection for Sexual Medicine Society of North America. Int J Impot Res 2001;13(Suppl 5):S35–8.
21. Mulcahy JJ. Surgical management of penile prosthesis complications. Int J Impot Res 2000; 12(Suppl 4):S108–11.
22. Knoll LD. Penile prosthetic infection: management by delayed and immediate salvage techniques. Urology 1998;52:287–90.
23. Wilson SK, Salem EA, Costerton W. Anti-infection dip suggestions for the coloplast titan inflatable penile prosthesis in the era of the infection retardant coated implant. J Sex Med 2011;8:2647–54.
24. Serefoglu EC, Mandava SH, Gokce A, et al. Long-term revision rate due to infection in hydrophilic-coated inflatable penile prostheses: 11-year follow-up. J Sex Med 2012;9:2182–6.
25. Carson CC 3rd, Mulcahy JJ, Harsch MR. Long-term infection outcomes after original antibiotic impregnated inflatable penile prosthesis implants: up to 7.7 years of followup. J Urol 2011;185:614–8.
26. Mulcahy JJ, Carson CC 3rd. Long-term infection rates in diabetic patients implanted with antibiotic-impregnated versus nonimpregnated inflatable penile prostheses: 7-year outcomes. Eur Urol 2011;60:167–72.

27. Raad I, Darouiche R, Dupuis J, et al. Central venous catheters coated with minocycline and rifampin for the prevention of catheter-related colonization and bloodstream infections. A randomized, double-blind trial. The Texas Medical Center Catheter Study Group. Ann Intern Med 1997;127:267–74.

28. Darouiche RO, Bella AJ, Boone TB, et al. North American consensus document on infection of penile prostheses. Urology 2013;82:937–42.

29. Wolf JS Jr, Bennett CJ, Dmochowski RR, et al. Best practice policy statement on urologic surgery antimicrobial prophylaxis. J Urol 2008;179:1379–90.

30. Katz DJ, Stember DS, Nelson CJ, et al. Perioperative prevention of penile prosthesis infection: practice patterns among surgeons of SMSNA and ISSM. J Sex Med 2012;9:1705–12 [quiz: 712–4].

31. Katz BF, Gaunay GS, Barazani Y, et al. Use of a preoperative checklist reduces risk of penile prosthesis infection. J Urol 2014;192:130–5.

32. Bode LG, Kluytmans JA, Wertheim HF, et al. Preventing surgical-site infections in nasal carriers of *Staphylococcus aureus*. N Engl J Med 2010; 362:9–17.

33. Paocharoen V, Mingmalairak C, Apisarnthanarak A. Comparison of surgical wound infection after preoperative skin preparation with 4% chlorhexidine [correction of chlohexidine] and povidone iodine: a prospective randomized trial. J Med Assoc Thai 2009;92:898–902.

34. Yeung LL, Grewal S, Bullock A, et al. A comparison of chlorhexidine-alcohol versus povidone-iodine for eliminating skin flora before genitourinary prosthetic surgery: a randomized controlled trial. J Urol 2013; 189:136–40.

35. Litwiller SE, Kim KB, Fone PD, et al. Post-prostatectomy incontinence and the artificial urinary sphincter: a long-term study of patient satisfaction and criteria for success. J Urol 1996;156:1975–80.

36. Montague DK, Angermeier KW, Paolone DR. Long-term continence and patient satisfaction after artificial sphincter implantation for urinary incontinence after prostatectomy. J Urol 2001;166:547–9.

37. Montague DK. Artificial urinary sphincter: long-term results and patient satisfaction. Adv Urol 2012; 2012:835290.

38. Linder BJ, de Cogain M, Elliott DS. Long-term device outcomes of artificial urinary sphincter reimplantation following prior explantation for erosion or infection. J Urol 2014;191:734–8.

39. Magera JS Jr, Elliott DS. Artificial urinary sphincter infection: causative organisms in a contemporary series. J Urol 2008;180:2475–8.

40. de Cogain MR, Elliott DS. The impact of an antibiotic coating on the artificial urinary sphincter infection rate. J Urol 2013;190:113–7.

41. Brant WO, Erickson BA, Elliott SP, et al. Risk factors for erosion of artificial urinary sphincters: a multicenter prospective study. Urology 2014;84:934–8.

42. Catto JW, Natarajan V, Tophill PR. Simultaneous augmentation cystoplasty is associated with earlier rather than increased artificial urinary sphincter infection. J Urol 2005;173:1237–41.

43. Segal RL, Cabrini MR, Harris ED, et al. Combined inflatable penile prosthesis-artificial urinary sphincter implantation: no increased risk of adverse events compared to single or staged device implantation. J Urol 2013;190:2183–8.

44. Bryan DE, Mulcahy JJ, Simmons GR. Salvage procedure for infected noneroded artificial urinary sphincters. J Urol 2002;168:2464–6.

45. Raj GV, Peterson AC, Webster GD. Outcomes following erosions of the artificial urinary sphincter. J Urol 2006;175:2186–90 [discussion: 90].

46. Wiedemann L, Cornu JN, Haab E, et al. Transcorporal artificial urinary sphincter implantation as a salvage surgical procedure for challenging cases of male stress urinary incontinence: surgical technique and functional outcomes in a contemporary series. BJU Int 2013;112:1163–8.

47. Trost L, Elliott D. Small intestinal submucosa urethral wrap at the time of artificial urinary sphincter placement as a salvage treatment option for patients with persistent/recurrent incontinence following multiple prior sphincter failures and erosions. Urology 2012; 79:933–8.

Epidemiology and Management of Emerging Drug-Resistant Gram-Negative Bacteria
Extended-Spectrum β-Lactamases and Beyond

Daniel P. Boyle, MD*, Teresa R. Zembower, MD

KEYWORDS

- Antibiotic resistance • Extended-spectrum β-lactamases
- Carbapenem-resistant enterobacteriaceae • New Delhi metallo–β-lactamase
- Carbapenem-resistant *Acinetobacter baumannii* • Multidrug-resistant *Pseudomonas aeruginosa*

KEY POINTS

- Antibiotic resistance is increasing at an alarming rate primarily due to antibiotic overuse.
- The most common classes of resistance encountered in gram-negative bacteria include extended-spectrum β-lactamase (ESBL)–containing organisms, carbapenem-resistant Enterobacteriaceae (CRE), carbapenem-resistant *Acinetobacter baumannii* (CRAB), and multidrug-resistant (MDR) *Pseudomonas.*
- Urinary tract infections (UTIs) are the most commonly encountered infections with these MDR bacteria, and infections with these organisms result in increased morbidity and mortality.
- The antimicrobials used to treat these infections are termed, *drugs of last resort*, and often carry a high risk of adverse drug events.
- Antimicrobial stewardship and infection prevention programs are the most proved modalities used to stop the development and spread of antimicrobial resistance.

INTRODUCTION

In the past couple of decades, worldwide prevalence of antimicrobial resistance has increased at a startling rate. Many factors play a role in increasing drug resistance; however, the main driver remains antibiotic overuse. In addition, person-to-person spread of resistant bacteria and the passage of resistance genes between bacteria also play a large role. With the increase in global travel and trade, resistance mechanisms are easily transmitted worldwide.[1] Each year in the United States, it is estimated that more than 2 million individuals suffer an infection from a resistant bacteria and more than 23,000 deaths are attributed to these organisms.[2] Because of these alarming numbers, President Obama issued an Executive Order in 2014 outlining a national plan to detect, prevent, and control the spread and

Division of Infectious Diseases, Department of Medicine, Northwestern University Feinberg School of Medicine, 645 North Michigan Avenue, Suite 900, Chicago, IL 60611, USA
* Corresponding author. Division of Infectious Diseases, Northwestern University Feinberg School of Medicine, 645 North Michigan Avenue, Suite 900, Chicago, IL 60611.
E-mail address: daniel.boyle@northwestern.edu

Urol Clin N Am 42 (2015) 493–505
http://dx.doi.org/10.1016/j.ucl.2015.05.005

Abbreviations	
CAUTIs	Catheter associated urinary tract infections
CLABSIs	Central line associated bloodstream infections
CRAB	Carbapenem-resistant *Acinetobacter baumannii*
CRE	Carbapenem-resistant Enterobacteriaceae
ESBL	Extended spectrum β-lactamase
HAIs	Healthcare associated infection
KPC	*Klebsiella pneumoniae* carbapenemase
MDR	Multidrug-resistant
NDM-1	New Delhi metallo-β-lactamase
SSIs	Surgical site infections
UTI	Urinary tract infection
VAPs	Ventilator associated pneumonias

emergence of antimicrobial resistance. This plan emphasizes implementation of strong antimicrobial stewardship programs aimed at preventing antibiotic misuse and infection prevention programs aimed at decreasing person-to-person transmission of these resistant bacteria.[2]

When resistant bacteria are encountered in the clinical setting, decisions regarding management are difficult. The first decision to be made is whether the isolated bacteria represents a true infection versus colonization. In those who are colonized (have no signs or symptoms consistent with infection), treatment is not warranted, because treatment increases the risk for an adverse drug event and drives further resistance. When treatment is warranted, antibiotic options are often limited and many of the choices carry a significant risk of side effects (ie, polymyxins and renal failure).

This review discusses emerging gram-negative resistance patterns. For each resistance pattern, the mechanisms of resistance, risk factors, type of infections, treatment, and outcomes are highlighted. Common side effects associated with the antimicrobial therapies and the tools the medical community is using to combat the continued spread of resistant bacteria also are discussed.

EXTENDED-SPECTRUM β-LACTAMASE–CONTAINING BACTERIA
Definition and Types

ESBLs are plasmid-mediated enzymes that mediate resistance to extended-spectrum (third-generation) cephalosporins (eg, ceftazidime, cefotaxime, and ceftriaxone) and monobactams (eg, aztreonam) but do not affect cephamycins (eg, cefoxitin and cefotetan) or carbapenems (eg, meropenem or imipenem).[3] These enzymes disrupt the β-lactam antibiotics through hydrolysis, resulting in an opening of the β-lactam ring, rendering these

antibiotics inactive. In addition to β-lactam resistance, many organisms carrying these enzymes also have resistance to other classes of antibiotics, including fluoroquinolones, aminoglycosides, and sulfonamides through different mechanisms of resistance, further complicating therapeutic choices.[4] The first clinical case involving an ESBL-producing organism was reported in 1983 in Germany and occurred in a *Klebsiella* species found to have resistance to a newer class of antibiotics, oxyimino-cephalosporins, which had been specifically designed to combat β-lactam–producing organisms.[5] In 1988, the first cases of infections due to ESBL-producing organisms in the United States were discovered.[6] Today, ESBL-producing organisms are a problematic cause of infections worldwide.[3]

ESBLs are most commonly encountered in organisms belonging to the Enterobacteriaceae family, and *Klebsiella pneumoniae* and *Escherichia coli* are the most common species found to produce ESBLs.[4] The first ESBL enzyme was termed, *SHV-2*, and over time, researchers have identified numerous genetic mutations leading to multiple classes of ESBLs, the most common belonging to the SHV, TEM, CTX-M, and OXA classes of β-lactamases.[7]

Although these mutations are predominantly seen in bacteria recovered from patients in the health care setting, a growing body of literature supports the existence of these resistant bacteria in the community, especially in patients with UTIs. Numerous environmental reservoirs for these bacteria have been detected, including poultry and other meats,[8,9] drinking and river water,[10,11] and companion animals.[12]

Epidemiology and Risk Factors

Estimates of the prevalence of ESBL-producing organisms are difficult to perform because of the labor required to identify these organisms and the hospital-to-hospital variability of these rates. One study evaluated *K pneumoniae* isolates from different regions of the world for phenotypic evidence of ESBL production and found that 7.6% of the US isolates had evidence of ESBL production, compared with 4.9% in Canada, 23% in Europe, 25% in the Asia-Pacific region, and 45% in Latin America.[13] Numerous studies have examined risk factors for infection with an ESBL-producing organism. In hospitalized patients the most commonly cited risk factors include[7]

- Recent antibiotic use
- Residence in a long-term care facility
- Prolonged hospital stays
- Recent abdominal surgeries
- Hemodialysis
- Presence of a bladder catheter
- Presence of a gastrostomy or jejunostomy tube

In patients in the community, the most commonly cited risk factors include recent antibiotic use, chronic indwelling bladder catheter, poor functional status, and recent prolonged hospitalization.[14]

Infections and Treatment

Although ESBL-producing organisms can cause bacteremia, pneumonia, prostatitis, meningitis, and numerous other infections, UTIs are the most commonly encountered infection. It is well known that infections due to these resistant organisms are associated with poor outcomes, but virulence of ESBL-producing organisms is no different from the same species that do not contain an ESBL. The reason patients experience worse outcomes is the initial selection of antimicrobial agents to which the infecting organisms are resistant,[4] leading to a delay in initiation of effective therapy.

Carbapenems are the treatment of choice for patients with severe infections due to ESBL-producing organisms, but no randomized controlled trials have been performed to confirm this because of the practice challenges associated with such a study. There is, however, a large amount of observational data supporting use of a carbapenem over other antibiotics in the treatment of severe infections caused by ESBL-producing organisms.[4] The evidence investigating whether cefepime or piperacillin-tazobactam can be used to treat a severe infection due to an ESBL-producing organism has yielded mixed results. If a patient has an infection that is not severe, such as an uncomplicated UTI, then cefepime or piperacillin-tazobactam–susceptible organisms likely

are successfully treated with these antibiotics.[15–17] Some ESBL isolates also have in vitro susceptibility to fluoroquinolones, aminoglycosides, and sulfonamides, and in nonsevere infections, these antibiotics likely successfully treat these infections as well.[18] Nitrofurantoin can be used for uncomplicated UTIs due to susceptible ESBL-producers but should not be used in patients with signs of ascending infections.[19] In addition to these antibiotics, some ESBL-producing isolates have in vitro susceptibility to fosfomycin or tetracyclines, and these oral agents are good choices of therapy for uncomplicated UTIs.[20]

Outcomes

As discussed previously, patients with infections due to ESBL-producing organisms have poor outcomes. A meta-analysis evaluating mortality found that patients with bacteremia due to an ESBL-producing Enterobacteriaceae had significantly higher mortality rates than patients who were bacteremic from a non–ESBL-producing Enterobacteriaceae.[21] An additional concern in the management of ESBL-producing organisms is the development of further antibiotic resistance. With the increased use of carbapenems, clinicians are encountering carbapenemase-producing organisms. These organism are difficult to treat becasue the antimicrobials used in these cases often have toxic side effects, and in some instances, the resistance profiles are such that no adequate antimicrobial options exist.[22]

CARBAPENEM-RESISTANT ENTEROBACTERIACEAE AND *KLEBSIELLA PNEUMONIAE* CARBAPENEMASE–PRODUCING ORGANISMS
Definition and Types

CRE refers to a group of bacteria that produce carbapenemases, β-lactamases capable of hydrolyzing carbapenems and all other β-lactam antibiotics, rendering these classes of antibiotics inactive. These bacteria are often resistant to numerous other non–β-lactam antibiotics, especially fluoroquinolones, leading to difficult treatment decisions.[23] There are 4 different molecular classes (A, B, C, and D) of carbapenemases, of which classes A, B, and D are the most clinically relevant. Classes A, C, and D contain the amino acid serine at the active site, whereas class B carbapenemases (also known as metallo–β-lactamases) contains zinc at the active site. The most commonly encountered carbapenemase in the United States is *K pneumoniae* carbapenemase (KPC), which belongs to the group of carbapenemases designated class A, and the terms, CRE and KPC, are often incorrectly used interchangeably.[24] As the name suggests, KPCs are most commonly found in *Klebsiella* species, but these enzymes are also frequently found in *E.coli* and *Enterobacter cloacae*.[25] Class D carbapenemases are termed OXA carbapenemases, and these enzymes are increasingly reported as causes of infection in European hospitals. Of the metallo–β-lactamases (class B), the New Delhi metallo–β-lactamase (NDM-1) has garnered much attention because of the continued worldwide spread of the extreme resistance associated with this enzyme.[26]

Epidemiology and Risk Factors

The first reported cases of CRE were described in 1996 in a *K pneumoniae* isolate in North Carolina, and the enzyme responsible for this resistance was thus termed *KPC-1*.[27] Since that time, the Centers for Disease Control and Prevention (CDC) report that 42 US states have reported infections due to KPC-producing bacteria.[28] In 2010, the National Healthcare Safety Network (NHSN) at the CDC estimated that of the Enterobacteriaceae species causing health care–associated infections (HAIs), 4.2% were considered to be CRE. Of all HAIs caused by a *Klebsiella* species, 10.4% had evidence of carbapenem resistance.[29] Infections due to CRE are also a large problem worldwide and have become endemic in parts of the South America, Africa, Asia, and Europe.[30]

Several studies have examined risk factors for CRE infection, and although some community-based transmissions have occurred, these pathogens are most commonly encountered in individuals who have contact with a health care setting. The most agreed-on risk factor for infection or colonization with a CRE is receiving carbapenems or a broad-spectrum cephalosporin.[31] Other risk factors for infection or colonization include[31–34]

- Undergoing solid organ or stem cell transplantation
- Malignancy
- Poorly controlled diabetes
- Trauma
- Prolonged mechanical ventilation
- Residence in a long-term acute care facility
- Poor functional status
- Prolonged ICU stay
- Chronic indwelling Foley catheters

Infections and Treatment

CREs commonly cause UTIs, bloodstream infections, pneumonia, and wound infections, and they are often implicated in HAIs, leading to central line–associated bloodstream infections (CLABSIs), catheter-associated UTIs (CAUTIs), ventilator-associated pneumonias (VAPs), and surgical site infections (SSIs).[29] Health care–associated outbreaks due to CRE have also been reported. In 2011, the US National Institutes of Health Clinical Center experienced an outbreak of KPC involving 18 patients, 6 of whom died as a direct consequence of the infection.[35]

Like ESBL-producing organisms, CREs often have resistance to numerous non–β-lactam antibiotics, making treatment extremely difficult. No optimal treatment regimens exist, and, along with assistance from infectious diseases experts, therapy for infections due to CRE should be tailored to antimicrobial susceptibility reports. Up to 98% of KPC-producing bacteria also carry resistance to fluoroquinolones, and up to 50% are resistant to commonly used aminoglycosides (gentamicin and amikacin).[23] Additional antimicrobial testing often needs to be requested, and a clinician should assure that the following susceptibility testing has been performed: colistin, polymyxin B, tigecycline, aztreonam, and fosfomycin.

UTIs can typically be successfully treated with a single antimicrobial agent that has a favorable susceptibility.[36] For more complicated infections (eg, bloodstream infections and severe pneumonia), treatment with 2 antimicrobials is recommended to protect against further development of resistance and the higher mortality associated with antimicrobial monotherapy in these situations. There is also a limited amount of evidence that addition of a carbapenem as a third antimicrobial in the setting of a severe infections improves mortality.[37]

Outcomes

Because of limited treatment options, the mortality rate associated with CRE infections is 40% to 50%. As with ESBLs, CRE are not any more virulent than non-CRE, but delay in or lack of appropriate therapy contributes to the high mortality rate.[32,38] Other poor outcomes are related to the toxic effects of the antimicrobials used to treat CRE infections. The polymyxins (colistin [ie, polymyxin E] and polymyxin B) are nephrotoxic, and a large retrospective study found that 43% of patients receiving a polymyxin developed renal failure.[39] The aminoglycosides are also nephrotoxic, leading to renal failure in 10% to 20% of patients, and these drugs can result in irreversible ototoxicity.[40] Often polymyxins and aminoglycosides are used in combination to treat severe infections, leading to an even greater risk of adverse events from the antimicrobials.

New Delhi Metallo–β-Lactamase

NDM-1 was first reported in Sweden in 2008 after being recovered from a patient who had been transferred from a New Delhi hospital. This enzyme is of concern because of its increasing prevalence and, in many cases, resistance to all drugs except the polymyxins and occasionally tigecycline. Due to the ease of plasmid spread of this mutation, NDM-1 has now been detected in environmental bacteria, commonly recovered in water sources in India and other parts of Asia.[41] Although the majority of NDM-1 infections occurs in Asia, NDM-1–producing organisms are found worldwide.[30] In 2013, an outbreak of an NDM-1–producing *E.coli* was detected in a Chicago hospital, resulting in 39 patients colonized or infected with this organism.[42] Management guidelines for NDM-1 are the same as for CRE: consultation with infectious diseases experts, use of susceptibility reports to guide therapy, and treatment with at least 2 agents for severe infections.

CARBAPENEM-RESISTANT *ACINETOBACTER BAUMANNII*
Definition and Types

Worldwide nosocomial infections due to *A baumannii* have increased substantially in recent decades. With the recent emergence of MDR *A baumannii*, carbapenems have become the treatment of choice for these pathogens. Unfortunately, clinicians are encountering an increasing number of infections due to CRAB.[43] In the United States, *A baumannii* is less commonly identified as causing HAIs compared with the Enterobacteriaceae, but when it does lead to HAI, greater than 60% of these isolates are resistant to carbapenems.[29] The mechanisms of carbapenem resistance in CRAB include[44,45]

- Various carbapenemases (most commonly OXA and metallo–β-lactamases)
- AdeABC efflux system (efflux pump)
- Modifications of penicillin-binding proteins
- Modification of outer membrane proteins (porins)

Epidemiology and Risk Factors

Numerous environmental sources of *A baumannii* have been identified, including soil, meat, fish, and vegetables.[43] Carrier or colonization rates in healthy individuals are typically low, 1% in a European cohort, but may be higher in some Asian populations—a healthy Hong Kong cohort had a carrier rate of 32%.[46,47] Community-acquired infections due to CRAB are uncommon, but when they occur, pneumonia is the most common infection, typically occurring in patients with underlying pulmonary disease, renal failure, or diabetes or in those with excessive alcohol use.[48]

Most commonly, CRAB is seen as a nosocomial pathogen and can lead to difficult to control outbreaks. The most common mode of transmission is from the hands of hospital staff, but CRAB can also be spread through exposure to contaminated equipment/surfaces and, possibly, aerosolized water droplets. *A baumannii* can survive for prolonged periods of time on dry surfaces, and in many CRAB outbreaks, cultures obtained from computer keyboards, curtains, door handles, and furniture grow this pathogen.[44] Several risk factors have been identified for becoming colonized or infected with CRAB, notably[49,50]

- Major trauma (especially burn injuries) or surgery
- Prolonged ICU stay
- Prolonged mechanical ventilation
- Chronic indwelling devices (including bladder catheters)
- Receiving broad-spectrum antibiotics

Recently there has also been an increased number of deep wound infections, burns, and osteomyelitis due to CRAB among US service members injured in Iraq and Afghanistan, thought to be due to environmental contamination of field hospitals and other health care facilities.[51]

Infections and Treatments

CRAB is typically identified as a nosocomial pathogen. In 2009 to 2010, NHSN concluded that *A baumannii* was the infecting organism in 0.9% of CAUTIs, 2.1% of CLABSIs, 6.6% of VAPs, and 0.6% of SSIs. Of these isolates, carbapenem resistance was found in 74.2% of CAUTIS, 62.6% of CLABSIs, 61.2% of VAPs, and 37.3% of SSIs.[29]

A baumannii, in general, is an organism with remarkable ability to acquire resistance mechanisms, and resistance to most classes of antibiotics is common among CRAB isolates. As with CRE, antimicrobial therapy should be tailored to susceptibility reports, and susceptibility testing for the following should be requested if not routinely performed: colistin, polymyxin B, tigecycline, minocycline, and doxycycline.

Carbapenem susceptibility may vary; thus, both imipenem and meropenem susceptibilities should be performed on *A baumannii* isolates.[52] Occasionally fluoroquinolones can be used, but this is becoming uncommon.[44] Ampicillin/sulbactam is a good choice when in vitro susceptibility is observed, but resistance to this drug is also increasing.[53] Aminoglycosides and polymyxins are often the only therapeutic options. Based on animal studies and in vitro data, combination therapy is recommended for severe infections with the goals of improving outcomes and preventing emergence of further resistance.[44]

Outcomes

Patients with minor infections due to CRAB (ie, uncomplicated UTIs) typically do well and suffer low mortality and morbidity, but those with more severe infections tend to do poorly. The mortality rates for patients with bloodstream infections from CRAB have been estimated to be 34% to 41%,[54,55] and those with VAP also have substantial mortality.[56] Although severe infections with CRAB portend high mortality, debate exists on whether mortality can be attributed to the CRAB infection because the majority of patients with these infections has severe underlying disease. A matched cohort study performed in a Belgian ICU concluded that A baumannii bacteremia is not associated with a significant increase in attributable mortality (mortality rate for cases vs controls: 42%–34%).[57] Regardless of whether CRAB is the true cause of death or a surrogate marker for poor outcome, severe infections with CRAB are associated with high mortality rates.

MULTIDRUG-RESISTANT PSEUDOMONAS
Definition and Types

Pseudomonas aeruginosa was first identified as a unique pathogen in the mid-1800s after being recovered from bluish-green purulent fluid draining from a patient's surgical wound. This non–lactose-fermenting gram-negative aerobic bacillus is often identified as a water bug because it thrives in moist settings but has the ability to survive in a variety of environmental conditions.[58] It has been found on numerous surfaces throughout hospitals and is a major cause of HAIs.[29]

Due to the intrinsic resistance to many antibiotics and the ease with which this organism requires resistance mechanisms, clinicians are encountering increasing antimicrobial resistance in P aeruginosa.[58] The various resistance mechanisms in P aeruginosa are shown in **Box 1**.

In response to mounting resistance and the need for standardized definitions for use in medical literature, the CDC and the European Centre for Disease Prevention and Control established definitions for MDR, extensively drug-resistant, and pandrug-resistant P aeruginosa in 2011[59] (**Table 1**).

Epidemiology and Risk Factors

P aeruginosa is a ubiquitous organism that has been recovered from numerous environmental settings, including swimming pools, hot tubs, humidifiers, contact lens solution, animals, soil, plants, vegetables, and acrylic finger nails.[58] Despite the widespread presence of this organism, the colonization rate of a healthy individual is low (0%–2%)[60] but in hospitalized patients this rate often exceeds 50%.[58] Consistent with the low colonization rate seen in healthy individuals, a majority of infections caused by P aeruginosa are HAIs, and the most frequently encountered HAIs due to this organism are CAUTIs.[29] Risk factors associated with MDR Pseudomonas infections in the hospitalized patients include[61,62]

- Surgery
- Trauma (especially burn injuries)

Box 1
Mechanisms and enzymes associated with antimicrobial resistance in Pseudomonas aeruginosa

- Multidrug efflux pumps
- Change in outer membrane proteins/porins (ie, OprD, a carbapenem-specific porin)
- Change in membrane permeability (resulting in polymyxin resistance)
- AmpC β-lactamase
- Various ESBLs
- Carbapenemases (most commonly metallo–β-lactamases)
- Aminoglycoside-modifying enzymes
- Topoisomerase gene mutations (ie, gyrA)

Data from Bonomo RA, Szabo D. Mechanisms of multidrug resistance in Acinetobacter species and Pseudomonas aeruginosa. Clin Infect Dis 2006;43(Suppl 2):S49–56; and Lister PD, Wolter DJ, Hanson ND. Antibacterial-resistant Pseudomonas aeruginosa: clinical impact and complex regulation of chromosomally encoded resistance mechanisms. Clin Microbiol Rev 2009;22(4):582–610.

Table 1
Classifying drug-resistant *Pseudomonas aeruginosa*

Resistance Class	Definition
MDR	The isolate is nonsusceptible to at least 1 agent in 3 antimicrobial categories[a]
Extensively drug resistant	The isolate is nonsusceptible to at least 1 agent in all but 2 or fewer antimicrobial categories[a]
Pandrug resistant	Nonsusceptibility to all agents in all antimicrobial categories[a]

[a] Antimicrobial categories include aminoglycosides, antipseudomonal carbapenems, antipseudomonal cephalosporins (ceftazidime, cefepime), fluoroquinolones, antipseudomonal penicillins (ticarcillin-clavulanic acid, piperacillin-tazobactam), monobactams (aztreonam), polymyxins, and phosphonic acids (fosfomycin).

- Presence of indwelling catheters (including bladder catheters)
- Prior use of broad-spectrum antibiotics
- Poorly controlled diabetes
- Poor functional status
- Prolonged ICU stay

Hospital outbreaks of MDR *Pseudomonas* occur and patients infected during these outbreaks can have increased mortality rates.[63] Some of the commonly identified sources of outbreaks include bronchoscopes, endoscopes, water systems (eg, pipes and sinks), ventilators, and cleaning equipment.[64]

Infections and Treatments

MDR *Pseudomonas* is almost exclusively identified as a nosocomial pathogen. The NHSN found *P aeruginosa* to be the second most common cause of CAUTIs (11.3%) and VAPs (16.6%), the seventh most common cause of SSIs (5.5%), and the fifth most common cause of CLABSIs (7.9%). Of the isolates that lead to CAUTIs, 34% were fluoroquinolone resistant, 21% were carbapenem resistant, 11% were aminoglycoside resistant, 17% were piperacillin-tazobactam resistant, and 14% were MDR *Pseudomonas*.[29]

The approach to treating MDR *Pseudomonas* is similar to many other resistant pathogens. Therapy should be targeted to the susceptibility profile of the specific isolate. In the rare setting where an MDR *Pseudomonas* remains fluoroquinolone susceptible, ciprofloxacin and levofloxacin are good choices for treatment of UTIs. Susceptibility profiles to polymyxins, fosfomycin, and carbapenems should be performed when managing an MDR *Pseudomonas* infection. In the treatment of severe infections due to MDR *Pseudomonas*, there is much debate over whether combination therapy is warranted. There are no clinical data that suggest improved mortality outcomes with the use of combination therapy, but data suggest that combination therapy may prevent the

development of further resistance.[51] To help guide therapy for the treatment of MDR *Pseudomonas*, the expert opinion of an infectious diseases specialist should be obtained.

Outcomes

Patients with uncomplicated UTIs due to MDR *Pseudomonas* typically have good outcomes if the correct antimicrobial choices are made. These patients can do poorly if MDR *Pseudomonas* is not identified as the pathogen, leading to inappropriate antibiotic selection and progression to a complicated infection (ie, bacteremia due to UTI). Patients with severe infections due to MDR *Pseudomonas* have a significantly increased mortality rate compared with patients infected with non-MDR *Pseudomonas*. In a retrospective cohort study evaluating patients with *P aeruginosa* bacteremia, patients infected with MDR *Pseudomonas* had significantly longer hospital stays, significantly higher mortality rates, and a significantly shorter time to mortality than patients with non-MDR *Pseudomonas*.[65]

DRUGS OF LAST RESORT

Drugs of last resort refers to antibiotics that are some of the final drugs that can be used to successfully treat a resistant pathogen.[66] Unfortunately, many of these drugs carry significant side-effect profiles. **Table 2** outlines commonly prescribed drugs of last resort and the most commonly encountered side effects.

STRATEGIES TO PREVENT RESISTANCE

To combat the emergence and spread of resistance, attention has focused on the 2 most important factors contributing to the alarming spread of antimicrobial resistance: (1) inappropriate antibiotic use and (2) person-to-person spread of resistant bacteria. Antimicrobial stewardship programs are tasked with monitoring the antimicrobial use at

Table 2
Drugs of last resort and side effects

Class of Antibiotics	Drugs	Most Common Side Effects
Aminoglycosides	Amikacin Gentamicin Tobramycin	Renal toxicity (10%–20%) Ototoxicity (vestibular and cochlear)
Polymyxins	Colistin (polymyxin E) Polymyxin B	Nephrotoxicity (up to 40%) Neurotoxicity (confusion, vertigo, parasthesias)
Tetracyclines	Minocycline Doxycycline	Gastrointestinal discomfort Phototoxicity
Glycylcyclines	Tigecycline	Nausea/vomiting Diarrhea
Carbapenems	Meropenem Imipenem Doripenem Ertapenem (not effective against *Pseudomonas*)	Decreases seizure threshold
Other	Fosfomycin	Diarrhea Headache

Box 2
Commonly used techniques of effective antimicrobial stewardship programs

- Protocols and guidelines for clinicians to promote appropriate antibiotic use
- Hospital formulary restrictions on broad-spectrum antibiotics
- Mandatory infectious diseases consultation in the setting of resistant bacteria or for the use of broad-spectrum antibiotics
- Antibiotic evaluation committees who review the use of antibiotics at their institution
- Educating the medical staff on appropriate antibiotic use

Data from Centers for Disease Control and Prevention (CDC). Core elements of hospital antibiotic stewardship programs. Atlanta (GA): US Department of Health and Human Services, CDC; 2014. Available at: http://www.cdc.gov/getsmart/healthcare/implementation/core-elements.html. Accessed May 26, 2015; and Dellit TH, Owens RC, McGowan JE Jr, et al. Infectious Diseases Society of America and the Society for Healthcare Epidemiology of America guidelines for developing an institutional program to enhance antimicrobial stewardship. Clin Infect Dis 2007;44(2):159–77.

Box 3
Commonly used techniques of effective infection control and prevention programs

- Strict adherence to hand hygiene
- Contact precautions for patients colonized or infected with resistant bacteria
- Patient cohorting
- Chlorhexidine bathing
- Surveillance cultures for high-risk units or patients
- Environmental cleaning guidelines
- Early discontinuation of unnecessary equipment (ie, central venous catheter, bladder catheters, endotracheal intubation, etc.)
- Appropriate precautions used when performing medical procedures
- Appropriate cleaning of medical instruments (ie, bronchoscopes, endoscopes, etc.)

Table 3
Summary of classes of resistance

Class of Resistance	Mechanisms of Resistance*	Organisms Most Commonly Carrying Resistance	Potential Therapies for Urinary Tract Infection**	Risk Factors for Infection
ESBL	• SHV β-lactamase • TEM β-lactamase • CTX-M β-lactamase • OXA β-lactamase	• *Klebsiella pneumoniae* • *E.coli* • *P aeruginosa* • *Proteus mirabilis*	• Carbapenems • Cefepime • Piperacillin/tazobactam • Aminoglycosides • Fosfomycin • Tetracyclines • Fluoroquinolones	• Recent antibiotic use • Residence in a long-term care facility • Prolonged hospital stays • Recent abdominal surgeries • Hemodialysis • Presence of a bladder catheter • Presence of a gastrostomy or jejunostomy tube
CRE/KPC	• Class A (KPC, SME, NMC, IMI, GES) • Class B (metallo–β-lactamase) • Class C (Amp-C type carbapenemase) • Class D (OXA carbapenemases)	• *K pneumoniae* • *E.coli* • *Enterobacter cloacae* • *Serratia marcescens* • *P aeruginosa* • *A baumannii*	• Colistin • Tigecycline • Aztreonam • Fosfomycin	• Receiving carbapenem or broad-spectrum cephalosporin • Undergoing solid organ or stem cell transplantation • Malignancy • Poorly controlled diabetes • Trauma • Prolonged mechanical ventilation • Residence in a long-term acute care facility • Poor functional status, prolonged ICU stay • Chronic indwelling Foley catheters

(continued on next page)

Table 3
(continued)

Class of Resistance	Mechanisms of Resistance*	Organisms Most Commonly Carrying Resistance	Potential Therapies for Urinary Tract Infection**	Risk Factors for Infection
CRAB	• Various carbapenemases (outlined previously) • AdeABC efflux system • Modifications of penicillin-binding proteins • Modification of outer membrane proteins/porins	A baumannii	• Aminoglycosides • Polymyxins • Tigecycline • Minocycline/doxycycline Occasionally: • Ampicillin/sulbactam • Fluoroquinolones	• Major trauma (especially burn injuries) or surgery • Prolonged ICU stay • Prolonged mechanical ventilation • Chronic indwelling devices (including bladder catheters) • Receiving broad-spectrum antibiotics
MDR Pseudomonas	• Multidrug efflux pumps • Change in outer membrane proteins/porins (ie, OprD, a carbapenem-specific porin) • Change in membrane permeability (resulting in polymyxin resistance) • AmpC β-lactamase • Various ESBLs • Carbapenemases (most commonly metallo–β-lactamases) • Aminoglycoside-modifying enzymes • Topoisomerase gene mutations (ie, gyrA)	P aeruginosa	• Carbapenems • Polymyxins • Aminoglycosides • Fosfomycin Occasionally: • Cefepime • Piperacillin/tazobactam • Fluoroquinolones • Aztreonam	• Surgery • Trauma (especially burn injuries) • Presence of indwelling catheters (including bladder catheters) • Prior use of broad-spectrum antibiotics • Poorly controlled diabetes • Poor functional status • Prolonged ICU stay

* Most commonly encountered mechanisms of resistance for each class.
** Susceptibility testing should be performed on the organism investigating the listed medications, and treatment should be based upon the susceptibility results.

their institution. Some commonly used strategies to accomplish this are shown in **Box 2**. Effective stewardship programs can have drastic effects on rates of resistance. In 1 United States ICU, the rate of MDR gram negatives causing HAIs decreased from 37.4% to 8.5% from 2002 to 2008 after implementation of a rigorous antimicrobial stewardship program.[67]

Infection control and prevention programs are tasked with decreasing person-to-person transmission of resistant organisms, overall HAI rates, and control of outbreaks. Some commonly used techniques to accomplish these goals are shown in **Box 3**.

SUMMARY

The continued emergence and spread of antimicrobial resistance is one of the most concerning issues facing the medical community. Because the most common infections caused by resistant gram-negative organisms involve the urinary tract, urologists need to be well versed in the management of these difficult to treat pathogens. Therapeutic options are limited and those that do exist are associated with significant toxicities. Partnerships between clinicians, antimicrobial stewardship, and infection prevention programs will be vital to control the emerging resistance that will continue to present challenges for the foreseeable future (**Table 3**).

REFERENCES

1. Laxminarayan R, Duse A, Wattal C, et al. Antibiotic resistance-the need for global solutions. Lancet Infect Dis 2013;13(12):1057–98.
2. Available at: http://www.cdc.gov/drugresistance/index.html. Accessed April 1, 2015.
3. Paterson DL, Bonomo RA. Extended-spectrum beta-lactamases: a clinical update. Clin Microbiol Rev 2005;18(4):657–86.
4. Pitout JD, Laupland KB. Extended-spectrum beta-lactamase-producing Enterobacteriaceae: an emerging public-health concern. Lancet Infect Dis 2008;8(3):159–66.
5. Knothe H, Shah P, Krcmery V, et al. Transferable resistance to cefotaxime, cefoxitin, cefamandole and cefuroxime in clinical isolates of Klebsiella pneumoniae and Serratia marcescens. Infection 1983;11(6):315–7.
6. Jacoby GA, Medeiros AA, O'Brien TF, et al. Broad-spectrum, transmissible beta-lactamases. N Engl J Med 1988;319(11):723–4.
7. Jacoby GA, Munoz-Price LS. The new beta-lactamases. N Engl J Med 2005;352(4):380–91.
8. Wu G, Day MJ, Mafura MT, et al. Comparative analysis of ESBL-positive Escherichia coli isolates from animals and humans from the UK, the Netherlands and Germany. PLoS One 2013;8(9):e75392.
9. Vincent C, Boerlin P, Daignault D, et al. Food reservoir for Escherichia coli causing urinary tract infections. Emerg Infect Dis 2010;16(1):88–95.
10. De Boeck H, Miwanda B, Lunguya-Metila O, et al. ESBL-positive Enterobacteria isolates in drinking water. Emerg Infect Dis 2012;18(6):1019–20.
11. Dhanji H, Murphy NM, Akhigbe C, et al. Isolation of fluoroquinolone-resistant O25b:H4-ST131 Escherichia coli with CTX-M-14 extended-spectrum beta-lactamase from UK river water. J Antimicrob Chemother 2011;66(3):512–6.
12. Johnson JR, Miller S, Johnston B, et al. Sharing of Escherichia coli sequence type ST131 and other multidrug-resistant and Urovirulent E. coli strains among dogs and cats within a household. J Clin Microbiol 2009;47(11):3721–5.
13. Winokur PL, Canton R, Casellas JM, et al. Variations in the prevalence of strains expressing an extended-spectrum beta-lactamase phenotype and characterization of isolates from Europe, the Americas, and the Western Pacific region. Clin Infect Dis 2001; 32(Suppl 2):S94–103.
14. Ben-Ami R, Rodríguez-Baño J, Arslan H, et al. A multinational survey of risk factors for infection with extended-spectrum beta-lactamase-producing enterobacteriaceae in nonhospitalized patients. Clin Infect Dis 2009;49(5):682–90.
15. Chopra T, Marchaim D, Veltman J, et al. Impact of cefepime therapy on mortality among patients with bloodstream infections caused by extended-spectrum-beta-lactamase-producing Klebsiella pneumoniae and Escherichia coli. Antimicrob Agents Chemother 2012;56(7):3936–42.
16. Zanetti G, Bally F, Greub G, et al. Cefepime versus imipenem-cilastatin for treatment of nosocomial pneumonia in intensive care unit patients: a multicenter, evaluator-blind, prospective, randomized study. Antimicrob Agents Chemother 2003;47(11):3442–7.
17. Gavin PJ, Suseno MT, Thomson RB Jr, et al. Clinical correlation of the CLSI susceptibility breakpoint for piperacillin- tazobactam against extended-spectrum-beta-lactamase-producing Escherichia coli and Klebsiella species. Antimicrob Agents Chemother 2006;50(6):2244–7.
18. Rupp ME, Fey PD. Extended spectrum beta-lactamase (ESBL)-producing Enterobacteriaceae: considerations for diagnosis, prevention and drug treatment. Drugs 2003;63(4):353–65.
19. Tasbakan MI, Pullukcu H, Sipahi OR, et al. Nitrofurantoin in the treatment of extended-spectrum beta-lactamase-producing Escherichia coli-related lower urinary tract infection. Int J Antimicrob Agents 2012;40(6):554–6.

20. Falagas ME, Kastoris AC, Kapaskelis AM, et al. Fosfomycin for the treatment of multidrug-resistant, including extended-spectrum beta-lactamase producing, Enterobacteriaceae infections: a systematic review. Lancet Infect Dis 2010;10(1):43–50.

21. Rottier WC, Ammerlaan HS, Bonten MJ, et al. Effects of confounders and intermediates on the association of bacteraemia caused by extended-spectrum beta-lactamase-producing Enterobacteriaceae and patient outcome: a meta-analysis. J Antimicrob Chemother 2012;67(6):1311–20.

22. Paterson DL, Doi Y. A step closer to extreme drug resistance (XDR) in gram-negative bacilli. Clin Infect Dis 2007;45(9):1179–81.

23. Bratu S, Tolaney P, Karumudi U, et al. Carbapenemase-producing Klebsiella pneumoniae in Brooklyn, NY: molecular epidemiology and in vitro activity of polymyxin B and other agents. J Antimicrob Chemother 2005;56(1):128–32.

24. Queenan AM, Bush K. Carbapenemases: the versatile beta-lactamases. Clin Microbiol Rev 2007;20(3): 440–58. table of contents.

25. Sidjabat H, Nimmo GR, Walsh TR, et al. Carbapenem resistance in Klebsiella pneumoniae due to the New Delhi Metallo-beta-lactamase. Clin Infect Dis 2011;52(4):481–4.

26. Johnson AP, Woodford N. Global spread of antibiotic resistance: the example of New Delhi metallo-beta-lactamase (NDM)-mediated carbapenem resistance. J Med Microbiol 2013;62(Pt 4):499–513.

27. Yigit H, Queenan AM, Anderson GJ, et al. Novel carbapenem-hydrolyzing beta-lactamase, KPC-1, from a carbapenem-resistant strain of Klebsiella pneumoniae. Antimicrob Agents Chemother 2001; 45(4):1151–61.

28. Kuehn BM. "Nightmare" bacteria on the rise in US hospitals, long-term care facilities. JAMA 2013; 309(15):1573–4.

29. Sievert DM, Ricks P, Edwards JR, et al. Antimicrobial-resistant pathogens associated with healthcare-associated infections: summary of data reported to the National Healthcare Safety Network at the Centers for Disease Control and Prevention, 2009-2010. Infect Control Hosp Epidemiol 2013;34(1):1–14.

30. Nordmann P, Naas T, Poirel L, et al. Global spread of carbapenemase-producing enterobacteriaceae. Emerg Infect Dis 2011;17(10):1791–8.

31. Schwaber MJ, Klarfeld-Lidji S, Navon-Venezia S, et al. Predictors of carbapenem-resistant Klebsiella pneumoniae acquisition among hospitalized adults and effect of acquisition on mortality. Antimicrob Agents Chemother 2008;52(3):1028–33.

32. Patel G, Huprikar S, Factor SH, et al. Outcomes of carbapenem-resistant Klebsiella pneumoniae infection and the impact of antimicrobial and adjunctive therapies. Infect Control Hosp Epidemiol 2008; 29(12):1099–106.

33. Centers for Disease Control and Prevention (CDC). Vital signs: carbapenem-resistant Enterobacteriaceae. MMWR Morb Mortal Wkly Rep 2013;62(9): 165–70.

34. Won SY, Munoz-Price LS, Lolans K, et al. Emergence and rapid regional spread of Klebsiella pneumoniae carbapenemase-producing Enterobacteriaceae. Clin Infect Dis 2011;53(6):532–40.

35. Snitkin ES, Zelazny AM, Thomas PJ, et al. Tracking a hospital outbreak of carbapenem-resistant Klebsiella pneumoniae with whole-genome sequencing. Sci Transl Med 2012;4(148):148ra116.

36. Alexander BT, Marschall J, Tibbetts RJ, et al. Treatment and clinical outcomes of urinary tract infections caused by KPC-producing Enterobacteriaceae in a retrospective cohort. Clin Ther 2012;34(6):1314–23.

37. Tumbarello M, Viale P, Viscoli C, et al. Predictors of mortality in bloodstream infections caused by Klebsiella pneumoniae carbapenemase-producing K. pneumoniae: importance of combination therapy. Clin Infect Dis 2012;55(7):943–50.

38. Ben-David D, Kordevani R, Keller N, et al. Outcome of carbapenem resistant Klebsiella pneumoniae bloodstream infections. Clin Microbiol Infect 2012; 18(1):54–60.

39. Pogue JM, Lee J, Marchaim D, et al. Incidence of and risk factors for colistin-associated nephrotoxicity in a large academic health system. Clin Infect Dis 2011;53(9):879–84.

40. Moore RD, Smith CR, Lipsky JJ, et al. Risk factors for nephrotoxicity in patients treated with aminoglycosides. Ann Intern Med 1984;100(3):352–7.

41. Molton JS, Tambyah PA, Ang BS, et al. The global spread of healthcare-associated multidrug-resistant bacteria: a perspective from Asia. Clin Infect Dis 2013;56(9):1310–8.

42. Epstein L, Hunter JC, Arwady MA, et al. New Delhi metallo-beta-lactamase-producing carbapenem-resistant Escherichia coli associated with exposure to duodenoscopes. JAMA 2014;312(14):1447–55.

43. Karageorgopoulos DE, Falagas ME. Current control and treatment of multidrug-resistant Acinetobacter baumannii infections. Lancet Infect Dis 2008;8(12): 751–62.

44. Dijkshoorn L, Nemec A, Seifert H, et al. An increasing threat in hospitals: multidrug-resistant Acinetobacter baumannii. Nat Rev Microbiol 2007; 5(12):939–51.

45. Bonomo RA, Szabo D. Mechanisms of multidrug resistance in Acinetobacter species and Pseudomonas aeruginosa. Clin Infect Dis 2006;43(Suppl 2):S49–56.

46. Seifert H, Dijkshoorn L, Gerner-Smidt P, et al. Distribution of Acinetobacter species on human skin: comparison of phenotypic and genotypic identification methods. J Clin Microbiol 1997;35(11): 2819–25.

47. Chu YW, Leung CM, Houang ET, et al. Skin carriage of acinetobacters in Hong Kong. J Clin Microbiol 1999;37(9):2962–7.
48. Falagas ME, Karveli EA, Kelesidis I, et al. Community-acquired Acinetobacter infections. Eur J Clin Microbiol Infect Dis 2007;26(12):857–68.
49. Playford EG, Craig JC, Iredell JR, et al. Carbapenem-resistant Acinetobacter baumannii in intensive care unit patients: risk factors for acquisition, infection and their consequences. J Hosp Infect 2007;65(3):204–11.
50. Fournier PE, Richet H. The epidemiology and control of Acinetobacter baumannii in health care facilities. Clin Infect Dis 2006;42(5):692–9.
51. Scott P, Deye G, Srinivasan A, et al. An outbreak of multidrug-resistant Acinetobacter baumannii-calcoaceticus complex infection in the US military health care system associated with military operations in Iraq. Clin Infect Dis 2007;44(12):1577–84.
52. Reinert RR, Low DE, Rossi F, et al. Antimicrobial susceptibility among organisms from the Asia/Pacific Rim, Europe and Latin and North America collected as part of TEST and the in vitro activity of tigecycline. J Antimicrob Chemother 2007;60(5):1018–29.
53. Zalts R, Neuberger A, Hussein K, et al. Treatment of carbapenem-resistant acinetobacter baumannii ventilator-associated pneumonia: retrospective comparison between intravenous colistin and intravenous ampicillin-sulbactam. Am J Ther 2013. [Epub ahead of print].
54. Munoz-Price LS, Zembower T, Penugonda S, et al. Clinical outcomes of carbapenem-resistant Acinetobacter baumannii bloodstream infections: study of a 2-state monoclonal outbreak. Infect Control Hosp Epidemiol 2010;31(10):1057–62.
55. Wisplinghoff H, Bischoff T, Tallent SM, et al. Nosocomial bloodstream infections in US hospitals: analysis of 24,179 cases from a prospective nationwide surveillance study. Clin Infect Dis 2004;39(3):309–17.
56. Falagas ME, Bliziotis IA, Siempos II, et al. Attributable mortality of Acinetobacter baumannii infections in critically ill patients: a systematic review of matched cohort and case-control studies. Crit Care 2006;10(2):R48.
57. Blot S, Vandewoude K, Colardyn F, et al. Nosocomial bacteremia involving Acinetobacter baumannii in critically ill patients: a matched cohort study. Intensive Care Med 2003;29(3):471–5.
58. Lister PD, Wolter DJ, Hanson ND, et al. Antibacterial-resistant Pseudomonas aeruginosa: clinical impact and complex regulation of chromosomally encoded resistance mechanisms. Clin Microbiol Rev 2009;22(4):582–610.
59. Magiorakos AP, Srinivasan A, Carey RB, et al. Multidrug-resistant, extensively drug-resistant and pandrug-resistant bacteria: an international expert proposal for interim standard definitions for acquired resistance. Clin Microbiol Infect 2012;18(3):268–81.
60. Morrison AJ Jr, Wenzel RP. Epidemiology of infections due to Pseudomonas aeruginosa. Rev Infect Dis 1984;6(Suppl 3):S627–42.
61. Nakamura A, Miyake K, Misawa S, et al. Meropenem as predictive risk factor for isolation of multidrug-resistant Pseudomonas aeruginosa. J Hosp Infect 2013;83(2):153–5.
62. Aloush V, Navon-Venezia S, Seigman-Igra Y, et al. Multidrug-resistant Pseudomonas aeruginosa: risk factors and clinical impact. Antimicrob Agents Chemother 2006;50(1):43–8.
63. Bukholm G, Tannaes T, Kjelsberg AB, et al. An outbreak of multidrug-resistant Pseudomonas aeruginosa associated with increased risk of patient death in an intensive care unit. Infect Control Hosp Epidemiol 2002;23(8):441–6.
64. Kerr KG, Snelling AM. Pseudomonas aeruginosa: a formidable and ever-present adversary. J Hosp Infect 2009;73(4):338–44.
65. Tam VH, Rogers CA, Chang KT, et al. Impact of multidrug-resistant Pseudomonas aeruginosa bacteremia on patient outcomes. Antimicrob Agents Chemother 2010;54(9):3717–22.
66. Available at: http://www.cdc.gov/drugresistance/pdf/ar-threats-2013-508.pdf. Accessed April 1, 2015.
67. Dortch MJ, Fleming SB, Kauffmann RM, et al. Infection reduction strategies including antibiotic stewardship protocols in surgical and trauma intensive care units are associated with reduced resistant gram-negative healthcare-associated infections. Surg Infect (Larchmt) 2011;12(1):15–25.

Sexually Transmitted Infections

Lindsay Smith, MD, Michael P. Angarone, DO*

KEYWORDS

- STI • Syphilis • Gonorrhea • Chlamydia • HSV • HPV

KEY POINTS

- Sexually transmitted infections (STIs) continue to be a significant cause of morbidity and public health risk.
- Since 2011 the incidence of primary and secondary syphilis is increasing, particularly in men who have sex with men (MSM).
- Gonorrhea and chlamydia remain the main causes of bacterial urethritis and cervicitis.
- Human papillomavirus (HPV) can cause benign and malignant lesions and remains difficult to treat but can be prevented with vaccination.
- Primary prevention, behavior modification counseling, partner notification, and early treatment continue to be the mainstays in preventing the spread of STIs.

INTRODUCTION

STIs encompass a group of infections that can be spread or acquired through sexual contact. The Centers for Disease Control and Prevention (CDC) estimates approximately 20 million new STIs per year in the United States at a cost of approximately \$16 billion.[1] Half of these infections are in people between the ages of 15 and 24 years old. Each infection has the potential to pose significant immediate and long-term harm, affecting health and well-being. Primary prevention of STIs, through safe sex practices and partner awareness, can help decrease the incidence of many STIs. By far the most important tool to assist in the control of STIs is early diagnosis and treatment of these infected. This is evident in the decreased incidence in syphilis and gonorrhea seen from the 1980s to the early 2000s.[2,3] The most recent surveillance updates by the CDC have identified an overall decrease in the rates of Chlamydia and gonorrhea in the general population. In 2013 there were 1,401,906 cases of Chlamydia trachomatis infection in the United States, representing an infection rate of 446.6 cases per 100,000 population. This represented a decrease of 1.5% compared with the rate in 2012. In women, gonorrhea infection has also decreased by 5%; however, an increase of 4% was seen in men. In 2010 the rates of primary and secondary syphilis experienced their first decline in 10 years; however, from 2011 to 2013 the rates have increased by more than 20%.[1]

Individuals at the highest risk for contracting an STI are sexually active young adults between the ages of 18 and 25. Other important risk factors are the number of sexual partners, new sex partners, use of illicit drugs, admission to a correctional facility, and a prior history of STI.[3] A newly described risk factor for STI is the use of erectile dysfunction medications in older men. A review of men prescribed ED medication found a 2- to 3-fold increase in the rate of STIs in men taking erectile dysfunction medications compared with men not taking these medications.[4] Recent travel is also an important risk factor for the acquisition

Division of Infectious Diseases, Northwestern University Feinberg School of Medicine, 645 North Michigan Avenue, Suite 900, Chicago, IL 60611, USA
* Corresponding author.
E-mail address: m-angarone@northwestern.edu

Urol Clin N Am 42 (2015) 507–518
http://dx.doi.org/10.1016/j.ucl.2015.06.004
0094-0143/15/$ – see front matter © 2015 Elsevier Inc. All rights reserved.

of STIs and has been seen in approximately 2.9% of illnesses in returning travelers.[5]

Primary prevention of STIs begins with recognizing the risk behaviors of individual patients and counseling on changing these behaviors to prevent the acquisition of STIs. The US Preventive Services Task Force (USPSTF) recommends high-intensity behavioral counseling for all sexually active adolescents and adults.[6,7] This involves routinely obtaining a sexual history on all patients and a discussion of behavior modifications and changes to at-risk practices. These counseling interventions have demonstrated efficacy in reducing acquisition rates of syphilis, Chlamydia, gonorrhea, and trichomoniasis.[3,8] The CDC also promotes obtaining a sexual history focusing on the 5Ps: Partner(s), Prevention of pregnancy, Protection form STIs, sexual Practices, and Past history of STIs. These questions can lead to conversations about primary and secondary prevention. Prevention counseling should be provided in a safe, nonjudgmental, and empathetic environment.[3]

This review focuses on the common causes of STIs. The focus is on the causes of ulcerative and nonulcerative diseases, condyloma, and a discussion on partner notification and treatment.

INFECTIONS THAT CAUSE ULCERS
Syphilis

The incidence of syphilis in the United States peaked in the 1940s, with an incidence of 66.9 cases per 100,000 persons (**Table 1**). Aggressive public health interventions, including treatment with penicillin and contact tracing, led to a significant decrease in the incidence of primary and secondary syphilis. By the late 1990s, there was a significant decline in the incidence of syphilis, with a rate of 2.1 cases per 100,000 persons. Since 2011 there has been a steady increase in the incidence of syphilis, and in 2014 there was a rate of 5.5 cases per 100,000 persons. Approximately 75% of all primary and secondary syphilis cases have been diagnosed in MSM.[1]

Clinical presentation
Syphilis is caused by the spirochete, *Treponema pallidum pallidum*. Transmission occurs through contact with active lesions, infected body fluids, or blood transfusion or can be acquired in utero.

Once infection is established, there is rapid systemic dissemination, including to the central nervous system. The incubation period is approximately 21 days, at which time a single, painless chancre develops at the site of inoculation. These lesions often are unnoticed, particularly in women and MSM who are practicing receptive anal intercourse, where the lesions are in locations that are difficult to visualize. The lesion, which may be accompanied by regional lymphadenopathy, fever, or malaise, is often self-limited and resolves within a few days to weeks (3–90 days). Untreated, the infection may progress to a secondary and tertiary phase.[3]

Secondary syphilis presents as skin and mucous membrane lesions or rash, approximately 4 to 10 weeks after inoculation. The rash is macular and nonpruritic and may be associated with regional lymphadenopathy or systemic symptoms. Lesions are typically 5 to 10 mm and red in color and as they progress may become papular or papulosquamous (**Fig. 1**). Approximately 50% to 80% of cases have the rash on the palms and soles.[3] Like the primary chancre, the rash resolves with or without treatment and the infection enters a latent phase.

Latency is divided into early (infection acquired within the previous year) or late (infection acquired >1 y or unknown duration) phases. During this latent stage, most persons are not infectious, the major exception pregnant women who can pass the infection vertically to their fetus. Most patients with latent syphilis stay in this stage indefinitely; however, up to 25% of patients with untreated syphilis go on to develop tertiary manifestations.[9]

The primary manifestations of tertiary syphilis include cardiovascular disease, gummatous disease, and/or neurologic manifestations. Cardiovascular complications can present 10 to 30 years after infection and can lead to aoritis, angina from coronary ostitis, aortic regurgitation, or aortic aneurysm. Gummas can present in any organ and lead to serious complications depending on the organ involved, the most severe being the central and peripheral nervous systems.[3,9]

Neurosyphilis can occur at any stage of infection, including primary infection. Early neurosyphilis is characterized by meningovascular disease, including meningitis, strokes, seizures, myelopathy, cranial nerve palsy, and vestubular and ocular disease (retinitis). Late neurosyphilis affects the brain and spinal cord parenchyma, presenting as dementia, tabes dorsalis, general paresis, or sensory ataxia.[9]

Diagnostic testing
When a diagnosis of syphilis is suspected, a detailed sexual history and physical examination are necessary. Physical examination should focus on dermatologic, neurologic, ocular, auditory, and vestibular manifestations of syphilis. Diagnosis can be made using dark-field microscopy of a scraping of the ulcer or rash. This testing modality

Table 1
Comparison of causes of genital ulcerative sexually transmitted infections

Disease/Etiologic Agent	Ulcer Characteristics	Incubation	Pain	Adenopathy	Treatment	Alternative Treatment
Syphilis *T pallidum*	Indurated, smooth borders	9–90 d	Painless	Firm, painless; bilateral	See **Table 2**	See **Table 2**
HSV HSV-2: 85% HSV-1: 15%	Multiple small ulcers; erythematous base	2–7 d	Painful	Reactive Painful	See **Table 3**	See **Table 3**
Chancroid *Haemophilus ducreyi*	Sharply circumscribed, ragged edges; not indurated; gray, yellow base; multiple	3–10 d	Very painful	Usually unilateral; may suppurate or rupture	Azithromycin, 1g po × 1 Patients should be re-examined 3–7 d after treatment to ensure improvement in symptoms.	Ceftriaxone, 250 mg IM × 1
LGV *C trachomatis* L1-L3	Rare; small and shallow	5–21 d	Painless	Matted in clustered; unilateral or bilateral; sinus tracts	Doxycycline, 100 mg po bid × 21 days	Erythromycin, base 500 mg po q 6 h × 21 d
Granuloma inguinale *Klebsiella granulomatis*	Extensive, progressive granulation-like tissue; rolled edges	7–90 d	Usually painless	Pseudobuboes	Doxycycline, 100 mg po bid Treatment should be for at least 3 wk or until all lesions have completely healed, whichever is longer	Azithromycin, 1g po weekly OR Ciprofloxacin, 750 mg po bid OR Trimethoprim-suflamethoxazole, 1 DS tablet bid

Abbreviations: bid, twice daily; DS, double strength; IM, intramuscular; IV, intravenous; q, every.

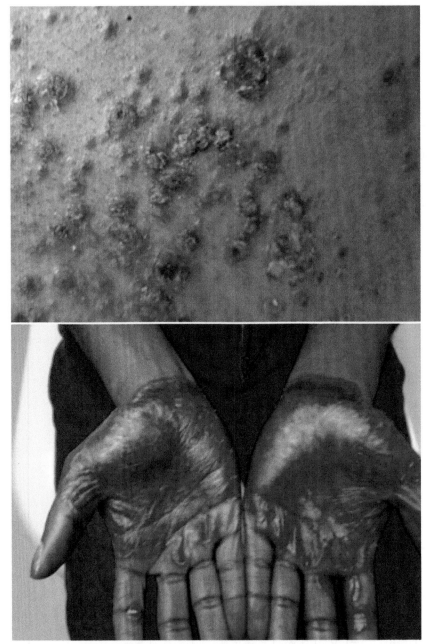

Fig. 1. Cutaneous rash of secondary syphilis. (*Courtesy of* J.L. Grant, MD, Chicago, IL.)

has 75% to 95% sensitivity, depending on the investigator, and requires specific staining and microscopes.[9]

Serologic testing remains the standard for diagnosis, and it is recommended that all patients with concern for syphilis undergo serologic testing. Most testing involves a 2-step process: first, nontreponemal testing with the rapid plasma reagin (RPR) or venereal disease research laboratory (VDRL), and second, followed by confirmatory

treponemal antibody testing of human IgM and IgG antibodies to *T pallidum* with, fluorescent treponemal antibody absorbed tests. Nontreponemal antibody titers peak during secondary syphilis without treatment and then gradually decline. Approximately 30% of patients become seronegative over their lifetimes without treatment.[9] Appropriate and successful treatment is considered if there is a 4-fold, or 2-dilution, decline in titers at 6 and 12 months post-treatment (example, RPR

1:16–1:4). A small percentage of patients become serofast with an RPR titer that fails to become nonreactive and stays detectable at 1:1 to 1:8 despite adequate therapy.[3,9] Treatment failure is defined as a lack of 4-fold decline in titers or recurrence of symptoms prior to the first follow-up period at 6 to 12 months. An initial RPR that is greater than or equal to 1:32 and/or the patient with concerning neurologic or ocular symptoms or physical examination inding is suggestive of neurosyphilis. Patients should be referred to an infectious diseases specialist for lumbar puncture with cerebrospinal fluid (CSF) analysis of cell count with differential, total protein, and CSF VDRL or treponemal antibody.[10] Regardless of disease stage, treponemal testing is positive for most patients infected with *T pallidum* and remains positive.

Treatment

Penicillin remains the first-line therapy for all stages of syphilis (**Table 2**).[3] Primary, secondary, and early latent syphilis are all treated with a single intramuscular dose of 2.4 million units of penicillin G benzathine. Late latent syphilis, syphilis of unknown duration, and tertiary syphilis are treated with 2.4 million units penicillin G benzathine intramuscularly, weekly, for 3 consecutive weeks. For patients with confirmed neurosyphilis, ocular syphilis, or auditory syphilis, treatment should be aqueous crystalline penicillin G intravenously, daily, for 10 to 14 days, followed by penicillin G benzathine 2.4 million units, intramuscularly, weekly, for 1 to 3 weeks. All patients should be warned about a possible Jarisch-Herxheimer reaction 2 to 24 hours after treatment.[3]

If patients are known to have an allergy to penicillin, treatment of primary, secondary, or early latent syphilis should be with doxycycline for 14 days or ceftriaxone for 8 to 10 days, but treatment failure rates may be high.[3,11] For late latent syphilis, treatment with doxycycline is extended for a total of 28 days. Pregnant patients should undergo desensitization to penicillin in an intensive care unit and then complete therapy as indicated based on stage of disease.[3]

Herpes Simplex Virus

Epidemiology

It is estimated that more than 50 million people in the United States have genital herpes, caused most often by herpes simplex virus (HSV)-2 but increasingly by HSV-1. Infection is lifelong, and the spectrum of disease is broad, ranging from asymptomatic to recurrent ulcerative disease. Seroprevalence studies reveal an overall decrease in the prevalence of HSV-2; however, most people have never been clinically diagnosed with HSV-2 infection. Transmission is likely occurring from chronic shedding in asymptomatic individuals.[12]

Clinical presentation

Primary genital HSV infection has a broad range of clinical symptoms. Most often, primary infection presents with painful genital or anal vesicles or ulcers and may be associated with dysuria, fever, and tender inguinal lymphadenopathy. Some individuals may have mild symptoms or may be completely asymptomatic. The average incubation period after exposure is 4 days.

A minority of patients develop extragenital complications during primary infection. In 1 series, the most common extragenital complications were development of extragenital lesions, secondary yeast infections, aseptic meningitis, and sacral autonomic dysfunction.[13] Rarely, infection may

Table 2
Treatment of syphilis by stage

Stage	Treatment (Drug of Choice)	Treatment (Alternative)
Primary syphilis Secondary syphilis Early latent syphilis	PCN G benzathine, 2.4 million units IM once	Doxycyline, 100 mg bid × 14 d[a]
Late latent syphilis[a] Tertiary syphilis[a]	PCN G benzathine, 2.4 million units IM weekly for 3 wk	Doxycyline, 100 mg bid × 4 wk[a]
Neurosyphilis[b,c]	PCN G, 3–4 million units IV q 4 h for 14 d	PCN G procaine, 2.4 million units IM daily *PLUS* probenecid 500 mg qid × 10–14 d OR Ceftriaxone, 2g IV daily for 14 d

Abbreviations: bid, twice daily; IM, intramuscular; IV, intravenous; PCN, penicillin; q, every; qid, 4 times daily.
[a] Not recommended in pregnancy.
[b] Patients allergic to penicillin should be desensitized and treated with penicillin.
[c] Fourteen days of IV PCN should be followed by 1 to 3 doses of PCN G benzathine weekly for neurosyphilis.

result in viremia and disseminated disease manifesting as pneumonitis, hepatitis, meningitis, and/or encephalitis. Recurrent HSV-2 meningitis, called Mollaret meningitis, is associated with a lymphocytic pleocytosis and normal glucose in the CSF and is not associated with concomitant genital lesions. HSV can also cause proctitis, particularly in MSM or in those practicing receptive anal intercourse. In a series of proctitis in MSM in San Francisco, HSV was the cause of the proctitis in 13% of the individuals tested.[14]

Diagnostic testing

Diagnosis of genital herpes is most often made clinically. Painful vesicular lesions that do not follow a dermatomal distribution are pathognomonic. To confirm the diagnosis, and to distinguish between HSV-1 and HSV-2, a vesicular lesion can be unroofed and the base swabbed for HSV-1– and HSV-2–specific polymerase chain reaction, direct fluorescent antibody testing, or viral culture. Failure to detect HSV from a vesicle likely represents sampling error or low viral shedding and not absence of infection when clinical suspicion remains high. Serologic screening at time of primary infection has little utility in making the diagnosis of genital herpes. Serologic testing may be useful to aid in the diagnosis of recurrent genital ulcers that do not respond to antiviral therapy, determine susceptibility to infection in a sexual partner of a person with documented HSV infection, or identify asymptomatic infection in a pregnant women.[15] Routine serologic screening for HSV-2 infection is not recommended due to the possible high false-positive rate of testing in a low-prevalence population.[16]

Treatment

Primary infection can result in a prolonged clinical illness with severe genital ulcers and possible neurologic involvement. All patients with first episodes of genital herpes should receive oral antiviral therapy. Topical therapy is ineffective and not recommended. Oral antivirals approved for the treatment of HSV include acyclovir, valacyclovir, and famciclovir. These agents can be used to treat primary or recurrent infections and may also be used for suppressive therapy (**Table 3**).[3] Recurrent outbreaks are less frequent with HSV-1 infection. Intermittent asymptomatic shedding can occur with genital HSV-2 infection. Antiviral therapy taken at the onset of recurrent symptoms can ameliorate or shorten the duration of the outbreak. In those patients with frequent outbreaks, chronic suppression should be discussed.

Rare Causes of Genital Ulcer in the United States

Chancroid, caused by *Haemophilus ducreyi*, results in painful genital ulceration and is associated with tender, suppurative inguinal lymphadenopathy. The lesion begins as an erythematous papule, progressing to a pustule, which then ruptures to form a shallow ulcer, with a granulomatous base, purulent exudate, and ragged undermined edges.[17,18] This is a rare condition, with only 10 cases reported to the CDC in 2013.[1]

Lymphogranuloma venereum (LGV) is caused by *C trachomatis* serovars L1, L2, and L3. Clinical presentation is characterized by unilateral tender inguinal and/or femoral lymphadenopathy, or buboes. A self-resolving genital ulcer or papule occurs at the site of inoculation. Rectal exposure in MSM or women can result in proctitis with mucoid or hemorrhagic rectal discharge, pain, constipation, fever, and tenesmus.

Granuloma inguinale is a genital ulcerative disease caused by *Klebsiella granulomatis* (formerly *Calymmatobacterium granulomatis*). Painless, slowly progressive ulcers on the genitals or perineum without lymphadenopathy characterize clinical presentation. Subcutaneous granulomas (pseudobuboes) may occur. The lesions are highly vascular, have a bright red appearance, and bleed easily on contact. Infection can progress into the pelvis or disseminate to intra-abdominal organs,

Table 3
Treatment of herpes simplex virus infection

Antiviral	First Episode[a]	Episodic Therapy[b]	Suppressive Therapy[c]
Acyclovir	200 mg 5×/d for 7–10 d	200 mg 5×/d for 5 d	400 mg bid
Famciclovir	250 mg tid for 7–10 d	125 mg bid for 5 d	250 mg bid
Valacyclovir	1000 mg bid for 7–10 d	500 mg bid or 1000 mg daily for 5 d	500 mg daily

Abbreviations: bid, twice daily; tid, 3 times daily.
[a] Dose should be adjusted based on creatinine clearance.
[b] Treatment should be started within 24 hours of symptom onset.
[c] Greater than 6 episodes per year; shown to decrease probability of transmission by 50%.

bones, or the mouth. Lesions can also develop secondary to bacterial infections.

Diagnosis of these 3 infections is made clinically because these organisms are difficult to culture.

See **Table 1** for treatment guidelines.

INFECTIONS THAT CAUSE URETHRITIS, EPIDIDYMITIS, CERVICITIS, AND VAGINAL DISCHARGE
Clinical Presentation

Urethritis results from multiple infectious causes. When symptomatic, patients can experience purulent urethral discharge, dysuria, or urethral pruritus. Diagnosis can be confirmed by 1 of the following 3 criteria[3]:

1. Mucopurulent or purulent discharge found on physical examination
2. Gram stain of urethral secretions revealing greater than or equal to 5 white blood cells (WBCs) per oil immersion field. Intracellular gram-negative diplococci seen within the WBCs are consistent with gonorrhea infection.
3. Positive leukocyte esterase test on first-void urine or microscopic examination of first-void urine revealing greater than or equal to 10 WBC per high-power field

Acute epididymitis consists of pain, swelling, and inflammation of the epididymis of less than 6 weeks' duration. Physical examination typically reveals unilateral testicular pain and tenderness, hydrocele, and palpable swelling of the epididymis. Differential diagnosis should include testicular torsion and should prompt evaluation with scrotal ultrasound. It is traditionally thought that in men less than 35 years of age, acute epididymitis is most frequently caused by C trachomatis or Neisseria gonorrhoeae. For men who practice insertive anal intercourse, organisms, such as Escherichia coli and other enteric gram-negative flora, must be considered potential pathogens. In men greater than 35 years of age, sexually transmitted epididymitis occurs less frequently, and those bacteria related to obstructive urinary disease are more frequently found as pathogens. A small European study identified that the most frequent cause of acute epididymitis was E coli (56%), whereas only 14% of cases were caused by a traditional STI organisms, with no influence of etiology based on age.[19] Chronic epididymitis is characterized by symptoms lasting more than 6 weeks. The most frequently isolated organism causing chronic infectious epididymitis is Mycobacterium tuberculosis (TB). TB should be considered in those patients with recent TB exposure or

who have clinically worsening symptoms despite appropriate antibacterial therapy.[20]

Cervicitis is typically asymptomatic, but some women present with abnormal vaginal discharge and/or intermenstrual vaginal bleeding, particularly after sexual intercourse.

Physical examination may reveal purulent or mucopurulent endocervical exudate, sustained endocervical bleeding induced by gentle passage of a cotton swab, or cervical motion tenderness.

Diagnosis

The diagnostic test of choice is nucleic acid amplification testing (NAAT). For men, NAAT can be performed on urine specimens or urethral swabs. For women, NAAT can be performed on urine specimen, endocervical, or vaginal swabs, collected by the provider or by the patient. For those who participate in receptive anal intercourse or oral intercourse, rectal or oropharyngeal swabs can be obtained for NAAT; however, this testing methodology has not been FDA approved yet.

CHLAMYDIA

Chlamydial infection, caused by C trachomatis, is the most frequently reported bacterial STI in the United States and has the highest prevalence in persons less than 25 years of age. The sequelae of untreated infection can be most devastating in women, leading to pelvic inflammatory disease, ectopic pregnancy, and infertility.

Asymptomatic infection in both men and women is common. Due to the severity of untreated infection in women, it is recommended that all sexually active women less than 25 years of age receive annual testing for chlamydia.[3,21,22] Women older than 25 years of age should receive testing with new or multiple sexual partners or partners who have tested positive for chlamydia. Routine screening of asymptomatic men who have sex with women is not recommended; however, MSM should be screened for urethral infection with Chlamydia annually, and rectal screening should be performed on men who participate in anal receptive intercourse.[3,21,22]

Treatment

Treatment should be given to those with positive NAAT or empirically for those with significant risk and symptoms. The standard regimens for treatment are azithromycin, 1 g for 1 dose, or doxycycline, 100 mg twice daily for 7 days.

For those who have poor treatment adherence or unpredictable follow-up, directly observed therapy with azithromycin is recommended. Test of cure is not recommended except for pregnant women and should be performed no earlier than 3 weeks from treatment. Routine retesting for men and women is recommended at 3 months regardless if the partner was treated.[3]

GONORRHEA

Gonorrhea, caused by N gonorrhoeae, is the second most commonly reported bacterial STI in the United States. In 2013, 333,004 cases were reported with a rate of 106.1 per 100,000 people, which has remained stable.[1] In men, symptoms usually present within several days of infection, prompting them to seek treatment; however, they may have already spread the infection to other partners prior to treatment. In women, similar to chlamydia, infection may be asymptomatic. At this time, the USPSTF recommends routine screening for those considered high risk: women who have previously tested positive for gonorrhea, women with multiple current partners, patients with a new sexual partner, patients with inconsistent condom usage, patients having sex while under the influence of drugs or alcohol, or patients having sex in exchange for money or drugs.[22,23]

Treatment

Ceftriaxone and cefixime have been the treatment of choice since 2007.[3] In July 2013, the CDC released an update to the treatment guidelines for gonorrhea based on increased resistance to cefixime noted in specimens tested in the western United States. The new treatment guideline recommends the use of ceftriaxone, 250 mg intramuscular, combined with either azithromycin, 1 g in a single dose, or doxycycline, 100 mg twice daily for 7 days.[24,25] If ceftriaxone is unavailable, cefixime, 400 mg, can be used in combination with azithromycin or doxycycline. For individuals with an allergy to cephalosporins, azithromycin, 2-g single dose, can be used. For the 2 alternate regimens, a test for cure should be performed 1 week after treatment.[24] Patients who have persistent symptoms after treatment should be retested with culture, and isolates should be submitted for resistance testing.

TRICHOMONIASIS

Trichomoniasis, caused by Trichomonas vaginalis, results in symptoms of urethritis or vaginitis. Women present with diffuse, malodorous, yellow-green vaginal discharge. Diagnosis is usually made by microscopy of vaginal secretions, revealing motile organisms. If diagnosis is not made by microscopy, culture is highly specific. In men, wet prep has low sensitivity and no point-of-care test is available. Culture and NAAT are diagnostic options, although not all facilities have NAAT available for T vaginalis.[3]

Treatment

Recommended treatment regimens are either metronidazole, 2 g as a single dose, or tinidazole, 2 g as a single dose. An alternative regimen is metronidazole, 500 mg, orally, twice daily for 7 days. Patients should be counseled to avoid consuming alcohol for up to 24 hours after completion of therapy with metronidazole or 72 hours after completing therapy with tinidazole.[3]

Other Organisms Causing Urethritis/ Epididymitis or Vaginitis/Cervicitis

Ureaplasma urealyticum, Mycoplasma hominis, or Mycoplasma genitalium may be the etiologic agent causing ongoing urethritis or cervicitis after negative testing for C trachomatis and N gonorrheae.[26] At this time, NAAT is not available and these organisms are difficult to grow in culture. First-line therapy for these organisms is azithromycin, 1 g as a single dose. If symptoms persist after empiric treatment, moxifloxacin, 400 mg orally daily for 7 days, can be used.[27] Doxycycline is no longer recommended as first-line therapy due to increasing resistance by Mycoplasma.[3]

HUMAN PAPILLOMA VIRUS

HPV is the cause of genital and anal warts in both women and men. There are more than 100 types of HPV, with more than 40 causing genital infection. Many of these infections are asymptomatic, unrecognized, or self-limited. It is estimated that more than 50% of sexually active persons become infected during their lifetime, with a peak incidence between the ages of 20 to 24 years old.[28,29] One prospective study followed female college students for 3 years. The incidence of new HPV infection of 43%; it was also found that the incidence decreased with time. The risk of HPV detection was associated with the more than 2 sex partners, younger age, and increased alcohol consumption.[30]

HPV has been associated with both benign and malignant genital tract disease in women and men. Most infections tend to be transient, with a median duration of 8 months, and 70% of women no longer infected by 12 months.[30] Genital warts, or condyloma accuminata, are the most common STIs in the United States, with 500,000 to 1 million new cases per year. The incidence of condyloma is estimated at approximately 3.4% (0.87 cases per 100 person years at risk) and the prevalence in the United States is estimated at approximately 1%.[31,32] HPV is a contagious virus spread by contact with infected skin. The risk factors for infection include high numbers of sexual partners, unprotected intercourse, a history of STI, use of oral contraceptives, and immunodeficiency.

HPV 6 and 11 are the most common causes of condyloma of the anogenital tract and are not associated with cervical cancer. Condyloma can occur anywhere in the genital tract, vagina, vulva, perineum, penis, and anal skin and mucosa. The lesions appear as flat, popular, or pedunculated growths. The lesions are most often asymptomatic but may be associated with pruritus or burning. Diagnosis of condyloma is based on the typical appearance of the condyloma. If there is uncertainty, a biopsy can be performed to confirm the diagnosis. Acetowhitening, with 3% to 5% acetic acid placed in the skin, cervix, or anal mucosa, can aid in the identification of subclinical or flat lesions. Cervical infection is typically diagnosed using cervical tissue sampling and a Papanicolaou smear.[3,33]

The oncogenic subtypes of HPV are associated with a majority of cervical cancers and anal cancers. The most common HPV types associated with dysplasia and cancer are HPV 16 and 18 (other types have been associated with cancer as well). It is important for women evaluated for STIs and condyloma to also be evaluated for the presence of these high-risk HPV subtypes. It has been estimated that up to 27% of women attending an STD clinic are positive for high-risk HPV, with the highest prevalence between the ages of 14 and 19.[34] More than half of these women are risk for cervical cancer based on their HPV infection, cervical disease, or a history of cervical disease.[35,36]

Treatment

Treatment of condyloma is divided into 2 main categories: those treatments that directly destroy wart tissue and those that use a patient's immune system to clear the wart. The choice of therapy depends on the wart size and location and patient preference. Many warts resolve with time, and observation is an appropriate treatment option. Treatment does not eradicate HPV but may reduce infectivity. The choice to pursue treatment is based on the relief of symptoms, including relief of cosmetic symptoms, of the wart. There is no evidence that 1 therapy is superior to another.

Patient-applied treatments include podofilox solution or gel and imiquimod cream.[37] Podofilox works as a cytodestructive agent, preventing cell division and leading to cell death. The medication is applied to the wart using a cotton swab twice daily for 3 days and care should be taken that no more than 0.5 mL of solution is used per day.[3,38] Imiquimod is a toll-like receptor-7 agonist that stimulates local cytokine production, thus reducing local HPV viral load.[39] The cream is applied to the dry warty area at bedtime and washed off 6 to 10 hours later. Sexual contact should be avoided while the medication is on the skin. There are 2 formulations available, a 5% cream and a 3.75% cream. The 5% cream is applied 3 times per week for 4 to 16 weeks, whereas the 3.75% cream is applied daily for 8 weeks. The patient experiences a mild local inflammatory reaction at the site of administration (erythema, induration, and vesicles), which indicates the medication is working.[3,40,41] With podofilox, approximately 50% of patients have reduction in the size of the wart and 29% have resolution of the wart.[38] With imiquimod treatment, approximately 50% of those treated have resolution of the wart.[40,42] A botanic product, sinecatechin, has been shown effective in treating external warts and is patient administered. Clinical efficacy has been demonstrated with this product, with approximately a 55% efficacy for wart resolution compared with 35% for placebo.[43,44]

Provider-applied therapy includes cryotherapy with liquid nitrogen, surgical removal (laser, electrosurgery, or scissor excision), podophyllin resin, trichloracetic acid (TCA), or bichloroacetic acid (BCA). Treatment with podophyllin resin 10% to 25% is applied to the wart once weekly. It is necessary for the area to be washed 1 to 4 hours after the application of the product to avoid skin irritation or systemic absorption. To decrease the likelihood of toxicity, less than 0.5 mL of the solution should be used on warts that have an area less than 10 cm^2 and the product should not be applied to skin that is ulcerated.[3] TCA and BCA are caustic agents that destroy the wart via chemical coagulation. There is a potential for the solution to spread and damage adjacent tissues; therefore, care should be taken when applying these solutions. Cryotherapy uses liquid nitrogen to cause a thermal cytolysis. It is important for the provider to be trained in effective use of cryotherapy to avoid complications and under-treatment, leading to low efficacy. Surgical treatment has the advantage of treating larger warts in a single visit; however, substantial clinical training and equipment are required.

For further treatment recommendations, see selected national organization guidelines: CDC,[3] European guideline for the management of anogenital warts,[45] and the American College of Obstetricians and Gynecologists' practice guidelines.[46]

Human Papillomavirus Vaccine

Currently there are 3 available HPV vaccines: a bivalent vaccine, a quadrivalent vaccine, and a 9-valent vaccine. The vaccines consist of virus-like particles that induce an immune response to the particular virus subtype targeted.[47] The bivalent (HPV 16/18) and the quadrivalent (HPV 6/11/16/18) have both demonstrated efficacy in preventing the development of carcinoma in situ 2 or 3, adenocarcinoma in situ, and cervical cancer related to HPV 16 and 18 in female patients.[48–50] The quadrivalent vaccine is also effective in reducing the development of condyloma related to HPV 6 and 11.[48,49] The quadrivalent vaccine has also demonstrated efficacy in reducing genital warts in male recipients as well as anal intraepithelial neoplasm related the HPV 6/11/16/18.[51,52] In December 2014, the FDA approved the licensing for a new 9-valent HPV vaccine that targets HPV 6/11/16/18 as well as 31/33/45/52/58. Approval of this vaccine was based on study data of more than 14,000 women, which demonstrated reduction in high-grade genital lesions comparable to the quadrivalent vaccine.[53] Currently the Advisory Committee on Immunization Practices (ACIP) recommends that all girls and boys receive the HPV vaccine at age 11. Vaccination can be started at age 9 and is recommended for female patients between 13 and 26 years and male patients between 13 and 22 years. For MSM the vaccine can be given up to the age of 26. All 3 of the evaluable vaccines can be used and the ACIP does not prefer 1 formulation to another.[54]

PARTNER NOTIFICATION AND TREATMENT

Important components to control STIs are identifying and treating those infected, counseling on behavior modification, and identifying sexual partners to interrupt transmission. Intensive counseling on behavior modification has been demonstrated effective at reducing bacterial STIs.[55,56] This process can be time-consuming and should not replace direct treatment and screening strategies.[57] Partner notification and treatment is an effective tool in identifying cases of STI within the community. Treatment of sexual partners reduces the rate at which the index case becomes reinfected.[58,59] Providers can offer patient-delivered partner therapy (PDPT), in which a prescription for treatment is given to partner(s) of the index case. This can be done without the provider giving a medical evaluation of the partner; however, some states may prohibit this practice and providers should visit www.cdc.gov/std/ept for information about their individual state.[3] Most of the data supporting PDPT are based on trials of heterosexual men and women with Chlamydia and gonorrhea. When PDPT was used, there was a 25% to 62% reduction in reinfection of the index case.[58,59] The ideal approach to management of sex partners is physician evaluation, counseling, and treatment. This approach is frequently unsuccessful due to the burden on the index case identifying recent sex partners and having those individuals follow-up. Use of public health workers is costly and time-consuming and the practice of using patients to notify their partners has not been successful. Newer identification procedures (including use of the Internet to notify partners and enhanced referral instructions) are innovative and promising and require further study.[60]

Currently the CDC recommends that index patients be instructed to refer their sex partners for evaluation, testing, and treatment. For many of the STIs, any sex partner within 60 days of diagnosis should be notified and referred for evaluation and treatment. For syphilis, transmission is thought to occur only in the presence of mucocutaneous lesions; therefore, persons exposed to an individual with primary, secondary, or early latent syphilis within 90 days should be evaluated and treated.[3]

REFERENCES

1. Centers for Disease Control and Prevention. Sexually transmitted infections surveillance 2013. Atlanta (GA): U.S. Department of Health and Human Services; 2014.
2. Aral SO, Holmes KK, Padian NS, et al. Overview: individual and population approaches to the epidemiology and prevention of sexually transmitted diseases and human immunodeficiency virus infection. J Infect Dis 1996;174(Suppl 2):S127–33.
3. Workowski KA, Berman S, Centers for Disease Control Prevention. Sexually transmitted diseases treatment guidelines, 2010. MMWR Recomm Rep 2010; 59(RR-12):1–110.
4. Jena AB, Goldman DP, Kamdar A, et al. Sexually transmitted diseases among users of erectile dysfunction drugs: analysis of claims data. Ann Intern Med 2010;153(1):1–7.
5. Leder K, Torresi J, Libman MD, et al. GeoSentinel surveillance of illness in returned travelers, 2007–2011. Ann Intern Med 2013;158(6):456–68.
6. U.S. Preventive Services Task Force. Behavioral counseling to prevent sexually transmitted infections: U.S. Preventive Services Task Force recommendation statement. Ann Intern Med 2008;149(7): 491–6. W95.
7. Lin JS, Whitlock E, O'Connor E, et al. Behavioral counseling to prevent sexually transmitted

infections: a systematic review for the U.S. Preventive Services Task Force. Ann Intern Med 2008; 149(7):497–508. W96–9.

8. Perez G, Skurnick JH, Denny TN, et al. Herpes simplex type II and Mycoplasma genitalium as risk factors for heterosexual HIV transmission: report from the heterosexual HIV transmission study. Int J Infect Dis 1998;3(1):5–11.

9. Zetola NM, Engelman J, Jensen TP, et al. Syphilis in the United States: an update for clinicians with an emphasis on HIV coinfection. Mayo Clin Proc 2007;82(9):1091–102.

10. Marra CM, Maxwell CL, Smith SL, et al. Cerebrospinal fluid abnormalities in patients with syphilis: association with clinical and laboratory features. J Infect Dis 2004;189(3):369–76.

11. Ghanem KG, Erbelding EJ, Cheng WW, et al. Doxycycline compared with benzathine penicillin for the treatment of early syphilis. Clin Infect Dis 2006; 42(6):e45–9.

12. Xu F, Sternberg MR, Kottiri BJ, et al. Trends in herpes simplex virus type 1 and type 2 seroprevalence in the United States. JAMA 2006;296(8): 964–73.

13. Corey L, Adams HG, Brown ZA, et al. Genital herpes simplex virus infections: clinical manifestations, course, and complications. Ann Intern Med 1983; 98(6):958–72.

14. Klausner JD, Kohn R, Kent C. Etiology of clinical proctitis among men who have sex with men. Clin Infect Dis 2004;38(2):300–2.

15. Scoular A. Using the evidence base on genital herpes: optimising the use of diagnostic tests and information provision. Sex Transm Infect 2002;78(3): 160–5.

16. Krantz I, Lowhagen GB, Ahlberg BM, et al. Ethics of screening for asymptomatic herpes virus type 2 infection. BMJ 2004;329(7466):618–21.

17. Lewis DA. Chancroid: clinical manifestations, diagnosis, and management. Sex Transm Infect 2003; 79(1):68–71.

18. Lewis DA, Ison CA. Chancroid. Sex Transm Infect 2006;82(Suppl 4):iv19–20.

19. Pilatz A, Hossain H, Kaiser R, et al. Acute epididymitis revisited: impact of molecular diagnostics on etiology and contemporary guideline recommendations. Eur Urol 2014. [Epub ahead of print].

20. Tracy CR, Steers WD, Costabile R. Diagnosis and management of epididymitis. Urol Clin North Am 2008;35(1):101–8, vii.

21. U.S. Preventive Services Task Force. Screening for chlamydial infection: U.S. Preventive Services Task Force recommendation statement. Ann Intern Med 2007;147(2):128–34.

22. Meyers D, Wolff T, Gregory K, et al. USPSTF recommendations for STI screening. Am Fam Physician 2008;77(6):819–24.

23. U.S. Preventive Services Task Force. Screening for gonorrhea: recommendation statement. Ann Fam Med 2005;3(3):263–7.

24. Centers for Disease Control and Prevention. Update to CDC's Sexually transmitted diseases treatment guidelines, 2010: oral cephalosporins no longer a recommended treatment for gonococcal infections. MMWR Morb Mortal Wkly Rep 2012; 61(31):590–4.

25. Kirkcaldy RD, Bolan GA, Wasserheit JN. Cephalosporin-resistant gonorrhea in North America. JAMA 2013;309(2):185–7.

26. Bradshaw CS, Tabrizi SN, Read TR, et al. Etiologies of nongonococcal urethritis: bacteria, viruses, and the association with orogenital exposure. J Infect Dis 2006;193(3):336–45.

27. Bradshaw CS, Chen MY, Fairley CK. Persistence of Mycoplasma genitalium following azithromycin therapy. PLoS One 2008;3(11):e3618.

28. Dunne EF, Unger ER, Sternberg M, et al. Prevalence of HPV infection among females in the United States. JAMA 2007;297(8):813–9.

29. Myers ER, McCrory DC, Nanda K, et al. Mathematical model for the natural history of human papillomavirus infection and cervical carcinogenesis. Am J Epidemiol 2000;151(12):1158–71.

30. Ho GY, Bierman R, Beardsley L, et al. Natural history of cervicovaginal papillomavirus infection in young women. N Engl J Med 1998;338(7):423–8.

31. Garland SM, Steben M, Sings HL, et al. Natural history of genital warts: analysis of the placebo arm of 2 randomized phase III trials of a quadrivalent human papillomavirus (types 6, 11, 16, and 18) vaccine. J Infect Dis 2009;199(6):805–14.

32. Koutsky L. Epidemiology of genital human papillomavirus infection. Am J Med 1997;102(5A):3–8.

33. Nelson EL, Stockdale CK. Vulvar and vaginal HPV disease. Obstet Gynecol Clin North Am 2013; 40(2):359–76.

34. Datta SD, Koutsky LA, Ratelle S, et al. Human papillomavirus infection and cervical cytology in women screened for cervical cancer in the United States, 2003–2005. Ann Intern Med 2008;148(7):493–500.

35. Jones RW, Rowan DM, Stewart AW. Vulvar intraepithelial neoplasia: aspects of the natural history and outcome in 405 women. Obstet Gynecol 2005; 106(6):1319–26.

36. Rodriguez AC, Schiffman M, Herrero R, et al. Rapid clearance of human papillomavirus and implications for clinical focus on persistent infections. J Natl Cancer Inst 2008;100(7):513–7.

37. Perry CM, Lamb HM. Topical imiquimod: a review of its use in genital warts. Drugs 1999;58(2):375–90.

38. Bonnez W, Elswick RK Jr, Bailey-Farchione A, et al. Efficacy and safety of 0.5% podofilox solution in the treatment and suppression of anogenital warts. Am J Med 1994;96(5):420–5.

39. Tyring SK, Arany I, Stanley MA, et al. A randomized, controlled, molecular study of condylomata acuminata clearance during treatment with imiquimod. J Infect Dis 1998;178(2):551–5.

40. Garland SM, Waddell R, Mindel A, et al. An open-label phase II pilot study investigating the optimal duration of imiquimod 5% cream for the treatment of external genital warts in women. Int J STD AIDS 2006;17(7):448–52.

41. Gotovtseva EP, Kapadia AS, Smolensky MH, et al. Optimal frequency of imiquimod (aldara) 5% cream for the treatment of external genital warts in immunocompetent adults: a meta-analysis. Sex Transm Dis 2008;35(4):346–51.

42. Edwards L, Ferenczy A, Eron L, et al. Self-administered topical 5% imiquimod cream for external anogenital warts. HPV Study Group. Human PapillomaVirus. Arch Dermatol 1998;134(1):25–30.

43. Stockfleth E, Beti H, Orasan R, et al. Topical Polyphenon E in the treatment of external genital and perianal warts: a randomized controlled trial. Br J Dermatol 2008;158(6):1329–38.

44. Tatti S, Swinehart JM, Thielert C, et al. Sinecatechins, a defined green tea extract, in the treatment of external anogenital warts: a randomized controlled trial. Obstet Gynecol 2008;111(6):1371–9.

45. Lacey CJ, Woodhall SC, Wikstrom A, et al. 2012 European guideline for the management of anogenital warts. J Eur Acad Dermatol Venereol 2013;27(3): e263–70.

46. American College of Obstetricians and Gynecologists. ACOG Practice Bulletin. Clinical Management Guidelines for Obstetrician-Gynecologists. Number 61, April 2005. Human papillomavirus. Obstet Gynecol 2005;105(4):905–18.

47. Zhou J, Sun XY, Stenzel DJ, et al. Expression of vaccinia recombinant HPV 16 L1 and L2 ORF proteins in epithelial cells is sufficient for assembly of HPV virion-like particles. Virology 1991;185(1):251–7.

48. Garland SM, Hernandez-Avila M, Wheeler CM, et al. Quadrivalent vaccine against human papillomavirus to prevent anogenital diseases. N Engl J Med 2007; 356(19):1928–43.

49. FUTURE II Study Group. Quadrivalent vaccine against human papillomavirus to prevent high-grade cervical lesions. N Engl J Med 2007; 356(19):1915–27.

50. Paavonen J, Naud P, Salmeron J, et al. Efficacy of human papillomavirus (HPV)-16/18 AS04-adjuvanted vaccine against cervical infection and precancer caused by oncogenic HPV types (PATRICIA): final analysis of a double-blind, randomised study in young women. Lancet 2009; 374(9686):301–14.

51. Giuliano AR, Palefsky JM, Goldstone S, et al. Efficacy of quadrivalent HPV vaccine against HPV Infection and disease in males. N Engl J Med 2011;364(5):401–11.

52. Palefsky JM, Giuliano AR, Goldstone S, et al. HPV vaccine against anal HPV infection and anal intraepithelial neoplasia. N Engl J Med 2011;365(17): 1576–85.

53. Joura EA, Giuliano AR, Iversen OE, et al. A 9-valent HPV vaccine against infection and intraepithelial neoplasia in women. N Engl J Med 2015;372(8): 711–23.

54. Petrosky E, Bocchini JA Jr, Hariri S, et al. Use of 9-Valent Human Papillomavirus (HPV) Vaccine: updated HPV vaccination recommendations of the Advisory Committee on Immunization Practices. MMWR Morb Mortal Wkly Rep 2015;64(11):300–4.

55. LeFevre ML, U.S. Preventive Services Task Force. Behavioral counseling interventions to prevent sexually transmitted infections: U.S. PreventiveServices Task Force recommendation statement. Ann Intern Med 2014;161(12):894–901.

56. O'Connor EA, Lin JS, Burda BU, et al. Behavioral sexual risk-reduction counseling in primary care to prevent sexually transmitted infections: a systematic review for the U.S. Preventive Services Task Force. Ann Intern Med 2014;161(12):874–83.

57. Haukoos JS, Thrun MW. Eliminating prevention counseling to improve HIV screening. JAMA 2013; 310(16):1679–80.

58. Golden MR, Whittington WL, Handsfield HH, et al. Effect of expedited treatment of sex partners on recurrent or persistent gonorrhea or chlamydial infection. N Engl J Med 2005;352(7):676–85.

59. Kissinger P, Mohammed H, Richardson-Alston G, et al. Patient-delivered partner treatment for male urethritis: a randomized, controlled trial. Clin Infect Dis 2005;41(5):623–9.

60. Hogben M. Partner notification for sexually transmitted diseases. Clin Infect Dis 2007;44(Suppl 3): S160–74.

Work-up of Pediatric Urinary Tract Infection

Bogdana Schmidt, MD, MPH, Hillary L. Copp, MD, MS*

KEYWORDS

- Pediatric • UTI • Guidelines • Uropathogen • Suprapubic aspiration • Vesicoureteral reflux
- Antibiotic resistance

KEY POINTS

- Given the high false-positive rate of urinary tests it is important to test a population with a high pre-test probability of infection.
- The sensitivity and specificity of a catheterized specimen is significantly better than those of a bagged sample, and has a specificity of 83% to 89% compared with a suprapubic sample; in samples with greater than 100,000 colony-forming units/mL approaches 99%.
- Comparing a positive urine dipstick and positive microscopic analysis showed no difference between the two methods when correlating with urine culture.
- Pediatric UTIs are treated with 2 goals: to eliminate the infection and prevent severe systemic illness; and to prevent and/or reduce possible long-term complications, such as renal scarring and hypertension.

INTRODUCTION

Pediatric urinary tract infection (UTI) is a common cause of presentation to health care providers and is an area of concern for parents and clinicians alike. There is a broad spectrum of presentations ranging from asymptomatic infection to mild lower urinary tract symptoms, to febrile and systemic illness.

The prevalence and incidence of pediatric UTI varies by age, race/ethnicity, sex, and circumcision status (**Table 1**).[1] Although calculating the true cumulative incidence is challenging given the varied reporting in different clinical settings, it is likely to be at least 2% in boys and 7% in girls in the first 6 years of life, with 2.2% of boys and 2.1% of girls having had a UTI before reaching 2 years of age.[2,3] Controlling for other clinical parameters, Hispanic and white children are more likely to be diagnosed with a UTI than black children.[4] After the first 12 months, girls are more likely to be diagnosed with a UTI. About half of boys with UTI are diagnosed within the first 12 months of life;

however, 80% of girls are diagnosed at a later age.[2] Circumcision has been shown to have a protective effect on UTI, reducing the odds of infection by 87%, with an even greater effect for boys with recurrent infections or posterior urethral valves.[5,6]

Pediatric UTI costs the health care system more than $180 million annually, and accounts for more than 1.5 million clinician visits per year.[3] Accurate and timely diagnosis of these infections is important for determining appropriate treatment and preventing long-term complications, such as renal scarring, hypertension, and end-stage renal disease.[7]

HISTORY AND PHYSICAL

Clinicians must have a high index of suspicion for UTI in the pediatric population, especially in infants and children less than 2 years of age. The evaluation must include a thorough history and the importance of the physical examination in pediatric patients cannot be overstated.

Disclosures: The authors have nothing to disclose.
University of California – San Francisco, San Francisco, CA 94143, USA
* Corresponding author. Box: 1695, Building: 550 16th Street, 5th Floor, San Francisco, CA 94143.
E-mail address: hillary.copp@ucsf.edu

Urol Clin N Am 42 (2015) 519–526
http://dx.doi.org/10.1016/j.ucl.2015.05.011

urologic.theclinics.com

Table 1
Uropathogen prevalence by sex and visit setting

Organism	Male		Female	
	Outpatient (%)	Inpatient (%)	Outpatient (%)	Inpatient (%)
Escherichia coli	50 (48–52)	37 (35–39)	83 (83–84)	64 (63–66)
Enterobacter	5 (5–6)	10 (8–11)	1 (1–1)	4 (4–5)
Enterococcus	17 (16–18)	27 (25–29)	5 (5–5)	13 (12–14)
Klebsiella	10 (9–11)	12 (10–13)	4 (4–5)	10 (9–11)
Pseudomonas aeruginosa	7 (6–8)	10 (8–11)	2 (2–2)	6 (5–7)
Proteus mirabilis	11 (10–12)	5 (4–6)	4 (4–4)	2 (2–3)

Based on national data from The Surveillance Network (TSN). Prevalence varies based on region.

Children Less Than 2 Years of Age

This is the most challenging population in which to make the diagnosis of UTI. Presentations are often vague and include irritability, poor feeding, lethargy, jaundice, vomiting, and fever.[8] In evaluating risk factors among children less than 2 years old presenting to emergency rooms with an ill appearance, high fever (greater than 39°C); history of UTI; change in urine characteristics (malodor or hematuria); and distension and tenderness in the suprapubic area, abdomen, or flanks were associated with UTI.[9] History of a previous UTI, temperature greater than 40°C, and suprapubic tenderness are the most useful for diagnosing UTI in febrile infants.[10]

Children Aged 2 to 12 Years

Toddlers and verbal children are more able to describe their symptoms and localize them to the urinary tract; however, given the high prevalence of UTI, the lack of localizing symptoms does not rule out UTI in this population.

History
Descriptions of dysuria, frequency, urgency, and urinary incontinence (in a toilet-trained child) increase the likelihood of UTI diagnosis.

Examination
A thorough examination should include evaluation of external genitalia, with special attention to identifying any external lesions, discharge, or foreign bodies. Palpation of the abdomen, suprapubic region, and costovertebral angles to elicit tenderness is key.[10]

- Special considerations for girls include evaluation for labial adhesions, foreign bodies, vulvovaginitis, and signs of sexually transmitted diseases.[11]

- Special considerations for boys include evaluation for phimosis, meatal stenosis, and tenderness in the testes to suggest epididymitis and/or orchitis.[12]

Adolescent Children

Although adolescents are better able to provide history and participate in physical examinations, sexual activity is a special consideration for this population that requires additional diagnostic attention. Among surveyed high-school students in 2013, 47% had had sexual intercourse and 34% reported having sexual activity in the last 3 months.[13] Sexually transmitted infections (STIs) are an important consideration for adolescents with urinary symptoms.

ADOLESCENT GIRLS AND URINARY TRACT INFECTION

- Adolescent girls with urinary symptoms often present with a UTI, STI, or both. Statistics on STI rates vary, with a prospective study finding that 29% of adolescent girls with urinary symptoms had had an STI.[14] Among sexually active girls with urinary symptoms, history of STI, more than 1 partner in the last 3 months, and urinalysis with blood and leukocyte esterase were predictive of STI.
- No specific symptoms or history findings have been shown to reliably predict which adolescent girls with urinary symptoms are at increased risk for either UTI or STI.[15,16]
- Current recommendations suggest testing sexually active girls with urinary symptoms for UTI as well as STIs including *Neisseria gonorrhoeae*, *Chlamydia*, and *Trichomonas*, especially in those with sterile pyuria.[15] Patients being evaluated or treated for STI should be offered HIV testing.[17]

ADOLESCENT BOYS AND URINARY TRACT INFECTION

- Although the prevalence of UTI in this age group is low, several risk factors have been identified, including sexual activity and lack of circumcision.[18]
- In adolescent boys with urinary symptoms it is also important to evaluate for balanitis xerotica obliterans, with nearly 35% incidence reported globally.[19,20] In pubertal boys, prostatitis can also present with symptoms of voiding dysfunction.[21]

URINE TESTING

Clinical and demographic factors should be used to determine the probability of an infection and guide the decision-making process to obtain a specimen for analysis. Given the high false-positive rate of urinary tests it is important to test a population with a high pretest probability of infection.[22,23]

URINE SPECIMEN COLLECTION IN NON–TOILET-TRAINED CHILDREN
Bag Specimen

- The simplest method of using a taped sterile bag to collect the urine is the least reliable, and has been consistently shown to have the greatest contamination rate.[24–26]
- A positive urine culture from a bag specimen has up to a 75% rate of false-positives, with periurethral organisms being isolated more than 98% of the time. Given its low positive predictive value, this method of collection has the lowest diagnostic utility in the clinical setting.
- If a bag specimen is negative, this can be used to rule out UTI without the need for confirmatory culture; however, positive urinalysis tests from bag specimens warrant further investigation with a catheterized specimen or suprapubic aspiration.

Urethral Catheterization

- Obtaining a catheterized specimen is a safe, fast, reliable way of collecting urine for analysis in the non–toilet-trained population.[26,30]
- The success of specimen collection depends on the specific anatomy and cooperation of the patient and the technical skill of the medical provider.
- Success rates in the literature have been quoted from 23% to 99%.

- The possible complications, including trauma and hematuria, have been shown to be minimal.
- The sensitivity and specificity of a catheterized specimen are significantly better than those of bagged samples, and have a specificity of 83% to 89% compared with a suprapubic sample, and in samples with greater than 100,000 colony-forming units (CFU)/mL approaches 99%.

Suprapubic Aspiration

- Arguably the most invasive method of urine collection, suprapubic aspiration is the most accurate. It is the least likely to be contaminated and any presence of bacteria indicates infection.[27–30]
- Suprapubic aspiration has an advantage for uncircumcised boys with phimosis, or girls with labial adhesions in whom catheterized specimens are more technically challenging to obtain.
- Despite its advantages, in the clinic or emergency room setting, suprapubic aspiration may prove more challenging to perform in a timely manner, given the requirement for physician participation and variable success rate per attempt (46%–97%), although this is improved with the use of ultrasonography.

URINE TESTS
Dipstick Urinalysis

This is the most clinically available, affordable, and accessible urine test, and the most widely used in the outpatient setting. The most clinically useful findings are the presence or absence of leukocyte esterase and nitrite in the urine specimen.[22,31,32]

- Positive leukocyte esterase is suggestive of inflammation in the urine and the presence of white blood cells (WBC). False-positives include other inflammatory conditions, such as Kawasaki disease; appendicitis; gastroenteritis; and presence of reactive inflammation, in the case of urinary stone disease. False-negatives include urine collected too early in the disease course or in a child with a suppressed immune response. Positive leukocyte esterase is 84% sensitive and 78% specific for diagnosing UTI.
- Positive nitrite is suggestive of the presence of gram-negative bacteria. False-negatives include urine collection that has been in the bladder less than 4 hours, which is the approximate conversion time from nitrate to nitrite; and infection with gram-positive

bacteria or non–nitrite-producing bacteria (namely enterococci and *Pseudomonas*). A positive nitrite test is up to 50% sensitive and 98% specific for diagnosing UTI.
- Combined positive nitrite-leukocyte esterase on dipstick analysis is 80% to 90% sensitive and 60% to 98% specific. When both are negative, the negative predictive value approaches 100%.

Microscopic Analysis

This method of analysis is more expensive and requires more equipment and skilled analysis than a urine dipstick. Analysis is performed to evaluate the presence of WBC, red blood cells, and bacteria in the sample.[26,33–35]

- Pyuria is the presence of greater than 5 WBC per high-power field on a centrifuged sample (10 WBC per high-power field in an uncentrifuged sample).
- Bacteriuria is the presence of any bacteria per high-power field.
- In a centrifuged sample, the presence of both pyuria and bacteriuria is up to 66% sensitive and 99% specific for diagnosing UTI.
- Comparing a positive urine dipstick and positive microscopic analysis showed no difference between the two methods when correlating with urine culture.

Urine Culture

This is the gold standard for diagnosing UTI and should be processed as soon as possible after collection to maximize diagnostic accuracy.[34,36]

- Greater than 50,000 CFU on a catheterized specimen or suprapubic aspiration indicate the presence of a UTI.
- Greater than 100,000 CFU on a voided specimen is considered a positive culture.
- Diagnosis of UTI in children 2 to 24 months old is made based on the presence of both pyuria and at least 50,000 colonies per milliliter of a single organism obtained via suprapubic aspiration or catheterization.

Serum Tests

Serum markers, including complete blood count, blood cultures, serum creatinine, C-reactive protein, erythrocyte sedimentation rate, and procalcitonin, have been evaluated as measures for UTI severity; however, none has been shown to be clinically useful or to alter management.[37,38]

IMAGING

There is no consensus on the need and optimal strategy for imaging in the setting of UTI in the pediatric population. The role and timing of imaging to evaluate for anatomic abnormalities and renal scarring, after a febrile UTI, is an area of debate. Renal bladder ultrasonography (RBUS), voiding cystourethrogram (VCUG), and dimercaptosuccinic acid (DMSA) scan are the most commonly used imaging modalities in this population; however, their role in diagnosis and management is controversial.

Renal Bladder Ultrasonography

- Noninvasive, relatively inexpensive, and safe in any age group.[39–41]
- Most commonly used modality to evaluate for anatomic abnormalities such as duplication, dilatation, and obstruction in the genitourinary tract.
- It is an unreliable modality to evaluate for vesicoureteral reflux (VUR), but has been shown to be useful in identifying pyelonephritis.
- For young children with a first UTI, RBUS is unlikely to alter clinical management and is not universally recommended.
  - National Institute for Health and Care Excellence (NICE) guidelines recommend RBUS after the first febrile UTI in children less than 6 months of age or older than 6 months with atypical or recurrent UTI.
  - American Academy of Pediatrics (AAP) guidelines recommend RBUS for children 2 to 24 months of age after their first febrile UTI.

Voiding Cystourethrogram

- Invasive, expensive, and exposes patients to radiation.[37,42]
- Most commonly used modality to evaluate for VUR.
  - NICE guidelines recommend VCUG for children less than 6 months of age with atypical or recurrent UTI and children 6 months to 3 years of age with atypical or recurrent UTI and abnormalities on RBUS, poor urine flow, or family history of VUR.
  - AAP guidelines recommend VCUG for children 2 to 24 months of age after the second febrile UTI, and after the first for patients with abnormalities on RBUS or high-grade VUR.

Dimercaptosuccinic Acid Scan

- Time intensive, invasive, expensive, and exposes patients to radiation.[41,43–45]

- Can provide information about extent of renal inflammation and renal scarring.
- Children with acute DMSA changes are at increased risk for VUR grade III to V on VCUG.
- Both NICE and AAP guidelines do not recommend using DMSA in routine evaluation of a first febrile UTI in children.
- The role of DMSA in evaluation of clinically significant renal scarring following infection is still controversial.
  - NICE guidelines recommend DMSA 4 to 6 months after:
    - Atypical or recurrent infection in children less than 3 years of age.
    - Recurrent infection in children more than 3 years of age.
  - AAP guidelines do not include the use of DMSA in their recommendations.

TREATMENT

Pediatric UTIs are treated with 2 goals: to eliminate the infection and prevent severe systemic illness; and to reduce possible long-term complications, such as renal scarring and hypertension.[41]

The decision to initiate empiric treatment should be based on clinical suspicion of infection based on history and physical examination and positive urinalysis on an appropriately collected urine specimen. Most patients can be treated as outpatients if the child appears nontoxic, can tolerate oral medications, and can comply with recommendations.[46] For some patients in whom a urinalysis and clinical picture are concerning for infection, antibiotics can be started empirically without awaiting culture results. Alternatively, if the diagnosis is uncertain and the child appears nontoxic, treatment can be delayed until urine culture results are obtained; in both cases, medication should be tailored to the antibiotic sensitivities of the urine culture results.[10]

The choice of treatment therapy depends on numerous factors, including the child's age, underlying medical problems, illness severity, ability to tolerate oral medications, and most importantly the local resistance patterns to uropathogens (**Table 2**).

Treatment Course

A 7-day to 14-day outpatient treatment course is an appropriate regimen.[46–48]

Table 2
Uropathogen resistance rates

Antibiotics	E coli	Enterobacter	Enterococcus	Klebsiella	P mirabilis	P aeruginosa
			Antibiotic Resistance (%)			
Narrow Spectrum						
TMP/SMX	24	18	—	15	11	94
Ampicillin	45	78	3	81	12	—
Nitrofurantoin	<1	23	<1	17	94	0
Cephalothin	16	96	—	7	4	—
Cefazolin	4	91	—	7	4	—
Gentamicin	4	2	—	3	5	10
Vancomycin	—	—	<1	—	—	—
Broad Spectrum						
Amox-clav	5	91	—	4	1	—
Cefuroxime	2	33	—	7	0	—
Ceftriaxone	<1	12	—	2	<1	31
Ceftazidime	<1	15	—	2	<1	4
Ciprofloxacin	5	1	5	3	3	5
Pip-tazo	1	7	—	3	<1	5
Imipenem	<1	<1	—	<1	2	3
Aztreonam	<1	13	—	3	<1	4

Based on national data from TSN. Resistance rates vary based on region. Blanks indicate that testing was not performed for antibiotics to which uropathogens are known to be nonsusceptible.
Abbreviations: Amox-clav, amoxicillin-clavulanate; Pip-tazo, piperacillin/tazobactam; TMP/SMX, trimethoprim/sulfamethoxazole.

- NICE guidelines: oral antibiotics for 7 to 10 days or intravenous antibiotics for 2 to 4 days followed by oral antibiotics for a total duration of 10 days.
- AAP guidelines: oral or intravenous antibiotics for 7 to 14 days.

Oral Antibiotics

Escherichia coli is the most common pathogen, being found in more than 80% of pediatric UTIs. Empiric antibiotics should be based on local resistance patterns, because certain widely used choices are becoming increasingly resistant.[49–51] Narrow-spectrum antibiotics, such as nitrofurantoin and first-generation cephalosporins, are more likely to be effective than trimethoprim-sulfamethoxazole, in many communities; however, nitrofurantoin should not be used in febrile UTI treatment or when renal involvement is suspected. Therapy should ultimately be based on the culture organism with the most narrow-spectrum agent.

Parenteral Antibiotics

For patients who are more ill appearing, have underlying urologic conditions, have had recent urinary infections or have taken antibiotics, immunocompromised patients, as well as those with intractable nausea and vomiting, inpatient admission and parenteral therapy is appropriate. Empiric choices include ampicillin and gentamicin, third-generation or fourth-generation cephalosporins, broad-spectrum penicillins, carbapenems, macrolides, and fluoroquinolones.[46,50,52]

Renal Scarring

It remains controversial whether initiation of treatment within the first 24 to 72 hours prevents renal damage.[46,48,53–55] In patients who present with ascending infection and renal involvement, there are conflicting data as to whether early treatment can prevent subsequent scarring, because the presence of pyelonephritis has been shown to be associated with scarring, independent of treatment timing. There is evidence to suggest that early treatment helps prevent acute pyelonephritis, and both AAP and NICE guidelines recommend early initiation of treatment.

REFERENCES

1. Shaikh N, Morone NE, Bost JE, et al. Prevalence of urinary tract infection in childhood: a meta-analysis. Pediatr Infect Dis J 2008;27:302–8.
2. National Collaborating Centre for Women's and Children's Health (UK). Urinary tract infection in children: diagnosis, treatment and long-term management [Internet]. London: RCOG Press; 2007. Available at: http://www.ncbi.nlm.nih.gov/books/NBK50606/. Accessed April 13, 2015.
3. Freedman AL, Urologic Diseases in America Project. Urologic diseases in North America Project: trends in resource utilization for urinary tract infections in children. J Urol 2005;173:949–54.
4. Chen L, Baker MD. Racial and ethnic differences in the rates of urinary tract infections in febrile infants in the emergency department. Pediatr Emerg Care 2006;22:485–7.
5. Singh-Grewal D, Macdessi J, Craig J. Circumcision for the prevention of urinary tract infection in boys: a systematic review of randomised trials and observational studies. Arch Dis Child 2005;90:853–8.
6. Mukherjee S, Joshi A, Carroll D, et al. What is the effect of circumcision on risk of urinary tract infection in boys with posterior urethral valves? J Pediatr Surg 2009;44:417–21.
7. Jacobson SH, Eklöf O, Eriksson CG, et al. Development of hypertension and uraemia after pyelonephritis in childhood: 27 year follow up. BMJ 1989;299:703–6.
8. Zorc JJ, Levine DA, Platt SL, et al. Clinical and demographic factors associated with urinary tract infection in young febrile infants. Pediatrics 2005;116:644–8.
9. Shaw KN, Gorelick M, McGowan KL, et al. Prevalence of urinary tract infection in febrile young children in the emergency department. Pediatrics 1998;102:e16.
10. Shaikh N, Morone NE, Lopez J, et al. Does this child have a urinary tract infection? JAMA 2007;298:2895–904.
11. Piippo S, Lenko H, Vuento R. Vulvar symptoms in paediatric and adolescent patients. Acta Paediatr 2000;89:431–5.
12. Merlini E, Rotundi F, Seymandi PL, et al. Acute epididymitis and urinary tract anomalies in children. Scand J Urol Nephrol 1998;32:273–5.
13. CDC. Sexual behaviors - adolescent and school health [Internet]. Available at: http://www.cdc.gov/health yyouth/sexualbehaviors/. Accessed April 13, 2015.
14. Demetriou E, Emans SJ, Masland RP. Dysuria in adolescent girls: urinary tract infection or vaginitis? Pediatrics 1982;70:299–301.
15. Huppert JS, Biro F, Lan D, et al. Urinary symptoms in adolescent females: STI or UTI? J Adolesc Health 2007;40:418–24.
16. Huppert JS, Biro FM, Mehrabi J, et al. Urinary tract infection and *Chlamydia* infection in adolescent females. J Pediatr Adolesc Gynecol 2003;16:133–7.
17. Branson BM, Handsfield HH, Lampe MA, et al. Revised recommendations for HIV testing of adults, adolescents, and pregnant women in health-care settings. MMWR Recomm Rep 2006;55:1–17 [quiz: CE1–4].

18. Horowitz M, Cohen J. Review of adolescent urinary tract infection. Curr Urol Rep 2007;8:319–23.

19. Gargollo PC, Kozakewich HP, Bauer SB, et al. Balanitis xerotica obliterans in boys. J Urol 2005;174: 1409–12.

20. Celis S, Reed F, Murphy F, et al. Balanitis xerotica obliterans in children and adolescents: a literature review and clinical series. J Pediatr Urol 2014;10:34–9.

21. Li Y, Qi L, Wen JG, et al. Chronic prostatitis during puberty. BJU Int 2006;98:818–21.

22. Whiting P, Westwood M, Bojke L, et al. Clinical effectiveness and cost-effectiveness of tests for the diagnosis and investigation of urinary tract infection in children: a systematic review and economic model. Health Technol Assess 2006;10:iii–iv, xi–xiii, 1–154.

23. Bachur R, Harper MB. Reliability of the urinalysis for predicting urinary tract infections in young febrile children. Arch Pediatr Adolesc Med 2001;155:60–5.

24. Schlager TA, Hendley JO, Dudley SM, et al. Explanation for false-positive urine cultures obtained by bag technique. Arch Pediatr Adolesc Med 1995; 149:170–3.

25. Schlager TA, Lohr JA. Urinary tract infection in outpatient febrile infants and children younger than 5 years of age. Pediatr Ann 1993;22:505–9.

26. Whiting P, Westwood M, Watt I, et al. Rapid tests and urine sampling techniques for the diagnosis of urinary tract infection (UTI) in children under five years: a systematic review. BMC Pediatr 2005;5:4.

27. Tobiansky R, Evans N. A randomized controlled trial of two methods for collection of sterile urine in neonates. J Paediatr Child Health 1998;34:460–2.

28. Hardy JD, Furnell PM, Brumfitt W. Comparison of sterile bag, clean catch and suprapubic aspiration in the diagnosis of urinary infection in early childhood. Br J Urol 1976;48:279–83.

29. Kiernan SC, Pinckert TL, Keszler M. Ultrasound guidance of suprapubic bladder aspiration in neonates. J Pediatr 1993;123:789–91.

30. Pollack CV, Pollack ES, Andrew ME. Suprapubic bladder aspiration versus urethral catheterization in ill infants: success, efficiency and complication rates. Ann Emerg Med 1994;23:225–30.

31. Gorelick MH, Shaw KN. Screening tests for urinary tract infection in children: a meta-analysis. Pediatrics 1999;104:e54.

32. Huicho L, Campos-Sanchez M, Alamo C. Metaanalysis of urine screening tests for determining the risk of urinary tract infection in children. Pediatr Infect Dis J 2002;21:1–11, 88.

33. Hoberman A, Wald ER. Urinary tract infections in young febrile children. Pediatr Infect Dis J 1997; 16:11–7.

34. Finnell SM, Carroll AE, Downs SM, et al. Technical report—Diagnosis and management of an initial UTI in febrile infants and young children. Pediatrics 2011;128:e749–70.

35. Mori R, Yonemoto N, Fitzgerald A, et al. Diagnostic performance of urine dipstick testing in children with suspected UTI: a systematic review of relationship with age and comparison with microscopy. Acta Paediatr 2010;99:581–4.

36. Hoberman A, Wald ER, Reynolds EA, et al. Pyuria and bacteriuria in urine specimens obtained by catheter from young children with fever. J Pediatr 1994;124:513–9.

37. Shaikh N, Craig JC, Rovers MM, et al. Identification of children and adolescents at risk for renal scarring after a first urinary tract infection: a meta-analysis with individual patient data. JAMA Pediatr 2014; 168:893–900.

38. Shaikh N, Borrell JL, Evron J, et al. Procalcitonin, C-reactive protein, and erythrocyte sedimentation rate for the diagnosis of acute pyelonephritis in children. Cochrane Database Syst Rev 2015;(1):CD009185.

39. Massanyi EZ, Preece J, Gupta A, et al. Utility of screening ultrasound after first febrile UTI among patients with clinically significant vesicoureteral reflux. Urology 2013;82:905–9.

40. Nelson CP, Johnson EK, Logvinenko T, et al. Ultrasound as a screening test for genitourinary anomalies in children with UTI. Pediatrics 2014;133: e394–403.

41. Hoberman A, Charron M, Hickey RW, et al. Imaging studies after a first febrile urinary tract infection in young children. N Engl J Med 2003;348:195–202.

42. Shaikh N, Ewing AL, Bhatnagar S, et al. Risk of renal scarring in children with a first urinary tract infection: a systematic review. Pediatrics 2010;126:1084–91.

43. Craig JC, Wheeler DM, Irwig L, et al. How accurate is dimercaptosuccinic acid scintigraphy for the diagnosis of acute pyelonephritis? A meta-analysis of experimental studies. J Nucl Med 2000;41:986–93.

44. Paterson A. Urinary tract infection: an update on imaging strategies. Eur Radiol 2004;14(Suppl 4): L89–100.

45. La Scola C, De Mutiis C, Hewitt IK, et al. Different guidelines for imaging after first UTI in febrile infants: yield, cost, and radiation. Pediatrics 2013; 131:e665–71.

46. Subcommittee on Urinary Tract Infection, Steering Committee on Quality Improvement and Management, Roberts KB. Urinary tract infection: clinical practice guideline for the diagnosis and management of the initial UTI in febrile infants and children 2 to 24 months. Pediatrics 2011;128:595–610.

47. Newman TB. The New American Academy of Pediatrics urinary tract infection guideline. Pediatrics 2011;128:572–5.

48. Baumer JH, Jones RW. Urinary tract infection in children, National Institute for Health and Clinical Excellence. Arch Dis Child Educ Pract Ed 2007;92: 189–92.

49. Edlin RS, Shapiro DJ, Hersh AL, et al. Antibiotic resistance patterns of outpatient pediatric urinary tract infections. J Urol 2013;190:222–7.

50. Allen UD, MacDonald N, Fuite L, et al. Risk factors for resistance to "first-line" antimicrobials among urinary tract isolates of *Escherichia coli* in children. CMAJ 1999;160:1436–40.

51. Paschke AA, Zaoutis T, Conway PH, et al. Previous antimicrobial exposure is associated with drug-resistant urinary tract infections in children. Pediatrics 2010;125:664–72.

52. Jones ME, Karlowsky JA, Draghi DC, et al. Rates of antimicrobial resistance among common bacterial pathogens causing respiratory, blood, urine, and skin and soft tissue infections in pediatric patients. Eur J Clin Microbiol Infect Dis 2004;23:445–55.

53. Hewitt IK, Zucchetta P, Rigon L, et al. Early treatment of acute pyelonephritis in children fails to reduce renal scarring: data from the Italian Renal Infection Study Trials. Pediatrics 2008;122:486–90.

54. Doganis D, Siafas K, Mavrikou M, et al. Does early treatment of urinary tract infection prevent renal damage? Pediatrics 2007;120:e922–8.

55. Fernández-Menéndez JM, Málaga S, Matesanz JL, et al. Risk factors in the development of early technetium-99m dimercaptosuccinic acid renal scintigraphy lesions during first urinary tract infection in children. Acta Paediatr 2003;92:21–6.

Urinary Tract Infection and Neurogenic Bladder

Maxim J. McKibben, MD[a], Patrick Seed, MD, PhD[b], Sherry S. Ross, MD[a], Kristy M. Borawski, MD[a],*

KEYWORDS

- Neurogenic bladder • Spinal cord injury • Spina bifida • Urinary tract infection
- Bacterial interference • Probiotics • Antibiotic prophylaxis • Antimicrobial resistance

KEY POINTS

- Urinary tract infections (UTI) are frequent, recurrent, and lifelong for patients with neurogenic bladder (NGB) and present challenges in diagnosis and treatment.
- Failure to recognize and treat infections can quickly lead to life-threatening autonomic dysreflexia or sepsis, whereas overtreatment contributes to antibiotic resistance.
- Widely accepted diagnostic criteria for UTI in NGB are lacking.
- Multiple UTI prevention methods are used, but evidence-based practices are few.
- Current research is aimed at understanding the dysfunctional immune response in NGB, the role of probiotics and avirulent bacteria in prevention, and judicious antibiotic use.

INTRODUCTION

Normal micturition requires proper function of the bladder and urethral sphincter complex. This process requires coordination between the central and the peripheral nervous systems. Disruption of this pathway caused by damage or disease interferes with this coordinated effort and can lead to neurogenic bladder (NGB) with abnormal bladder storage and emptying. Management of NGB is a challenging long-term issue for both patients and providers. Improper management of NGB and pyelonephritis can result in renal injury and eventually renal failure. Recurrent pyelonephritis results in renal scarring and contributes to deterioration of the kidney. Although advances in medical care have significantly reduced the morbidity and mortality of urinary tract infection (UTI) in NGB, currently 10% to 15% of patients with NGB die from sepsis of urinary origin.[1]

Because of the causal and functional heterogeneity of NGB, each patient must be approached individually, because risk factors vary significantly between patients. This article addresses UTI in the general NGB population and evaluates the epidemiology, pathogenesis, risk factors, evaluation, diagnosis, treatment, and prevention in these patients.

EPIDEMIOLOGY

Estimates of NGB in the United States include approximately 400,000 people with diagnoses of spina bifida (SB), spinal cord injury (SCI), cerebral palsy, multiple sclerosis (MS), and Parkinson disease.[2–4] UTIs are the most common infection in this population; 31% of patients with a new diagnosis of SCI were diagnosed with a UTI within the first year, and 21% required hospitalization.[5] In patients with SB, UTI is the most common complaint in the emergency room setting.[6] Patients with SCI average 2.5 symptomatic UTIs per year, with similar findings in other NGB populations.[7] With the increased frequency and severity

[a] Department of Urology, University of North Carolina at Chapel Hill, Chapel Hill, NC, USA; [b] Division of Infectious Disease, Department of Pediatrics, Duke University Medical Center, Durham, NC, USA
* Corresponding author. Department of Urology, University of North Carolina, 170 Manning Drive, 2115 Physicians Office Building, CB#7235, Chapel Hill, NC 27599-7235.
E-mail address: Kristy_borawski@med.unc.edu

Urol Clin N Am 42 (2015) 527–536
http://dx.doi.org/10.1016/j.ucl.2015.05.006

of infection, there is higher risk of morbidity and mortality secondary to urosepsis and end-stage renal disease relative to the general population.[8]

PATHOGENESIS

In the past, mechanical factors such as increased postvoid residuals (PVR), urinary stasis, and bladder stones were thought to be the primary causal factors in development of recurrent UTI in patients with NGB. However, emerging data suggest that the propensity to develop infections is much more complex (**Fig. 1**), and dysfunctional immune response in the bladder may be a strong contributor as well.[4]

BLADDER DYSFUNCTION

Abnormal urodynamic parameters in patients with NGB may correlate with increased risk of UTI. Prior studies showed that detrusor overactivity, decreased bladder compliance, and vesicoureteral reflux are significant risk factors for febrile UTI among patients with spinal dysraphism.[9] The mechanism by which these abnormalities lead to increased rate of UTI is not clear, but there are several theories. Evidence suggests that increased intravesical pressure results in bladder ischemia, which in turn may result in delayed or deficient immune response to pathogens.[10,11] Animal and human studies have found that increased intravesical pressure significantly reduces blood flow, in both the distended and empty bladder, suggesting global dysfunction.[12,13] Although most patients with NGB have abnormal urodynamic studies, many of these parameters can be mitigated successfully with medications or surgery.

URINARY STASIS/INCREASED POSTVOID RESIDUAL

Normal voiding is protective against development of UTI, because emptying greatly decreases overall bacterial count in the urine, which is then diluted by bladder filling.[10] Animal studies have shown that 99.9% of bacteria injected into the bladder are removed by voiding.[14] Based on these studies, inefficient voiding with residual urine in theory predisposes to development of UTI. Multiple studies have investigated the association between PVR urine volume and rate of developing UTI. Among patients with spinal cord injury and NGB, PVR of greater than 300 mL was associated with a 4 to 5 times greater rate of development of UTI.[15] Two studies of patients after stroke showed that PVR greater than 150 mL was an independent risk factor for development of UTI,[16] and PVR

greater than 100 mL resulted in 4.9-fold increase in UTI development compared with those with PVR less than 100 mL.[17] In a rat model of SCI and UTI, PVR did not correlate with UTI, suggesting other contributing factors.[18] Although the exact PVR necessary to predispose a patient with NGB to UTI is not clear, urinary stasis and increased PVR are risk factors associated with UTI.

CATHETER USE

Urinary catheters are a mainstay management strategy for patients with NGB. Significant research has examined indwelling catheterization and clean intermittent catheterization (CIC), as well as catheter material, with the primary outcome in most studies being frequency of UTI.

CIC is the preferred method of drainage in patients with NGB as long as their dexterity or caretaker support and body habitus allow access. However, CIC increases the risk for UTI caused by catheter contamination and the introduction of external microorganisms into the bladder environment.[19] A study comparing quadriplegic patients with NGB managed with either CIC or suprapubic catheter (SP) found an annual rate of symptomatic UTI of 26% for the CIC group, and 12% for the SP group, although SP was more often complicated by bladder stones (65% vs 30%).[20] In addition, patients with indwelling catheters have higher rates of bladder cancer and renal scarring.[21] In both groups the overall rate of infection remains high.

Catheters are generally made from silicon or other soft rubbers. Because of concerns for catheterization trauma as a contributing causal factor for development of UTI, hydrophilic coated catheters are under investigation. These catheters have a slippery, prelubricated surface and may cause less urethral trauma and irritation. In a randomized study of patients with recent SCI with initiation CIC, there was a 21% reduction in incidence of symptomatic UTI among the hydrophilic catheter group compared with the polyvinyl chloride catheter group at 3 months after initiation. However, this difference did not persist at 6 months.[22] A more recent meta-analysis of 5 studies (n = 462) comparing patients using hydrophilic or nonhydrophilic catheters in CIC found a significantly decreased rate of symptomatic UTI among the hydrophilic group (odds ratio [OR] = 0.36; $P<.0001$), as well as less gross hematuria (OR = 0.57; $P = .001$).[23] Although no clear consensus has been reached regarding the efficacy of hydrophilic catheters in prevention of UTI, they are favored by some patients because of comfort and convenience.

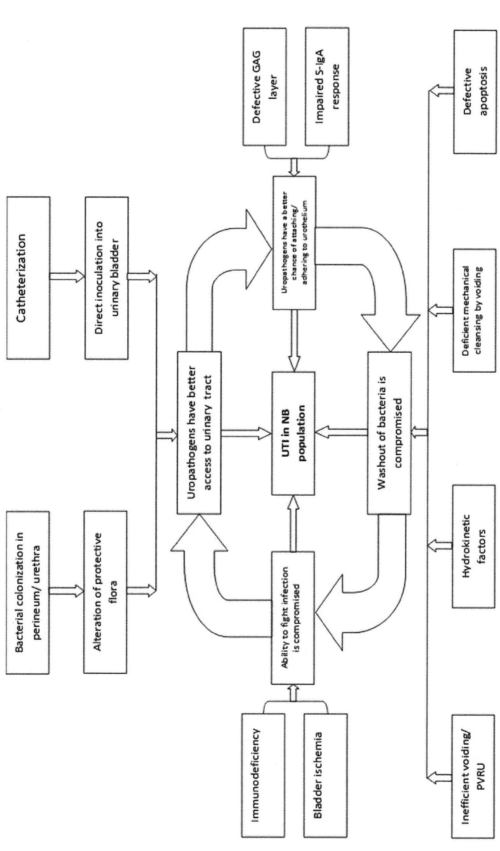

Fig. 1. Multifactorial causes of UTI in NGB. (*From* Vasudeva P, Madersbacher H. Factors implicated in pathogenesis of urinary tract infections in neurogenic bladders: Some revered, few forgotten, others ignored. Neurourol Urodyn 2014;33(1):95–100; with permission.)

Silver alloy–impregnated and antibiotic-coated catheters have been shown to decrease asymptomatic bacteriuria, but only for 1 week after initiation of use and are therefore not recommended in the NGB population at this time.[24]

External condom catheters have approximately the same rate of symptomatic UTI as CIC and are a reasonable management strategy in male patients with a low-resistance bladder outlet.[25] However, many patients with NGB do not drain optimally with a condom catheter with increased PVR, potentially leading to both bladder and upper tract damage.

IMMUNE DYSFUNCTION

A recent hypothesis under investigation is immune dysfunction incited by SCI. In a rat model of induced SCI-UTI, animals had decreased proinflammatory and antiinflammatory responses to uropathogenic Escherichia coli, and inflammation was not appropriately suppressed after the infection was eliminated.[4,18] This dysfunctional immunologic response may redispose to infection and hinder bacterial eradication.

Although the urine and urinary tract luminal space commonly contain bacteria during acute UTI, uropathogenic bacteria such as uropathogenic E coli (UPEC) and Klebsiella pneumoniae also invade urothelial cells.[26,27] Studies from murine UTI models show that UPEC can proliferate within the urothelium, which may not be easily eradicated with antibiotic treatment, providing a nidus of reinfection.[28,29] Using the rat model of SCI-UTI, intracellular replication of E coli in the bladder urothelium of the NGB has been observed and may underlie the challenge of effective treatment of UTI with NGB and be a risk factor for recurrent disease.

In addition to the immune dysfunction that seems to be inherent to NGB, pharmacologic immunosuppression in patients with MS and NGB may provide a further risk for recurrent UTI. Some centers test patients with MS for bacteriuria before initiation of steroid induction therapy and treat even asymptomatic bacteriuria to avoid potential development of invasive disease once steroid treatment is underway, although the degree of infection reduction is not clear.[30]

DIAGNOSIS

A key factor complicating the study and treatment of UTI in NGB is the lack of consensus definition of infection, both in study populations and in clinical practice. Impaired sensation with nonspecific infectious symptoms, as well as ubiquitous bacterial colonization of the bladder in patients with NGB, often leads to an unclear clinical picture.

MONITORING FOR INFECTION

There is universal agreement that renal and bladder function in patients with NGB should be monitored, but no consensus regarding monitoring frequency, studies that should be performed, or definition of UTI. A meta-analysis of studies evaluating follow-up among patients with SCI showed no clear definition of UTI and no demonstrable utility in routine screening with urinalysis or urine culture.[31] A systematic review of UTI in the pediatric SB literature found that only a third of studies provided a definition of UTI, and, of those, the definitions were heterogeneous.[32] After analysis of these studies, the investigators suggested the following definition for UTI in pediatric patients with SB: greater than or equal to 2 symptoms (fever>38°C, abdominal pain, new back pain, new or worse incontinence, pain with catheterization or urination, or malodorous/cloudy urine), and greater than 100,000 colony-forming units (CFU)/mL of a single organism, and greater than 10 white blood cells (WBC) per high-power field (HPF) on microscopy.[32] The National Institute on Disability and Rehabilitation Research provides guidelines for diagnosis of UTI in patients with SCI: greater than 10^2 CFU/mL from intermittent catheterized specimen, greater than 10^4 CFU/mL from condom catheter, and any value from indwelling and suprapubic catheters, along with pyuria and signs and symptoms of UTI.[33]

The typical symptoms of UTI in the general population, such as dysuria, urgency, and frequency, are rarely present in the NGB population. More common symptoms, especially in the SCI population, include autonomic dysreflexia, increased spasticity, new or worsening urinary incontinence, vague back or abdominal pain, or foul-smelling urine.[34,35] Patients with SCI are able to predict the presence of a UTI based on symptoms with an accuracy of only 61% to 66.2%,[36,37] although they are much better at predicting when they did not have a UTI (negative predictive value 82.8%) than when they did (positive predictive value 32.6%).[36] In the same study, cloudy urine had the highest accuracy (83.1%), whereas presence of pyuria had the highest sensitivity (82.8%) in predicting the presence of UTI. The absence of pyuria strongly suggests another cause for the symptoms.[38] In contrast, foul smell of the urine has a low sensitivity as a predictor for UTI (48.3%), with multiple noninfectious causes.[36,39]

Heterogeneous definitions of UTI in the NGB population have long hampered clinical and research efforts. Universally accepted diagnosis criteria will lead to less ambiguity in diagnosis and treatment, reduce overtreatment of asymptomatic bacteriuria, and allow researchers to design more robust studies with outcomes that can be generalized to better care for this population and develop preventive measures (Fig. 2).

TREATMENT

Treatment of UTI in NGB mirrors that in the general population, with some exceptions. Most importantly, urine cultures must be obtained before

antibiotic administration. Antibiotic choice should be tailored to the specific pathogen and sensitivities of the culture data, because pathogen and sensitivity trends in the NGB population differ from the general population. A study of patients with SCI found E coli to be the primary cause in 18% of symptomatic UTI, compared with 75% to 95% in the general population.[36,40] In addition, bacterial isolates may vary in the community versus hospital settings and have higher rates of resistance to commonly prescribed antibiotics, making broad-spectrum antibiotics necessary in severe cases.[41]

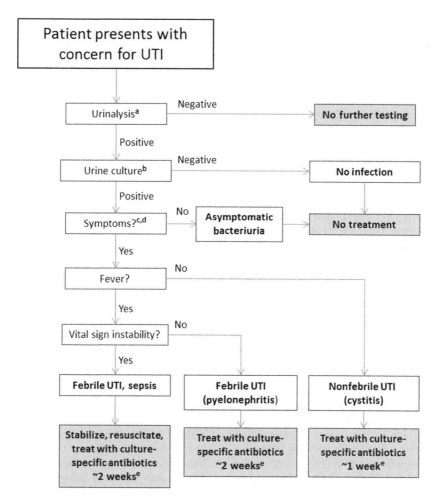

Fig. 2. Management algorithm for patients with NGB and suspected UTI. [a] Positive urinalysis: greater than 10 WBC/HPF on microscopy (not validated end point). [b] Positive urine culture: greater than 10^2 CFU/mL from intermittent catheterized specimen, greater than 10^4 CFU/mL from condom catheter, and any value from indwelling and suprapubic catheters (not validated). [c] Symptoms include 2 or more of: fever greater than 38°C, abdominal pain, new back pain, new or worse incontinence, pain with catheterization or urination, and malodorous/cloudy urine. [d] Urine culture should not be performed in the absence of symptoms, but often is, thus is included in this algorithm. [e] Treatment duration may vary based on other considerations. (Data from Madden-Fuentes RJ, Ross SS. Urinary tract infections in the spina bifida population. Novel Insights into Urinary Tract Infections and Their Management 2014:61; and Everaert K, Lumen N, Kerckhaert W, et al. Urinary tract infections in spinal cord injury: prevention and treatment guidelines. Acta Clin Belg 2009;64(4):335–40.)

Commonly, patients with NGB have a urinalysis or urine culture performed by providers who are not accustomed to caring for patients with NGB, and the identification of asymptomatic colonization prompts inappropriate antibiotic treatment. Avoiding treatment of asymptomatic bacteriuria in NGB is important, except in select populations such as those on immunosuppression, pregnant women, or patients undergoing a urologic procedure.[30,42] Recurrent courses of antibiotics result in higher rates of antibiotic-resistant isolates and antibiotic prophylaxis has limited efficacy and is associated with increased antibiotic resistance.[43–47] Education of both patients with NGB and providers who care for these patients is necessary to promote antibiotic stewardship and prevent inappropriate treatment of asymptomatic bacteriuria.

Choice of treatment duration is largely based on provider experience, because there are few data supporting specific treatment durations. A 60-patient study of those with SCI and symptomatic UTI randomized to either a 3-day or 14-day course of antibiotics found an increased rate of bacteriuria and symptomatic relapse in the 3-day group (37% and 23%, respectively), compared with the 14-day group (7% and 0%, respectively).[48] In patients with indwelling Foley catheters and catheter-associated UTIs, the Infectious Disease Society of America recommends early catheter exchange and a 7-day to 14-day treatment course with culture-specific antibiotics.[38] A recent study of patients with SCI with indwelling catheters evaluated a 5-day treatment course with early catheter exchange versus a 10-day course with catheter retention and found that the 5-day course was associated with more relapses, reinforcing the belief that long treatment durations are necessary in patients with NGB.[49]

A review of UTI in patients with SCI sought to determine optimal antibiotic choices and treatment durations. They recommend 5 days of antibiotic treatment of chronic SCI with no fever, 7 days for acute SCI with no fever, and 14 days for UTI with fever.[50] The investigators suggest nitrofurantoin or trimethoprim for UTI in chronic SCI, fluoroquinolones or cefuroxime in UTI in acute SCI, and broad-spectrum intravenous coverage with fever. However, this may vary depending on the local antibiogram.[50]

PREVENTION
Cranberry, D-Mannose, Ascorbic Acid

Cranberry juice, D-mannose, and other products have been used to prevent UTIs in the nonneurogenic population, although the studies are heterogeneous and the results are mixed. In a recent Cochrane Review, the routine use of cranberry products in patients with NGB performing CIC did not show any clear benefit, and it is not recommended for prevention of UTI in this population.[35,51] A study of women with normal bladders and recurrent UTIs found that daily D-mannose reduced the incidence of UTI over a 6-month period by 45%, comparable with nitrofurantoin prophylaxis, but similar studies have not been performed in the NGB population.[52] One possible mechanism for the seeming lack of efficacy of cranberry products seen in the neurogenic population is that cranberry primarily works to decrease the binding and invasion of E coli and Pseudomonas to the uroepithelial cell. Because patients with NGB tend to have more varied uropathogens, the binding may not be as efficient in the NGB. Future studies investigating the use of cranberry and D-mannose in patients with NGB with predominantly E coli or Pseudomonas UTIs may show a benefit.[34]

Ascorbic acid and other agents used to either acidify or alkalinize urine lack appreciable data in the prevention of UTI in the NGB population and are not recommended.

Bacterial Interference/Probiotics

There has been increased recent interest in probiotics and avirulent bacterial strains in prevention of UTI, termed bacterial interference. A study with avirulent 83972 E coli compared the frequency of UTI in subjects with SCI before and after bladder inoculation, and saw a dramatic reduction in frequency of symptomatic UTIs after colonization (zero infections in 18.4 patient years) compared with before (3.1 infections per year).[53] A more recent study randomized 65 patients with NGB to receive bladder inoculation with avirulent E coli HU2117 (a derivative of 83972 E coli) or placebo (sterile saline). The patients colonized with E coli HU2117 had significantly fewer symptomatic UTIs at 1 year (0.50) compared with the control group (1.68)[54]; however, the utility of bacterial interference may be limited by the propensity for colonization by these strains. In the later study, only 37% of subjects achieved sustained colonization with the therapeutic strain. A murine model of UTI suggests that 83972 E coli also has the potential to clear acute bacterial cystitis and reduce associated pelvic pain with efficacy similar to ciprofloxacin.[55] The mechanism of bacterial interference with avirulent E coli is not completely understood, but recent research shows that 83972 E coli causes broad suppression of host RNA-polymerase II gene expression, which is intimately involved in normal inflammatory and immune responses to pathogenic bacteria.[56]

Bacterial interference has several barriers to wide use: (1) inoculation is cumbersome, requiring multiple indwelling bacterial administrations over consecutive days; (2) maintenance of colonization is difficult; and (3) patients may be bothered by the foul smell of their urine.[57] Novel colonization strategies, such as use of avirulent *E coli*–coated catheters, have shown promise.[58] Further research is needed regarding optimal inoculation methods, monitoring, and the exact mechanism of symptomatic UTI prevention.

The vaginal tract is a reservoir for uropathogenic bacteria, which are normally kept in low numbers by commensal organisms. Alteration of the normal vaginal flora and pathogen invasion may precede recurrent UTI. A study of women with recurrent UTI showed that intravaginal *Lactobacillus* suppositories significantly decreased the risk of future UTI.[59] In postmenopausal women with recurrent UTI, oral *Lactobacillus* was compared with trimethoprim-sulfamethoxazole (TMP-SMX) prophylaxis. Both interventions reduced the rate of symptomatic UTI by more than 50%, although *Lactobacillus* did not meet predesignated noninferiority criteria compared with TMP-SMX.[60] Data regarding probiotics in prevention of UTI in NGB are scant, but there are several ongoing studies and a Cochrane Systematic Review pending, which may provide another nonantibiotic option for this population.

There are many unknowns regarding bacterial interference and probiotics, such as the optimal flora (eg, bacterial species, fungi), maintenance of colonization, and the possibility for conversion into virulent bacterial strains. Clinical use of probiotics and bacterial interference would provide a major advantage for patients with NGB, decreasing the reliance on antibiotics and delaying the development of antibiotic resistance.

Bladder Irrigation

Bladder irrigation in patients with NGB has been studied over the last several decades and, despite initial excitement, guidelines do not recommend bladder irrigation because of poor improvement rates of symptomatic UTI and increased mucosal irritation, possibly increasing susceptibility to infection.[61] A novel irrigant, iAluRil (1.6% hyaluronic acid and 2% chondroitin sulfate), has recently shown promise. In neurointact women with recurrent UTIs, the treatment group that underwent weekly and then monthly instillation saw an 86.6% reduction in infection, versus 9.6% with placebo.[62] A study of hyaluronic acid instillation

in patients with indwelling catheters secondary to spinal cord compression showed a 5.7-fold reduction in symptomatic infection,[63] but otherwise efficacy in the NGB population remains to be elucidated.

Onabotulinum Toxin A

Onabotulinum toxin A has seen increased use in urology since it was approved for use in overactive bladder in 2013. Increased detrusor pressures on urodynamics seem to be a risk factor for UTI in patients with NGB, thus decrease in pressures with botulinum toxin may decrease rates of infection. In a 41-patient study of patients with SCI in a rehabilitation facility, rates of symptomatic UTI (temperature>38°C, 2 or more symptoms, and 10^5 CFU/mL on culture) were monitored 6 months before and 6 months after 300-unit onabotulinum toxin injection. The total number of UTIs in the cohort decreased from 57 to 32 after injection ($P = .023$).[64] These results should be corroborated in a large, well-designed study, but, aside from the small risk of UTI immediately after instrumentation for administration of the therapeutic,[65] intravesical injection of onabotulinum toxin A may prove to be useful for UTI risk reduction in NGB.

Antibiotic Prophylaxis

Oral antibiotic prophylaxis in patients with NGB is controversial, with ongoing risk-benefit debates that weigh long-term efficacy against concern for development of antibiotic resistance. A meta-analysis of antibiotic prophylaxis in patients with SCI showed a reduction in incidence of asymptomatic bacteriuria, but no change in the rate of symptomatic infection, and an increase in antibiotic resistance.[44] In patients who have severe and frequent infections, there may be benefit to prophylaxis. Alternating antibiotic schedules are used in practice, with the theory that it may reduce the risk of resistance by continually challenging the bacterial flora with antimicrobials that target different mechanisms. In a study of patients with SCI, 2 different antibiotics were administered individually on a weekly basis based on each patient's cultures, which reduced the rate of symptomatic UTIs from 9.4 per year to 1.8 per year.[66] Although some studies have shown a decreased rate of symptomatic UTI with antimicrobial prophylaxis, the sustainability of this approach is questionable because of the finite effective life of antibiotics, constant selection pressure, and global increase of multidrug-resistant organisms (like *E coli* ST131)[67] that is likely to lead to more resistant pathogens in the long term.

SUMMARY

UTI in patients with NGB remains a challenge for urologists and other clinicians. Altered anatomy and bladder mechanics, frequent catheterization, impaired sensation, and immunologic dysfunction make patients with NGB uniquely prone to infections and difficult to diagnose and treat appropriately. A consensus states that asymptomatic bacteriuria should not be treated in most patients, but, given the absence of a standardized definition of UTI in this patient population, efforts to optimally diagnose, treat, and study recurrent UTI in patients with NGB have been significantly hampered. This area requires a major effort in future studies. Mechanical UTI prevention techniques such as use of hydrophilic or antibiotic-coated catheters, or bladder irrigation have not consistently shown a reduction in symptomatic infections and are not currently recommended. Pharmacologic prophylaxis with antibiotics and infection inhibitors (ie, cranberry and D-mannose) do not consistently reduce rates of symptomatic infections and are associated with a risk of emergence of resistant organisms. Research is ongoing to better understand the increased susceptibility to UTI in the NGB, and efforts are underway to study the use of probiotics and intentional colonization of the bladder with benign bacterial strains. Antibiotic choice for symptomatic infection is complicated by the variability of microorganisms in the NGB and the higher rates of antimicrobial resistance. Therefore, treatment should always be driven by culture sensitivities, because bacterial resistance patterns differ significantly from those in the general population.

REFERENCES

1. Garcia Leoni M, Esclarin De Ruz A. Management of urinary tract infection in patients with spinal cord injuries. Clin Microbiol Infect 2003;9(8):780–5.
2. Smith ED. Spina bifida and the total care of spinal myelomeningocele. Springfield (IL): 1965.
3. Burns AS, Rivas DA, Ditunno JF. The management of neurogenic bladder and sexual dysfunction after spinal cord injury. Spine 2001;26(24S):S129–36.
4. Chaudhry R, Madden-Fuentes RJ, Ortiz TK, et al. Inflammatory response to *Escherichia coli* urinary tract infection in the neurogenic bladder of the spinal cord injured host. J Urol 2014;191(5):1454–61.
5. Manack A, Motsko SP, Haag-Molkenteller C, et al. Epidemiology and healthcare utilization of neurogenic bladder patients in a US claims database. Neurourol Urodyn 2011;30(3):395–401.
6. Wang HS, Tejwani R, Zhang H, et al. Hospital surgical volume and associated post-operative complications of pediatric urologic surgery in the United States. J Urol 2015. [Epub ahead of print].
7. Siroky MB. Pathogenesis of bacteriuria and infection in the spinal cord injured patient. Am J Med 2002; 113(1):67–79.
8. Cameron AP, Wallner LP, Tate DG, et al. Bladder management after spinal cord injury in the United States 1972 to 2005. J Urol 2010;184(1):213–7.
9. Seki N, Masuda K, Kinukawa N, et al. Risk factors for febrile urinary tract infection in children with myelodysplasia treated by clean intermittent catheterization. Int J Urol 2004;11(11):973–7.
10. Vasudeva P, Madersbacher H. Factors implicated in pathogenesis of urinary tract infections in neurogenic bladders: some revered, few forgotten, others ignored. Neurourol Urodyn 2014;33(1):95–100.
11. Andriole VT, Lytton B. The effect and critical duration of increased tissue pressure on susceptibility to bacterial infection. Br J Exp Pathol 1965;46(3): 308–17.
12. Mehrotra R. An experimental study of the vesical circulation during distension and in cystitis. J Pathol Bacteriol 1953;66(1):79–89.
13. Kershen RT, Azadzoi KM, Siroky MB. Blood flow, pressure and compliance in the male human bladder. J Urol 2002;168(1):121–5.
14. Norden CW, Green GM, Kass EH. Antibacterial mechanisms of the urinary bladder. J Clin Invest 1968;47(12):2689–700.
15. Merritt JL. Residual urine volume: correlate of urinary tract infection in patients with spinal cord injury. Arch Phys Med Rehabil 1981;62(11):558–61.
16. Dromerick AW, Edwards DF. Relation of postvoid residual to urinary tract infection during stroke rehabilitation. Arch Phys Med Rehabil 2003;84(9):1369–72.
17. Kim B, Lim JH, Lee SA, et al. The relation between postvoid residual and occurrence of urinary tract infection after stroke in rehabilitation unit. Ann Rehabil Med 2012;36(2):248–53.
18. Balsara ZR, Ross SS, Dolber PC, et al. Enhanced susceptibility to urinary tract infection in the spinal cord-injured host with neurogenic bladder. Infect Immun 2013;81(8):3018–26.
19. Schlager TA, Dilks S, Trudell J, et al. Bacteriuria in children with neurogenic bladder treated with intermittent catheterization: natural history. J Pediatr 1995;126(3):490–6.
20. Mitsui T, Minami K, Furuno T, et al. Is suprapubic cystostomy an optimal urinary management in high quadriplegics? A comparative study of suprapubic cystostomy and clean intermittent catheterization. Eur Urol 2000;38(4):434–8.
21. Chao R, Clowers D, Mayo ME. Fate of upper urinary tracts in patients with indwelling catheters after spinal cord injury. Urology 1993;42(3):259–62.
22. Cardenas DD, Moore KN, Dannels-McClure A, et al. Intermittent catheterization with a hydrophilic-coated

catheter delays urinary tract infections in acute spinal cord injury: a prospective, randomized, multicenter trial. PM R 2011;3(5):408–17.

23. Li L, Ye W, Ruan H, et al. Impact of hydrophilic catheters on urinary tract infections in people with spinal cord injury: systematic review and meta-analysis of randomized controlled trials. Arch Phys Med Rehabil 2013;94(4):782–7.

24. Tenke P, Kovacs B, Johansen TE, et al. European and Asian guidelines on management and prevention of catheter-associated urinary tract infections. Int J Antimicrob Agents 2008;31:68–78.

25. Esclarín De Ruz A, García Leoni E, Herruzo Cabrera R. Epidemiology and risk factors for urinary tract infection in patients with spinal cord injury. J Urol 2000;164(4):1285–9.

26. Mulvey MA, Schilling JD, Hultgren SJ. Establishment of a persistent *Escherichia coli* reservoir during the acute phase of a bladder infection. Infect Immun 2001;69(7):4572–9.

27. Rosen DA, Pinkner JS, Jones JM, et al. Utilization of an intracellular bacterial community pathway in *Klebsiella pneumoniae* urinary tract infection and the effects of FimK on type 1 pilus expression. Infect Immun 2008;76(7):3337–45.

28. Berry RE, Klumpp DJ, Schaeffer AJ. Urothelial cultures support intracellular bacterial community formation by uropathogenic *Escherichia coli*. Infect Immun 2009;77(7):2762–72.

29. Blango MG, Mulvey MA. Persistence of uropathogenic *Escherichia coli* in the face of multiple antibiotics. Antimicrob Agents Chemother 2010;54(5): 1855–63.

30. Mahadeva A, Tanasescu R, Gran B. Urinary tract infections in multiple sclerosis: under-diagnosed and under-treated? A clinical audit at a large university hospital. Am J Clin Exp Immunol 2014;3(1):57.

31. Cameron AP, Rodriguez GM, Schomer KG. Systematic review of urological followup after spinal cord injury. J Urol 2012;187(2):391–7.

32. Madden-Fuentes RJ, Ross SS. Urinary tract infections in the spina bifida population. Novel Insights into Urinary Tract Infections and Their Management 2014;61.

33. The prevention and management of urinary tract infections among people with spinal cord injuries. National Institute on Disability and Rehabilitation research consensus statement. January 27–29, 1992. J Am Paraplegia Soc 1992;15(3):194–204.

34. Jahromi MS, Mure A, Gomez CS. UTIs in patients with neurogenic bladder. Curr Urol Rep 2014;15(9):1–7.

35. Wyndaele J, Brauner A, Geerlings SE, et al. Clean intermittent catheterization and urinary tract infection: review and guide for future research. BJU Int 2012;110(11c):E910–7.

36. Massa LM, Hoffman JM, Cardenas DD. Validity, accuracy, and predictive value of urinary tract infection signs and symptoms in individuals with spinal cord injury on intermittent catheterization. J Spinal Cord Med 2009;32(5):568–73.

37. Linsenmeyer TA, Oakley A. Accuracy of individuals with spinal cord injury at predicting urinary tract infections based on their symptoms. J Spinal Cord Med 2003;26(4):352–7.

38. Hooton TM, Bradley SF, Cardenas DD, et al. Diagnosis, prevention, and treatment of catheter-associated urinary tract infection in adults: 2009 international clinical practice guidelines from the Infectious Diseases Society of America. Clin Infect Dis 2010;50(5):625–63.

39. Nicolle LE. Consequences of asymptomatic bacteriuria in the elderly. Int J Antimicrob Agents 1994;4(2): 107–11.

40. Hooton TM. Uncomplicated urinary tract infection. N Engl J Med 2012;366(11):1028–37.

41. Yoon S, Lee B, Lee K, et al. Comparison of bacterial strains and antibiotic susceptibilities in urinary isolates of spinal cord injury patients from the community and hospital. Spinal Cord 2014;52(4):298–301.

42. Nicolle LE. Urinary tract infections in patients with spinal injuries. Curr Infect Dis Rep 2014;16(1):1–7.

43. Schlager TA, Anderson S, Trudell J, et al. Nitrofurantoin prophylaxis for bacteriuria and urinary tract infection in children with neurogenic bladder on intermittent catheterization. J Pediatr 1998;132(4):704–8.

44. Morton SC, Shekelle PG, Adams JL, et al. Antimicrobial prophylaxis for urinary tract infection in persons with spinal cord dysfunction. Arch Phys Med Rehabil 2002;83(1):129–38.

45. Zegers B, Uiterwaal C, Kimpen J, et al. Antibiotic prophylaxis for urinary tract infections in children with spina bifida on intermittent catheterization. J Urol 2011;186(6):2365–71.

46. Mohler JL, Cowen DL, Flanigan RC. Suppression and treatment of urinary tract infection in patients with an intermittently catheterized neurogenic bladder. J Urol 1987;138(2):336–40.

47. Craig JC, Williams GJ, Hodson EM. Antimicrobial prophylaxis for children with vesicoureteral reflux. N Engl J Med 2014;371(11):1070–3.

48. Dow G, Rao P, Harding G, et al. A prospective, randomized trial of 3 or 14 days of ciprofloxacin treatment for acute urinary tract infection in patients with spinal cord injury. Clin Infect Dis 2004;39(5): 658–64.

49. Darouiche RO, Al Mohajer M, Siddiq DM, et al. Short versus long course of antibiotics for catheter-associated urinary tract infections in patients with spinal cord injury: a randomized controlled noninferiority trial. Arch Phys Med Rehabil 2014;95(2):290–6.

50. Everaert K, Lumen N, Kerckhaert W, et al. Urinary tract infections in spinal cord injury: prevention and treatment guidelines. Acta Clin Belg 2009;64(4): 335–40.

51. Jepson RG, Craig JC. Cranberries for preventing urinary tract infections. Cochrane Database Syst Rev 2008;(1):CD001321.

52. Kranjčec B, Papeš D, Altarac S. D-mannose powder for prophylaxis of recurrent urinary tract infections in women: a randomized clinical trial. World J Urol 2014;32(1):79–84.

53. Hull R, Rudy D, Donovan W, et al. Urinary tract infection prophylaxis using *Escherichia coli* 83972 in spinal cord injured patients. J Urol 2000;163(3):872–7.

54. Darouiche RO, Green BG, Donovan WH, et al. Multicenter randomized controlled trial of bacterial interference for prevention of urinary tract infection in patients with neurogenic bladder. Urology 2011; 78(2):341–6.

55. Rudick CN, Taylor AK, Yaggie RE, et al. Asymptomatic bacteriuria *Escherichia coli* are live biotherapeutics for UTI. PLoS One 2014;9(11):e109321.

56. Lutay N, Ambite I, Gronberg Hernandez J, et al. Bacterial control of host gene expression through RNA polymerase II. J Clin Invest 2013;123(6): 2366–79.

57. Bao Y, Welk B, Reid G, et al. Role of the microbiome in recurrent urinary tract infection. Novel Insights into Urinary Tract Infections and Their Management 2014;49.

58. Prasad A, Cevallos ME, Riosa S, et al. A bacterial interference strategy for prevention of UTI in persons practicing intermittent catheterization. Spinal Cord 2009;47(7):565–9.

59. Stapleton AE, Au-Yeung M, Hooton TM, et al. Randomized, placebo-controlled phase 2 trial of a *Lactobacillus crispatus* probiotic given intravaginally for prevention of recurrent urinary tract infection. Clin Infect Dis 2011;52(10):1212–7.

60. ter Riet G, Nys S, van der Wal WM, et al. Lactobacilli vs antibiotics to prevent urinary tract infections: a randomized, double-blind, noninferiority trial in postmenopausal women. Arch Intern Med 2012;172(9): 704–12.

61. Elliott T, Reid L, Rao GG, et al. Bladder irrigation or irritation? Br J Urol 1989;64(4):391–4.

62. Damiano R, Quarto G, Bava I, et al. Prevention of recurrent urinary tract infections by intravesical administration of hyaluronic acid and chondroitin sulphate: a placebo-controlled randomised trial. Eur Urol 2011;59(4):645–51.

63. Mañas A, Glaría L, Peña C, et al. Prevention of urinary tract infections in palliative radiation for vertebral metastasis and spinal compression: a pilot study in 71 patients. Int J Radiat Oncol Biol Phys 2006;64(3):935–40.

64. Jia C, Liao L, Chen G, et al. Detrusor botulinum toxin A injection significantly decreased urinary tract infection in patients with traumatic spinal cord injury. Spinal Cord 2013;51(6):487–90.

65. Mouttalib S, Khan S, Castel-Lacanal E, et al. Risk of urinary tract infection after detrusor botulinum toxin A injections for refractory neurogenic detrusor overactivity in patients with no antibiotic treatment. BJU Int 2010;106(11):1677–80.

66. Salomon J, Denys P, Merle C, et al. Prevention of urinary tract infection in spinal cord-injured patients: safety and efficacy of a weekly oral cyclic antibiotic (WOCA) programme with a 2 year follow-up–an observational prospective study. J Antimicrob Chemother 2006;57(4):784–8.

67. Johnson JR, Johnston B, Clabots C, et al. *Escherichia coli* sequence type ST131 as the major cause of serious multidrug-resistant *E. coli* infections in the United States. Clin Infect Dis 2010;51(3):286–94.

Asymptomatic Bacteriuria in Noncatheterized Adults

Matthew Ferroni, MD, Aisha Khalali Taylor, MD*

KEYWORDS

- Asymptomatic bacteriuria • IDSA • Urinary tract infection • Translational barriers
- Antimicrobial overtreatment • Live biotherapeutics

KEY POINTS

- Asymptomatic bacteriuria (ASB) is defined by the presence of bacteria in an uncontaminated urine specimen collected from a patient without signs or symptoms referable to the urinary tract.
- ASB is highly prevalent among women over the age of 60, hospitalized and institutionalized patients, ambulatory elderly patients, and patients with diabetes mellitus.
- The Infectious Diseases Society of America (IDSA) has recommended against screening for and treating ASB with antimicrobials unless patients are undergoing invasive genitourinary procedures or are pregnant. Despite these clear guidelines, there remains significant overtreatment of ASB with antimicrobials, particularly in patients who are hospitalized or live in a nursing home setting, leading to deleterious consequences in this vulnerable patient population.
- Microbiologic evidence exists to support not treating ASB secondary to reduced virulence factors associated with ASB strains and may suggest that ASB may be beneficial in reducing symptomatic lower urinary tract infections (UTIs) in certain patient populations.
- Translational barriers to the implementation of IDSA recommendations for the management of ASB have been identified and addressed to some degree. In an era in which clinicians' face pay for performance concerns with current practice patterns not reflecting evidence-based recommendations, attention needs to be focused on eliminating these translational barriers on a global scale.

INTRODUCTION

Definition of Asymptomatic Bacteriuria and Infectious Diseases Society of America Recommendations

ASB is defined as the presence of bacteria in a noncontaminated urine specimen obtained from a patient without signs and symptoms of UTI.[1] In asymptomatic women, the diagnosis of ASB requires the isolation of the same organism in 2 consecutive voided urine specimens isolated in quantitative count greater than or equal to 100,000 colony-forming units (CFUs). In asymptomatic men, a single voided urine specimen with 1 bacterial species isolated in quantitative count greater than or equal to 100,000 CFUs/mL or a single catheterized specimen with 1 bacterial species isolated in quantitative count greater than or equal to 100 CFUs/mL in asymptomatic male or female patients constitutes the diagnosis of ASB (**Box 1**).[2] The significance of ASB and the effects of antimicrobial treatment on this condition are well established in some populations but remain unproved or uncertain in others.[3] In 2005, the IDSA published clear, evidence-based guidelines on the diagnosis and treatment of ASB in adults.[2] The only populations the IDSA

Department of Urology, University of Pittsburgh Medical Center, 300 Halket Street, Suite 4710, Pittsburgh, PA 15213, USA
* Corresponding author.
E-mail addresses: taylora10@upmc.edu; aishakhalalitaylor@gmail.com

Urol Clin N Am 42 (2015) 537–545
http://dx.doi.org/10.1016/j.ucl.2015.07.003
0094-0143/15/$ – see front matter © 2015 Elsevier Inc. All rights reserved.

Box 1
Diagnosis of asymptomatic bacteriuria

Lack of signs and symptoms of UTI

Diagnosis based on urine specimen collected in manner that minimizes contamination

For asymptomatic men – single voided urine specimen with 1 bacterial species isolated in quantitative count ≥100,000 CFUs/mL

For asymptomatic women – 2 consecutive voided urine specimens with isolation of same bacterial strain in quantitative counts ≥100,000 CFUs/mL

For men or women – single catheterized urine specimen with one bacterial species isolated in quantitative count ≥100 CFUs/mL

Based on ISDA guidelines.
  Data from Nicolle LE, Bradley S, Colgan R, et al. Infectious Disease Society of America Guidelines for the diagnosis and treatment of asymptomatic bacteriuria in adults. Clin Infect Dis 2005;40:643–54.

---

recommended for screening and treatment included pregnant patients to reduce the incidence of pyelonephritis and premature delivery and patients undergoing invasive genitourinary surgery to reduce the incidence of bacteremia and sepsis.[4] The IDSA strongly recommended against screening for ASB in premenopausal nonpregnant women, women with diabetes mellitus, hospitalized patients without UTI symptoms, ambulatory elderly adults, elderly institutionalized residents in long-term care facilities, patients with spinal cord injuries, or individuals with indwelling urethral catheters.[2,3] Despite these available clear guidelines from the IDSA, clinicians continue to misdiagnose and inappropriately manage ASB.[5–10] This article reviews the following:

- A review of the epidemiology and risk factors for ASB
- A review of the literature encompassing the management of ASB in patients with diabetes mellitus
- The basic science of ASB
- A discussion of translational barriers to the application of the IDSA recommendations and approaches to reducing these barriers

EPIDEMIOLOGY OF ASYMPTOMATIC BACTERIURIA

ASB is common among elderly patients in the community, patients in long-term care facilities, and patients in the hospital setting.[11] The prevalence of ASB increases with age, ranging from 0% in men aged 68 to 79 up to 5.4% in men aged 90 to 103.[12] The prevalence of ASB among women is even more pronounced, increasing from 13.6% among women aged 68 to 79 to 22.4% in among women aged 90 to 103.[13] ASB is more common in institutionalized patients, with

greater functional impairment compared with community dwellers (25%–50% of women and 15%–35% of men in institutionalized care).[11,14] In healthy young premenopausal nonpregnant women, the prevalence of ASB is 1% to 5%.[15] In hospitalized elderly patients, the prevalence of ASB is 32% to 50% among women and 30% to 34% among men.[12] Among community-dwelling older women, the predominant etiologic pathogens of ASB include *Escherichia coli* (51.4%), *Klebsiella pneumonia* (4.1%), *Proteus mirabilis* (3.3%), and *Enterococcus faecalis* (2.5%) (**Fig. 1**).[16] Among institutionalized patients and patients with long-term indwelling urinary catheters, polymicrobial bacteriuria is common, often including *Pseudomonas aeruginosa*, *Morganella morganii*, and *Providencia stuartii*.[2,17] Risk factors for ASB include older age, female gender, higher postvoid residuals in men, and genetic factors in certain women (**Table 1**).[15] Whether diabetes itself creates a predisposition to ASB is not entirely clear. A single-center study in 511

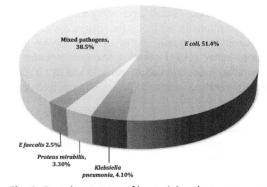

Fig. 1. Prevalence rates of bacterial pathogens among community-dwelling women with ASB.

Table 1
Factors associated with the presence asymptomatic bacteriuria

Physiologic	Pathologic
Age	Neurologic disease (eg, Alzheimer disease, Parkinson disease, stroke)
Gender (female more than male)	Diabetes mellitus Reduced mobility Urinary tract abnormality (eg, calculi, prostate enlargement, high post-void residual volume)
—	Indwelling urinary catheter

Data from Colgan R, Nicolle LE, McGlone A, et al. Asymptomatic bacteriuria in adults. Am Fam Physician 2006; 74:985–90.

diabetic and 97 nondiabetic subjects found a similar incidence of ASB in both groups.[18] The prevalence of ASB was higher in both women (14.2 vs 5.1%) and men (2.3 vs 0.8%) with diabetes than in healthy controls.[19] Taken together these data have confounded decision making regarding the management of ASB in this specific patient population; thus, the literature regarding this patient population is explored in depth.

ASYMPTOMATIC BACTERIURIA IN DIABETIC PATIENTS

UTIs occur more often in patients with diabetes mellitus than in nondiabetics and are associated with more severe infectious complications, such as emphysematous pyelonephritis and cystitis, and concurrent fungal infections.[20] ASB has also been found to have a 4-times higher incidence in diabetic women than nondiabetic women, with an overall prevalence of 26% compared with 6%.[21] Long-term carriage of bacteriuria in diabetics has revealed that up to 25% of diabetic women carry the same strain of E coli for up to 6 months compared with their nondiabetic female counterparts, in whom only 1% continue to carry the same bacterial strain beyond 2 months.[22] These differences have not been found to be bacterial strain specific, because the exact same virulence factor expression has been shown in E coli isolates in both diabetic and nondiabetic patients.[23] Thus, host factors contributing to bacterial growth as well as an impaired immune response for eradication of bacteria seem the primary drivers of these findings. Accelerated bacterial growth has been shown in vitro after the addition of glucose, mimicking concentrations found in the urine of poorly controlled diabetics, leading to speculation that glycosuria provides an additional substrate for bacterial proliferation.[24] Adherence of E coli type 1 fimbriae, a glycoprotein involved in bacterial cell attachment to urothelial cells, has also been demonstrated in vitro to be much greater in diabetic patients with poor glycemic control versus more optimal control.[25] In vivo studies, however, have not proved these factors to contribute to established higher rates of ASB colonization. In a large patient cohort of 636 diabetic women, poor glycemic control was not found a specific risk factor for either the development of ASB or symptomatic UTI.[26]

Concerning the host immune response, early speculation hypothesized that increased glucose in the urine would lead to glycosylation of a variety of immune cells in the urine and impede their bactericidal function. Granulocyte function testing, however, between diabetic and nondiabetic women with ASB has shown no differences in chemotaxis, opsonization, oxidation, phagocytosis, and killing, leading to the conclusion that impaired granulocyte dysfunction is not a factor in persistent bacteriuria.[27] Two proinflammatory cytokines, IL-6 and IL-8, have been found to have a significantly lower concentration in the urine of diabetic women with ASB compared with nondiabetic women with ASB and were correlated to an overall lower leukocyte count in diabetic patients.[28] Thus, the impaired immune response contributing to higher rates of ASB in diabetics seems not due to the qualitative function of leukocytes but rather a blunted quantitative immune cascade.

Untreated ASB in diabetic patients has not been shown to have any increased rates of complications compared with diabetic women without ASB. A long-term follow-up study of 6 years showed no difference in renal function deterioration, as measured by change in creatinine clearance over time, between diabetic woman with and without ASB.[29] Aimed at determining if ASB warranted treatment in diabetic patients to prevent conversion to symptomatic UTI as well as other complications, a prospective trial randomized women with both diabetes and ASB to continual antimicrobial agents to sterilize the urine and placebo. After 4 weeks, only 20% of patients receiving antimicrobials had continued bacteriuria, compared with 78% in the placebo group. At a mean follow-up of 27 months, however, there were no differences in the rate of symptomatic infection (40% vs 42%), or time to first symptomatic infection, pyelonephritis, and hospitalization due to infection.[30] This led the investigators to conclude that the treatment of ASB in diabetic women does not seem to increase complications and for this reason routine screening and treatment in this population is not recommended.

THE BASIC SCIENCE OF ASYMPTOMATIC BACTERIURIA

Two main factors distinguish acute symptomatic UTI from ASB colonization: (1) the virulence factors of the bacteria itself (fimbriae, lipopolysaccharides [LPSs], and toxins) and (2) the host factors implicated in disease susceptibility (urothelial receptor proteins and adequate immune system activation). These microbiologic factors are discussed in further detail.

Fimbriae

Perhaps the most studied factor in differentiating uropathogenic bacteria from ASB is the presence of specific fimbriae on the bacterial surface. Fimbriae are complex structures that mediate adherence to host epithelium through protein receptors.[31] Uropathogenic E coli has been found to express a markedly different fimbriae profile than ASB, including type 1, P, F1C, Dr, Auf, S, and M fimbriae.[32,33] Of all of these, P fimbriae expression has shown the strongest correlation to acute disease severity, found on the surface of more than 90% of E coli-causing pyelonephritis but on less than 20% of ASB strains.[34,35]

P fimbriae bind to Galα1-4Galβ epitopes of glycolipids on the urothelium, leading to the activation of the innate immune system promoting the release of cytokines and recruitment of neutrophils.[36,37] The expression of type 1 fimbriae, which bind to the mannosylated epitopes of bladder urolotheial integrin molecules, is also intimately involved in bacterial adherence and immune activation.[38] Although type 1 fimbriae are expressed by more than 90% of ASB strains, a cluster deletion has been identified in its coding gene, fimH, which may negate its ability to facilitate adherence and immune activation.[39] A recent study confirmed 26% of fimH-positive ASB strains were unable to express functional type 1 fimbriae.[40] This supports the hypothesis that many ASB strains may carry virulence genes but fail to express the associated phenotype for functional virulence.[41] Recently, the detection of 2 previously uncharacterized fimbriae, Yad and Ygi, were found more than twice as prevalent in uropathogenic E coli than ASB strains and associated with virulence-related activities including motility, biofilm formation, and cell adherence.[42] Although the expression of other fimbriae, such as F1C and Dr, have also been studied, their contribution

to virulence is much less clear but likely contributable to the overall pathogenetic profile.

Lipopolysaccharides

LPS is an endotoxin of gram-negative bacteria, containing the lipid type A anchored in the outer membrane, which activates Toll-like receptor (TLR) 4 on the urothelium and induces immune system activation.[43] This mechanism has proved responsible for significant fever and acute systemic illness associated with septicemia and is undoubtedly a contributor to the virulence of uropathogenic bacteria. Capsular polysaccharides surround bacteria and protect the organism from host defenses in blood and tissues.[43] Mutant bacteria with genetically altered capsular polysaccharide expression have shown significantly reduced virulence in experimental UTI animal models.[44] LPS from ASB E coli has biotherapeutic activity.[45]

Toxins

Two major toxins produced by uropathogenic E coli are hemolysin and cytotoxic necrotizing factor 1 (CNF1).[31] Hemolysin is a secreted protein found more commonly in uropathogenic strains than fecal strains, which inserts into host cell membranes leading to epithelial damage and hemorrhage.[46] Hemolysin activity has been shown to correlate to the severity of clinical infection, found in only 14% of ASB strains and in 47% and 31% of E coli-causing cystitis and pyelonephritis, respectively.[41] Although the actual expression of the hly A gene encoding for hemolysin was found in 58% of ASB, only 14% were functionally hemolytic compared with 100% functional hemolysis when found in E coli causing pyelonephritis.[41] Thus, genetic mutation leading to dysfunction of the toxin itself may significantly contribute to the benign nature of ASB strains. CNF1 is a cytokine released by uropathogenic E coli that leads to activation of the Rho family of GTP-binding proteins on the host urothelium and has been implicated in inducing bladder cell apoptosis.[47,48] CNF1-positive E coli strains have been shown to cause more inflammation than strains lacking production of this toxin.[49]

Host Factors

Fimbriae-mediated adhesion to the host urothelium activates TLR4 signaling, which triggers cytokine production and neutrophil recruitment for bacterial destruction and also determines the severity of signs and symptoms related to acute infection.[50] The loss of functional TLR4 signaling and activation promotes long-term bacterial colonization and can lead to ASB. Mutations in the TLR4 promotor, which significantly reduce the efficiency of TLR4 expression, have been shown in children with ASB compared with age-matched controls and those with acute pyelonephritis.[51] Thus, these mutations may be protective against recurrent acute UTIs and disease severity.

Growth Factors

The ASB strain E coli 83,972, initially isolated from a young Swedish girl who carried it asymptomatically for 3 years, is the most widely studied strain of nonvirulent E coli.[52] Despite the loss of functional fimbriae and inability to activate host innate immune response, this nonvirulent strain grows well in human urine and can outcompete uropathogenic E coli strains.[53] This property has led to its instillation as a prophylactic treatment method in patients with recurrent UTIs, refractory to traditional medical therapy.[54,55] The survival fitness of E coli 83,972 compared with uropathogenic bacteria was initially assumed related to unique biosynthetic pathways, enabling the nonvirulent strain to more efficiently utilize metabolic compounds, such as iron and amino acids for more rapid growth.[56] Genetic sequencing studies, however, have shown surprisingly little divergence of ASB strains from uropathogenic E coli in gene expression concerning metabolic pathways.[56] It is, therefore, speculated that the superior growth of E coli 83,972 may be due to overall energy conservation, because the production of virulent-factors, such as fimbriae, are costly to produce, but the exact fitness advantage mechanisms remain largely unknown.

Use as Biotherapeutics

The ability of ASB strains to outcompete uropathogenic E coli has led to the clinical study of its use a live biotherapeutic in patients with recurrent, symptomatic UTIs. Sundén and colleagues[57] in 2010 randomized 20 patients with incomplete bladder emptying and history of recurrent UTIs to intravesical inoculation with E coli 83,972 or saline. Patients who showed elimination of the bacterial strain by sterile urine culture underwent repeat inoculations. They showed a significantly longer time to first infection (11.3 vs 5.7 months) and fewer total numbers of symptomatic infections (13 vs 35 episodes) in patients who received ASB inoculation versus saline controls. Thus, a model for deliberate ASB as a protective mechanism for patients at high risk of recurrent UTI was established. Darouiche and colleagues[58] in 2011 performed a similar study on spinal cord injury patients with a history of recurrent UTIs, inoculating

17 patients with the ASB strain E coli HU2117 and comparing results to 10 patients receiving saline placebo. They showed a significant decrease in the average number of UTIs over 1-year follow-up (0.50 episodes in the treatment group vs 1.68 in the placebo group). In a murine model, Rudick and colleagues[59] in 2014 compared the use of ASB inoculation with E coli 83,972 to ciprofloxacin to treat acute UTI. Although both treatments showed equal clearance of uropathogenic bacteria, the ASB strain provided superior reduction in pain than ciprofloxacin, comparable to that of intravesical lidocaine. In addition to its analgesic benefit, ASB inoculation was also proved effective at clearance of a wide variety of bacterial pathogens, including Proteus mirabilis, Enterococcus faecalis, and Klebsiella pneumonia. Although promising, the complexity of administration and monitoring as well as the associated expense of ASB strain inoculation may continue to limit its clinical application.

TRANSLATIONAL BARRIERS TO THE APPLICATION OF THE INFECTIOUS DISEASES SOCIETY OF AMERICA RECOMMENDATIONS

Despite the clear recommendations per the IDSA regarding diagnosing and screening of ASB, many physicians still believe that bacteriuria should be treated with antimicrobials irrespective of the lacking presence of symptoms.[60] It is uncertain whether this belief indicates clinicians' lack of awareness of the IDSA recommendations or simply their disagreement with the evidence. It has been well established that treatment of ASB with antimicrobials has been associated with higher rates of resistance, reinfection, and significant collateral damage, including Clostridium difficile–associated disease, bacterial vaginosis, and vaginal candidiasis.[7,8,61–64] The decision to order a urine culture should be guided by the presence or suspicion of symptoms related to UTI.[2] Several studies evaluating physicians attitudes toward practice recommendations indicate that up to two-thirds of clinicians are unaware of practice guidelines, perceive adopting the practice guidelines as a challenge to autonomy, have diminished confidence in the professional organization, are confused regarding the guidelines, and in some instances have a greater concern with the adverse outcomes associated with not prescribing an antimicrobial more than with the risk of downstream complications of inappropriate prescribing.[65–70] Some investigators have suggested a multifaceted approach coupled with appropriate process outcome measures to address the issue of translational barriers to the acceptance of the IDSA ASB recommendations. The foundation of this multifaceted approach is the support by administrators and medical staff leadership. Second it has been suggested that intensive education be provided, including a review of clinical practice guidelines, identification of symptoms suggestive of UTI, use of diagnostic and therapeutic algorithms for providing feedback, documentation of reasons for obtaining urine specimens, improved collection techniques, and avoiding the pitfalls of pyuria as a marker of symptomatic UTI.[3] Although sound in concept, this multifaceted approach is daunting because it is resource (time and cost) intensive. Leis and colleagues[71] reported their results of a proof-of-concept study whereby a much more simplistic approach was used. All positive noncatheterized urine culture results from hospitalized patients in their study were not reported unless the primary managing clinician made a telephone call request. Through this simple intervention, the investigators were able to demonstrate a significant reduction in antimicrobial therapy for ASB from 48% at baseline to 12% postintervention ($P = .002$). Although promising, this study can only be extrapolated to medical and surgical inpatients. Larger studies are needed to confirm its generalizability, safety, and sustainability of this model of care.

SUMMARY

ASB is a common finding and is frequently detected in premenopausal nonpregnant women, institutionalized patients, patients with diabetes mellitus, and the ambulatory elderly population. Despite clear recommendations regarding the diagnosis and management of ASB in these populations from the IDSA, there remains an alarming rate of antimicrobial overuse, which has led to issues of increasing antimicrobial resistance of bacterial pathogens and significant deleterious consequences in the form of collateral damage among this already vulnerable patient population. Despite an increased prevalence of ASB among patients with diabetes mellitus and the concern for increased risk of symptomatic UTI, pyelonephritis, and sepsis, the literature does not support screening for or treating ASB in this patient population. To date there exist microbiological evidence to support not treating ASB secondary to reduced virulence factors associated with ASB strains. Some ASB strains have been shown beneficial in reducing symptomatic lower UTIs in certain patient populations.

Despite the existence of translational barriers to the implementation of IDSA recommendations for the management of ASB among a vast array of clinicians, there have been promising data to support the implementation of simplistic strategies to address these barriers. In an era in which clinicians' face pay for performance concerns with current practice patterns not reflecting evidence based recommendations, attention needs to be focused on eliminating these translational barriers in a safe, feasible, and sustainable manner.

REFERENCES

1. Hooton TM, Bradley SF, Cardenas DD, et al. Diagnosis, prevention, and treatment of catheter-associated urinary tract infection in adults: 2009 International Clinical Practice Guidelines from the Infectious Disease Society of America. Clin Infect Dis 2010;50:625–63.
2. Nicolle LE, Bradley S, Colgan R, et al. Infectious Disease Society of America Guidelines for the diagnosis and treatment of asymptomatic bacteriuria in adults. Clin Infect Dis 2005;40:643–54.
3. Dull RB, Friedman SK, Risoldi ZM, et al. Antimicrobial treatment of asymptomatic bacteriuria in noncatheterized adults: a systematic review. Pharmacotherapy 2014;34:941–60.
4. Nicolle LE. Asymptomatic bacteriuria: when to screen and when to treat. Infect Dis Clin North Am 2003;17:367–94.
5. Zabarsky TF, Sethis AK, Donskey CJ. Sustained reduction in inappropriate treatmet of asymptomatic bacteriuria n along term care facility through and education intervention. Am J Infect Control 2008;36:476–80.
6. Loeb M, Brazil K, Lohfeld L, et al. Effect of a multifaceted intervention on number of antimicrobial prescriptions for suspected urinary tract infections in resident of nursing homes: cluster randomized controlled trial. BMJ 2005;331:669–73.
7. Linares LA, Thornton DJ, Strymish J, et al. Electronic memorandum decreases unnecessary antimicrobial use for asymptomatic bacteriuria and culture-negative pyuria. Infect Control Hosp Epidemiol 2011;32:644–8.
8. Chowdhury F, Sarkar K, Branche A, et al. Preventing the innapropriate treatment of asymptomatic bacteriuria at a community teaching hospital. J Community Hosp Intern Med Perspect 2012;2:17814.
9. Kelley D, Aaronson P, Poon E, et al. Evaluation of an antimicrobial stewardship approach to minimize overuse of antibiotics in patients with asymptomatic bacteriuria. Infect Control Hosp Epidemiol 2014;35:193–5.
10. Pavese P, Saurel N, Labarere J, et al. Does an educational session with an infectious diseas physician reduce the use of inappropriate antibiotic therapy for inpatiens with positive urine culture

results? A controlled before and after study. Infect Control Hosp Epidemiol 2009;30:596–9.

11. Ariathianto Y. Asymptomatic bacteriuria: prevalence in the elderly population. Aust Fam Physician 2011; 40:805–9.

12. Kaye D, Boscia J, Abrutyn E, et al. Asymptomatic bacteriuria in elderly. Trans Am Clin Climatol Assoc 1989;100:155–62.

13. Boscia JA, Kobasa WD, Knight RA, et al. Epidemiology of bacteriuria in an elderly ambulatory population. Am J Med 1986;80:208–14.

14. Juthani-Mehta M. Asymptomatic bacteriuria and urinary tract infection in older adults. Clin Geriatr Med 2007;23:585–94.

15. Colgan R, Nicolle LE, McGlone A, et al. Asymptomatic bacteriuria in adults. Am Fam Physician 2006; 74:985–90.

16. Linhares I, Raposo T, Rodrigues A, et al. Frequency and antimicrobial resistance patterns of bacteria implicated in community urinary tract infections. BMC Infect Dis 2013;13:19.

17. Nicolle LE. Topics in long term care: urinary tract infections in long term facilities. Infect Control Hosp Epidemiol 1993;14:220–5.

18. Matteucci E, Trolio A, Leonetti P, et al. Significant bacteriuria in outpatient diabetic and non-diabetic persons. Diabet Med 2007;24:1455–9.

19. Renko M, Tapananinen P, Tossavainen P, et al. Meta-analysis of the significance of asymptomaic bacteriuria in diabetes. Diabetes Care 2011;4: 230–5.

20. Stapleton A. Urinary tract infections in patients with diabetes. Am J Med 2002;113:80S–4S.

21. Geerlings SE, Stolk RP, Camps MJ, et al. Asymptomatic bacteriuria may be considered a complication in women with diabetes. Diabetes Mellitus Women Asymptomatic Bacteriuria Utrecht Study Group. Diabetes Care 2000;23(6):744–9.

22. Dalal S, Nicolle L, Marrs CF, et al. Long-term Escherichia coli asymptomatic bacteriuria among women with diabetes mellitus. Clin Infect Dis 2009;49(4): 491–7.

23. Geerlings SE, Brouwer EC, Gaastra W, et al. Virulence factors of Escherichia coli isolated from urine of diabetic women with asymptomatic bacteriuria: correlation with clinical characteristics. Antonie Van Leeuwenhoek 2001;80(2):119–27.

24. Geerlings SE, Brouwer EC, Gaastra W, et al. Effect of glucose and pH on uropathogenic and non-uropathogenic Escherichia coli: studies with urine from diabetic and non-diabetic individuals. J Med Microbiol 1999;48(6):535–9.

25. Geerlings SE, Meiland R, van Lith EC, et al. Adherence of type 1-fimbriated Escherichia coli to uroepithelial cells: more in diabetic women than in control subjects. Diabetes Care 2002; 25(8):1405–9.

26. Geerlings SE, Stolk RP, Camps MJ, et al. Risk factors for symptomatic urinary tract infection in women with diabetes. Diabetes Care 2000;23(12):1737–41.

27. Balasoiu D, van Kessel KC, van Kats-Renaud HJ, et al. Granulocyte function in women with diabetes and asymptomatic bacteriuria. Diabetes Care 1997;20(3):392–5.

28. Geerlings SE, Brouwer EC, Van Kessel KC, et al. Cytokine secretion is impaired in women with diabetes mellitus. Eur J Clin Invest 2000;30(11): 995–1001.

29. Meiland R, Geerlings SE, Stolk RP, et al. Asymptomatic bacteriuria in women with diabetes mellitus: effect on renal function after 6 years of follow-up. Arch Intern Med 2006;166(20):2222–7.

30. Harding GK, Zhanel GG, Nicolle LE, et al, Manitoba Diabetes Urinary Tract Infection Study Group. Antimicrobial treatment in diabetic women with asymptomatic bacteriuria. N Engl J Med 2002;347(20): 1576–83.

31. Nielubowicz GR, Mobley HL. Host-pathogen interactions in urinary tract infection. Nat Rev Urol 2010;8: 430–41.

32. Mobley HL, Donnenberg MS, Hagan EC. EcoSal – Escherichia coli and Salmonella: cellular and molecular biology. Washington, DC: ASM Press; 2009.

33. Welsh RA, Burland V, Plunkett G, et al. Extensive mosaic structure revealed by the complete genome sequence of uropathogenic Escherichia coli. Proc Natl Acad Sci U S A 2002;99:17020–4.

34. Plos K, Connell H, Jodal U, et al. Intestinal carriage of P fimbriated Escherichia coli and the susceptibility to urinary tract infection in young children. J Infect Dis 1995;3:625–31.

35. Vaisanen V, Elo J, Tallgren LG, et al. Mannose-resistant haemagglutination and P antigen recognition are characteristic of Escherichia coli causing primary pyelonephritis. Lancet 1981;2(8260–61): 1366–9.

36. Leffler H, Svanborg-Eden C. Chemical identification of a glycosphingolipid receptor for Escherichia coli attaching to human urinary tract epithelial cells and agglutinating human erythrocytes. FEMS Microbiol Lett 1980;8:127–34.

37. Mulvey MA, Schilling JD, Martinez JJ, et al. Bad bugs and beleaguered bladders: interplay between uropathogenic Escherichia coli and innate host defenses. Proc Natl Acad Sci U S A 2000;97(16): 8829–35.

38. Pak J, Pu Y, Zhang ZT, et al. Tamm-Horsfall protein binds to type 1 fimbriated Escherichia coli and prevents E. coli from binding to uroplakin Ia and Ib receptors. J Biol Chem 2001;276(13): 9924–30.

39. Schembri MA, Ussery DW, Workman C, et al. DNA microarray analysis of fim mutations in Escherichia coli. Mol Genet Genomics 2002;267(6):721–9.

40. Bergsten G, Wullt B, Svanborg C. Escherichia coli, fimbriae, bacterial persistence and host response induction in the human urinary tract. Int J Med Microbiol 2005;295(6–7):487–502.

41. Mabbett AN, Ulett GC, Watts RE, et al. Virulence properties of asymptomatic bacteriuria Escherichia coli. Int J Med Microbiol 2009;299(1):53–63.

42. Spurbeck RR, Stapleton AE, Johnson JR, et al. Fimbrial profiles predict virulence of uropathogenic Escherichia coli strains: contribution of ygi and yad fimbriae. Infect Immun 2011;79(12):4753–63.

43. Ragnarsdóttir B, Svanborg C. Susceptibility to acute pyelonephritis or asymptomatic bacteriuria: host-pathogen interaction in urinary tract infections. Pediatr Nephrol 2012;27(11):2017–29.

44. Svanborg-Edén C, Hagberg L, Hull R, et al. Bacterial virulence versus host resistance in the urinary tracts of mice. Infect Immun 1987;55(5):1224–32.

45. Rudick CN, Billips BK, Pavlov VI, et al. Host-pathogen interactions mediating pain of urinary tract infection. J Infect Dis 2010;201:1240–9.

46. Smith YC, Rasmussen SB, Grande KK, et al. Hemolysin of uropathogenic Escherichia coli evokes extensive shedding of the uroepithelium and hemorrhage in bladder tissue within the first 24 hours after intraurethral inoculation of mice. Infect Immun 2008;76(7):2978–90.

47. Boquet P. The cytotoxic necrotizing factor 1 (CNF1) from uropathogenic Escherichia coli. Adv Exp Med Biol 2000;485:45–51.

48. Mills M, Meysick KC, O'Brien AD. Cytotoxic necrotizing factor type 1 of uropathogenic Escherichia coli kills cultured human uroepithelial 5637 cells by an apoptotic mechanism. Infect Immun 2000;68(10):5869–80.

49. Rippere-Lampe KE, O'Brien AD, Conran R, et al. Mutation of the gene encoding cytotoxic necrotizing factor type 1 (cnf(1)) attenuates the virulence of uropathogenic Escherichia coli. Infect Immun 2001;69(6):3954–64.

50. Hedlund M, Duan RD, Nilsson A, et al. Sphingomyelin, glycosphingolipids and ceramide signalling in cells exposed to P-fimbriated Escherichia coli. Mol Microbiol 1998;29(5):1297–306.

51. Ragnarsdóttir B, Samuelsson M, Gustafsson MC, et al. Reduced toll-like receptor 4 expression in children with asymptomatic bacteriuria. J Infect Dis 2007;196(3):475–84.

52. Lindberg U, Hanson LA, Jodal U, et al. Asymptomatic bacteriuria in schoolgirls. II. Differences in escherichia coli causing asymptomatic bacteriuria. Acta Paediatr Scand 1975;64(3):432–6.

53. Roos V, Ulett GC, Schembri MA, et al. The asymptomatic bacteriuria Escherichia coli strain 83972 outcompetes uropathogenic E. coli strains in human urine. Infect Immun 2006;74(1):615–24.

54. Darouiche RO, Donovan WH, Del Terzo M, et al. Pilot trial of bacterial interference for preventing urinary tract infection. Urology 2001;58(3):339–44.

55. Hull R, Rudy D, Donovan W, et al. Urinary tract infection prophylaxis using Escherichia coli 83972 in spinal cord injured patients. J Urol 2000;163(3):872–7.

56. Vejborg RM, Hancock V, Schembri MA, et al. Comparative genomics of Escherichia coli strains causing urinary tract infections. Appl Environ Microbiol 2011;77(10):3268–78.

57. Sundén F, Håkansson L, Ljunggren E, et al. Escherichia coli 83972 bacteriuria protects against recurrent lower urinary tract infections in patients with incomplete bladder emptying. J Urol 2010;184(1):179–85.

58. Darouiche RO, Green BG, Donovan WH, et al. Multicenter randomized controlled trial of bacterial interference for prevention of urinary tract infection in patients with neurogenic bladder. Urology 2011;78(2):341–6.

59. Rudick CN, Taylor AK, Yaggie RE, et al. Asymptomatic bacteriuria Escherichia coli are live biotherapeutics for UTI. PLoS One 2014;9(11):1–9.

60. Midthun S, Paur R, Bruce AW, et al. Urinary tract infections in the elderly: a survey of physicians an nurses. Geriatr Nurs 2005;26:245–51.

61. Asscher AW, Sussman M, Waters WE, et al. The clinical significance of asymptomatic bacteriuria in the nonpregnant woman. J Infect Dis 1969;120:17–26.

62. Giamarellou H, Iakovou M, Pistoni M, et al. Kinetics and comparative efficacy of ofloxacin verus co-trimoxazole in the asymptomatic bacteriuria of elderly subjects. Chemotherapy 1991;37:19–24.

63. Nicolle LE, Mayhew WJ, Bryan L. Prospective randomized comparison of therapy and no therapy for asymptomatic bacteriuria in institutionalized elderly women. Am J Med 1987;83:27–33.

64. Giamarellou H, Iakovou M, Pistoni M, et al. Kinetics and comparative efficacy of ofloxacin versus co-trimoxazole in the asymptomatic bacteriuria of elderly subjects. Chemotherapy 1991;37:19–24.

65. Wolfe RM, Sharp L, Wang RM. Family physicians' opinions and attitudes to three clinical practice guidelines. J Am Board Fam Pract 2004;17:150–7.

66. Wolff SH, Grol R, Hutchinson A, et al. Clinical guidelines: potential benefits, limitations, and harms of clinical guidelines. BMJ 1999;318:527–30.

67. James PA, Cowan TM, Graham RP, et al. Family physician's attitudes about and use of clinical practice guidelines. Fam Pract 1997;45:341–7.

68. Borowski NM, Allen WR. Does attribution theory explain physicians's nonacceptance of clinical practice guidelines? Hosp Top 2003;81:9–21.

69. Mueller KL, Harris JS, Low P, et al. Acceptance and self-reported use of national occupational medicine practice guidelines. J Occup Environ Med 2000; 42:362–9.

70. James PA, Cowan TM, Graham RP. Patient-centered clinical decisions and their impact on physician adherence to clinical guidelines. J Fam Pract 1998;46:311–8.

71. Leis JA, Rebick GW, Daneman N, et al. Reducing antimicrobial therapy for asymptomatic bacteriuria among noncatheterized inpatients: a proof-of-concept study. Clin Infect Dis 2014;58:980–3.

Urinary Tract Infection and Bacteriuria in Pregnancy

Alexander P. Glaser, MD, Anthony J. Schaeffer, MD*

KEYWORDS

- Urinary tract infection • Bacteriuria • Antimicrobials • Urinary tract infection • Pyelonephritis
- Pregnancy

KEY POINTS

- Antimicrobial choice in pregnancy should reflect safety for both the mother and the fetus.
- During pregnancy, asymptomatic bacteriuria (ASB) significantly increases the risk of pyelonephritis and subsequent maternal and fetal complications. Treatment of ASB significantly reduces these risks.
- Pregnant patients should be screened for ASB at least once early in pregnancy, and, if culture is positive, treated for 3 to 7 days. These patients should be followed with serial cultures throughout pregnancy, and prophylactic antimicrobial therapy should be considered.
- Pregnant patients with cystitis should also be treated for 3 to 7 days. These patients should be followed with serial cultures throughout pregnancy, and prophylactic antimicrobial therapy should be considered.
- Pregnant patients with pyelonephritis should initially be admitted for intravenous antimicrobial therapy and receive a total of 7 to 14 days of culture-directed treatment. These patients should be followed with serial cultures throughout pregnancy, and prophylactic antimicrobial therapy should be strongly considered.

INTRODUCTION

Urinary tract infections (UTIs) during pregnancy may be classified as asymptomatic bacteriuria (ASB), infections of the lower urinary tract (cystitis), or infections of the upper urinary tract (pyelonephritis). Lower tract bacteriuria (ASB or cystitis) is associated with a 20% to 30% increased risk of developing pyelonephritis in pregnancy, likely due to the physiologic changes of the urinary tract during pregnancy.[1–3] Both lower and upper urinary tract bacteriuria, including ASB, are associated with adverse maternal and fetal outcomes, including preterm birth.[4–10] Therefore, screening and treatment of bacteriuria during pregnancy have become standard of care recommended by multiple professional organizations.[2,11–15]

A.P. Glaser has nothing to disclose. A.J. Schaeffer has the following relationships to disclose: Advanstar Communications Inc (author honorarium); Boehringer Ingelheim International GmbH (advisory board participant); ClearView Healthcare Partners (consultant honorarium); Hollister Incorporated (consultant honorarium); KLJ Associates, Inc (consultant honorarium); Melinta Therapeutics, Inc (advisory board participant); Navigant Consulting, Inc (consultant honorarium); Philadelphia Urological Society (speaker honorarium); UpToDate, Inc (royalty payments for author contribution).
Department of Urology, Northwestern University, 303 East Chicago Avenue, Tarry 16-703, Chicago, IL 60611, USA
* Corresponding author. Department of Urology, Northwestern University, Tarry Building Room 16-703, 300 East Superior, Chicago, IL 60611.
E-mail address: ajschaeffer@northwestern.edu

Urol Clin N Am 42 (2015) 547–560
http://dx.doi.org/10.1016/j.ucl.2015.05.004
0094-0143/15/$ – see front matter © 2015 Elsevier Inc. All rights reserved.

PATHOGENESIS

The urinary tract is sterile under normal circumstances. Bacteriuria generally occurs because of ascending bacteria from a fecal reservoir or vaginal/perineal skin flora.[16] Pathogenic organisms in pregnant women are similar to those found in the nonpregnant population. *Escherichia coli* is the most common pathogen, representing 70% to 80% of all UTIs in pregnancy.[7,8,16–19] Enterobacteriaceae, including *Klebsiella* and *Enterobacter*, are also common pathogens, and infections with other gram-negative organisms such as *Proteus*, *Pseudomonas*, and *Citrobacter* can occur.[7,8,16–20] Gram-positive organisms, mostly group B *Streptococci* (GBS), are also common pathogens and are the cause of up to 10% of UTIs in pregnant women.[17,20] Infection with other microorganisms, including *Mycoplasma hominis*, *Ureaplasma parvum*, *Gardnerella vaginalis*, lactobacilli, and *Chlamydia trachomatis*, have also been described.[21–23]

URINARY TRACT CHANGES IN PREGNANCY

The entire urinary tract is anatomically and physiologically altered in pregnant women (**Table 1**).[1] Together, these upper and lower urinary tract changes are thought to increase the risk of development of pyelonephritis from ASB and lower UTIs.[4,7] During pregnancy, renal length increases by approximately 1 cm and glomerular filtration rate increases by approximately 30% to 50%.[1] Mild hydroureteronephrosis is observable as early as the seventh week of gestation.[5] This dilation is due to the overall decreased peristalsis in the collecting system and ureters, attributable to both the muscle-relaxing effects of progesterone and the progressive mechanical obstruction from the gravid uterus.[1,3,5,24] During pregnancy, the bladder also experiences progressive superior and anterior displacement as well as hypertrophy and smooth muscle relaxation, leading to increased capacity and urinary stasis.[1,3,24–26]

ANTIMICROBIALS IN PREGNANCY
Choice of Treatment

Choice of antimicrobials during pregnancy must reflect safety considerations for both the mother and the fetus. In the mother, physiologic changes in pregnancy can alter pharmacokinetics and decrease serum drug concentrations; changes include increased maternal fluid intravascular and extravascular fluid volumes, increased renal blood flow, increased glomerular filtration rate, and drug distribution to the fetus.[27,28] Most antimicrobials cross the placenta, and drugs that can cause teratogenesis or other harm to the fetus should be avoided. Despite this known risk, few large-scale trials on antimicrobial use during pregnancy have been performed because of logistical and ethical issues. Much of the known drug safety data derives from studies when pregnant women were not excluded from new therapies,[29,30] or from data extracted from animal models and observational studies.[27,28,31]

The US Food and Drug Administration (FDA) previously published a classification system for drugs in pregnancy, labeling medications either class A, B, C, D, or X. This system was widely panned as being unhelpful because of a lack of high-quality data, therefore leading to classification of most drugs, including antimicrobials, as category C ("animal studies have shown an adverse effect on the fetus and there are no adequate and well-controlled studies in humans, but potential benefits may warrant use of the drug in pregnant women despite potential risks").[28,32] In December 2014, the FDA approved a rule to remove the pregnancy categories A, B, C, D, and X from drug product labeling and instead instituted a new system for labeling medications in pregnancy that is intended to be more practical and help guide decision-making by physicians and patients.[33] Labeling changes go into effect in June 2015.

Despite a lack of high-quality safety data, many antimicrobials have been used in pregnancy for years without adverse maternal or fetal outcomes, including penicillins, cephalosporins, clindamycin, and macrolides (**Table 2**).[27,28] Recent meta-analyses found no evidence to support one particular antimicrobial over another for either ASB[34] or symptomatic UTIs.[35] Therefore, after reviewing safety profiles of antimicrobials, choice of empiric treatment should reflect local antibiograms and

Table 1 Urinary tract changes in pregnancy	
Kidneys	Increased renal length Increased glomerular filtration rate by 30%–50%
Collecting System	Decreased peristalsis
Ureters	Decreased peristalsis Mechanical obstruction
Bladder	Displaced anteriorly and superiorly Smooth muscle relaxation Increased capacity

Data from Waltzer WC. The urinary tract in pregnancy. J Urol 1981;125(3):271–6.

Table 2
Antimicrobials in pregnancy

Drug	Fetal Toxicity	Comments	Prior FDA Category
Penicillins			
Penicillin G	Low risk	Commonly used	B
Amoxicillin	Low risk	Commonly used	B
Ampicillin	Low risk	Commonly used	B
Cephalosporins			
Cephalexin	Low risk	1st generation; commonly used	B
Cefuroxime	Low risk	2nd generation; commonly used	B
Ceftriaxone	Low risk	3rd generation; commonly used	B
Ceftazidime	Low risk (limited data)	3rd generation with antipseudomonal coverage	B
Cefepime	Low risk (limited data)	4th generation with antipseudomonal coverage	B
Monobactams			
Aztreonam	Low risk (limited data)	Limited data; consider ID consultation	B
Carbapenems			
Imipenem	Very limited data	Limited data; must be administered with cilastatin; consider ID consultation	C
Meropenem	Very limited data	Limited data; consider ID consultation	B
Lincosamides			
Clindamycin	Low risk	Commonly used; useful in penicillin-allergic patients	B
Macrolides			
Azithromycin	Low risk	Commonly used	B
Erythromycin	Low risk	More gastrointestinal side effects than azithromycin	
Nitrofurans			
Nitrofurantoin	Controversial teratogenic risk; risk of hemolytic anemia in G6PD deficiency during third trimester	Commonly used; use for only for lower UTIs	B
Phosphonics			
Fosfomycin	Low risk (limited data)	Use for only for lower UTIs	B
Sulfonamides			
Sulfadiazine	Risk of antifolate teratogenesis; risk of hyperbilirubinemia in third trimester	Avoid if alternatives available	C
Trimethoprim-sulfamethoxazole	Risk of antifolate teratogenesis	Avoid in pregnancy	C
Glycopeptides			
Vancomycin	Very limited data	Limited data; consider ID consultation	B

(continued on next page)

Table 2
(continued)

Drug	Fetal Toxicity	Comments	Prior FDA Category
Oxazolidinones			
Linezolid	Only case reports available	Limited data; consider ID consultation	C
Lipopeptides			
Daptomycin	Only case reports available	Limited data; consider ID consultation	B
Aminoglycosides			
Gentamycin	Potential risks of ototoxicity and nephrotoxicity	Commonly used; useful for pyelonephritis	C
Fluoroquinolones			
Ciprofloxacin	Theoretic risk of arthropathy	Avoid in pregnancy	C
Tetracyclines			
Tetracycline	Risk of teratogenicity and discoloration of teeth/bones	Avoid in pregnancy	D
Doxycycline	—	Avoid in pregnancy	D

Abbreviations: G6PD, glucose-6-phosphate dehydrogenase; ID, infectious disease.
Data from Refs.[18,27,28,44]

susceptibility patterns, and final treatment should be tailored to culture-directed data.[11] Cost-effective choices should also be considered.[36] Finally, as with all patients, health care providers should prescribe antimicrobials for pregnant patients only for appropriate indications and duration, and after discussing the benefits and potential risks of treatment.

Antimicrobial Resistance

The prevalence of multi-drug-resistant (MDR) organisms is increasing at an alarming pace in the general population.[37–40] In addition, few drugs are being developed to combat the spread of resistance.[37,39] Although the spread of MDR organisms to the pregnant population has not been widely reported, it is likely that this challenge will be encountered in the future,[41] stressing the need for culture-directed therapy and clinician-driven antimicrobial stewardship.[42]

Penicillins

Penicillins are one of the oldest groups of antimicrobials and have been used for many years in pregnancy without known adverse effects.[43,44] Their safety profile has been confirmed in multiple studies.[31,44–47] These β-lactams include penicillin G, ampicillin, and amoxicillin. Although resistance is common, these drugs are considered first-line therapy for susceptible bacteria, especially for GBS.[28,31,36,43,48]

Cephalosporins

Cephalosporins are also a group of β-lactam antimicrobials with a well-established safety profile in pregnancy.[27,28,31,36,43,44,48,49] Susceptible bacteria vary with the different generations. Third-generation cephalosporins are particularly useful because of their excellent coverage of gram-negative organisms as well as some gram-positive organisms and are often used empirically in the treatment of pyelonephritis. In addition, certain third-generation cephalosporins such as ceftazidime have antipseudomonal activity. It is important to remember that none of the cephalosporins are effective against Enterococcus. More data in pregnancy are available for the earlier generations of cephalosporins, including cephalexin and cefuroxime, yet overall the cephalosporins are considered generally safe in pregnancy.[28,48]

Monobactams

Aztreonam is the only monocyclic β-lactam antimicrobial currently commercially available. It is effective against many gram-negative organisms and has low cross-reactivity in penicillin-allergic patients, but must be administered intravenously or intramuscularly. Limited data are available on the use of aztreonam in pregnancy, yet the risk of adverse events or teratogenicity is considered low.[27,50]

Carbapenems

Carabenems are a class of β-lactam antimicrobials that are resistant to the extended-spectrum β-lactamase enzymes made by MDR gram-negative bacteria.[40,51] They are available in intravenous form only. Because of their limited indications for use and relatively recent development, data on safety of these drugs in pregnancy are scarce.[27,36]

Clindamycin

Clindamycin, a lincosamide antimicrobial, is useful in penicillin-allergic patients for treatment of infections caused by Staphylococcus and GBS. It is not active against Enterococcus or most aerobic gram-negative bacteria. Clindamycin can cause diarrhea in up to 10% of patients, and rarely, pseudomembranous colitis, but there are no known studies associating clindamycin with teratogenicity.[27,28,36,44,52]

Macrolides

The macrolide antimicrobials, such as erythromycin, azithromycin, and clarithromycin, are useful for treatment of Staphylococcus infections, with limited activity against gram-negative pathogens. The most common side effect is gastrointestinal upset, especially with erythromycin. Macrolide antimicrobials have a long safety record in pregnancy, and large studies have not found associations between macrolide use and teratogenic risk.[27,28,36,53,54]

Nitrofurantoin

Nitrofurantoin is a unique antimicrobial specifically useful for lower UTIs. It achieves therapeutic levels in the urine but not in tissue and therefore should not be used to treat pyelonephritis. For lower UTIs, nitrofurantoin is useful because of limited resistance and bactericidal activity against many common uropathogens, including E coli, Enterococcus faecalis, Klebsiella spp, Staphylococcus saprophyticus, and Staphylococcus aureus, although it does not have activity against Proteus, Serratia, or Pseudomonas.[36,55]

Safety data for nitrofurantoin are conflicting. The National Birth Defects Prevention Study recently demonstrated an association between nitrofurantoin and congenital malformations, such as anophthalmia, microphthalmia, atrial septal defects, and cleft lip and palate.[31] However, results from this retrospective case-control study should be interpreted with caution because of recall bias and other flaws associated with this study design (for example, only 35% of patients could recall the drug name they were given).[31,48] Two recent population-based studies demonstrated no increase in teratogenicity in patients exposed to nitrofurantoin.[56,57] The American Congress of Obstetricians and Gynecologists (ACOG) supports appropriate use of nitrofurantoin in the first trimester when no suitable alternatives are available, and as a first-line agent in the second and third trimesters.[48]

Aside from potential teratogenic risks, there are known rare but serious risks, including pulmonary toxicity[58] and hemolytic anemia, in patients with glucose-6-phosphate dehydrogenate deficiency; nitrofurantoin should therefore be avoided in these patients.[59] Nitrofurantoin is also contraindicated at term and in the neonate less than 1 month of age because neonates have immature enzymatic activity and insufficient quantities of reduced glutathione in circulating neonatal red blood cells, leading to risk of hemolytic anemia.[60,61]

Fosfomycin

Fosfomycin, a phosphonic acid derivative, is a broad-spectrum antimicrobial not commonly used in clinical practice in the United States that may see resurgence in use because of increasing antimicrobial resistance.[62,63] It has no structural analogues to other antimicrobials and is useful against many MDR organisms, including extended-spectrum β-lactamase-producing organisms, Pseudomonas, methicillin-resistant S aureus, and vancomycin-resistant Enterococcus.[62,63] Use of fosfomycin in pregnancy has been studied primarily because it achieves high concentrations in the urine for up to 3 days, making it an attractive choice for treatment of uncomplicated lower UTIs.[62–64] Gastrointestinal upset is the most common adverse event.[63] Although there are no adequate studies specifically examining teratogenic risk, several trials have examined the use of single-dose fosfomycin for treatment of ASB and lower UTIs in pregnancy with no reported adverse outcomes.[34,62,65–68] Overall, fosfomycin has a broad spectrum of activity against many MDR organisms, and it may have an increasing role in the antimicrobial armamentarium for treatment of lower UTIs.

Sulfonamides and Trimethoprim

Sulfonamides and the combination drug trimethoprim-sulfamethoxasole are not recommended as first-line agents in pregnancy. Sulfonamides inhibit folate synthesis and therefore have been implicated in antifolate teratogenicity.[27,28,36,69] In the National Birth Defects Prevention Study, sulfonamides were associated with more congenital defects than any other antimicrobial.[31] However, other studies have not demonstrated this risk,[70] and ACOG states that sulfonamide treatment remains appropriate in the first trimester when no other suitable antimicrobial alternatives are available.[48] Aside from teratogenic risk, sulfonamides have also been reported to cause hyperbilirubinemia and kernicterus when used in the third trimester.[27]

Trimethoprim, a dihydrofolate reductase inhibitor, is also associated with antifolate teratogenicity and should be avoided in pregnancy.[69]

Aminoglycosides

The aminoglycosides, gentamycin, amikacin, and tobramycin, are effective for treating gram-negative bacilli and are often useful in the treatment of pyelonephritis in combination with ampicillin.[28,70] However, aminoglycosides have potential risks of ototoxicity and nephrotoxicity in both the mother and the fetus.[27,28,71,72] Gentamycin is the preferred aminoglycoside in obstetrics, if needed, because of its comparatively superior safety profile and low cost.[36] Despite potential risks, no teratogenicity or neonatal ototoxicity or nephrotoxicity has been reported after administration of gentamycin in pregnancy, and gentamycin is widely used.[28,44]

Quinolones

Quinolones, including ciprofloxacin and levofloxacin, achieve high tissue concentrations, making them effective choices for pyelonephritis in nonpregnant patients, yet they are generally avoided during pregnancy because of possible arthropathies and teratogenicity.[27,28] Quinolone exposure in animal models can induce abnormal cartilage development.[73] Interestingly, despite this risk, when pregnant women were exposed to quinolones, adverse events have not been consistently demonstrated.[31,74,75] Overall, this class of antimicrobials should be avoided in pregnancy if suitable alternatives are available.

Tetracyclines

Tetracycline and doxycycline should not be used in pregnancy, because they are associated with teratogenicity as well as discoloration of the bones and teeth.[27–30]

Vancomycin

Vancomycin is a glycopeptide antimicrobial useful for treatment of methicillin-resistant S aureus and other resistant gram-positive organisms such as Enterococcus. Its use is associated with potential nephrotoxicity and ototoxicity,[76] although these effects have not been demonstrated in the few published reports of vancomycin use in pregnancy.[44,77,78] Because of the very limited evidence of vancomycin use in pregnancy, it should be used with caution only when no alternatives exist.

Linezolid, Daptomycin, and Newer Antimicrobials

Even less is known about the use of newer antimicrobials in pregnancy at this time. Only case reports of linezolid, an oxazolidone antimicrobial,[79,80] and daptomycin, a lipopeptide antimicrobial,[81] have been published in the literature to date. Fittingly, these drugs should be used with extreme caution in pregnancy and with consideration of infectious disease consultation.

ASYMPTOMATIC BACTERIURIA IN PREGNANCY
Definition

ASB is the presence of significant bacteriuria without symptoms, such as dysuria, urgency, frequency, hematuria, or suprapubic discomfort. The Infectious Diseases Society of America (IDSA) defines ASB as 2 consecutive voided cultures with 10^5 or more colony-forming units of the same bacteria, or a single catheterized urine specimen with 10^2 or more colony-forming units of one bacterium.[2] This definition is based on observations from asymptomatic nonpregnant women who, when screened for ASB with urine cultures, only had confirmed bacteriuria in a second culture 80% of the time.[4,82–84] The United States Preventative Services Task Force (USPTF), ACOG, and others recommend screening with one urine culture and do not clarify whether this culture should be repeated to confirm the diagnosis of ASB.[12–15] Although a single culture may overestimate the prevalence of bacteriuria, it is reasonable to treat ASB without a confirmatory culture in the pregnant population.

Epidemiology

Pregnancy alone is not a risk factor for ASB; ASB occurs in 2% to 10% of pregnant and nonpregnant women (see **Table 3**).[2,85–87] The incidence of ASB in nonpregnant women increases with advancing age, the presence of diabetes, sexual activity, history of prior UTI, and anatomic or functional urinary tract abnormalities.[2,85,88–90] In pregnant women, socioeconomic status and parity have been inconsistently associated with prevalence of ASB.[91–95]

Table 3
Incidence, diagnosis, and recommended treatment and follow-up of asymptomatic bacteriuria, cystitis, and pyelonephritis

	Incidence (%)	Diagnosis	Treatment Duration (d)	Follow-up
ASB	2–10	• No symptoms • Bacteriuria	3–7	• Periodic screening for recurrent bacteriuria • Consider antimicrobial prophylaxis
Lower UTI (cystitis)	1–2	• Dysuria • Urgency • Frequency • Hematuria • Suprapubic discomfort • Bacteriuria	3–7	• Periodic screening for recurrent bacteriuria • Consider antimicrobial prophylaxis
Upper UTI (pyelonephritis)	≤1	• Fever • Chills • Flank pain • Nausea • Vomiting • Bacteriuria	7–14	• Periodic screening for recurrent bacteriuria • Strongly consider antimicrobial prophylaxis

Data from Refs.[2,12,34,35,124]

Significance

Unlike in the general population, ASB should be screened for and treated in pregnant women. If left untreated, up to 40% of pregnant women with ASB may develop pyelonephritis.[2,4–6] Treatment of ASB with antimicrobials significantly decreases the risk of symptomatic infection and pyelonephritis.[6,96,97] Untreated bacteriuria is also associated with preterm birth and low birth weight, likely due to association with pyelonephritis,[20,21,96,98–102] although this link remains controversial due to possible confounders and has not been consistently reported.[103–105]

Because of the outdated nature of much of the data linking ASB to pyelonephritis from the early antibiotic era, unclear methodology in these publications, and the possible consequences of antimicrobial overuse in the era of MDR organisms, a study is currently re-examining the significance of ASB. This trial is examining the benefits and cost-effectiveness of screening low-risk pregnant women for ASB at 16 and 22 weeks' gestation and then randomizing patients with a positive culture to treatment with either placebo or 5 days of nitrofurantoin (Netherlands Trial Registry NTR3068).[106] Primary outcomes are maternal pyelonephritis and preterm delivery. This study is being performing in the Netherlands, one of the few countries where screening and treatment of ASB in pregnancy is not currently standard of care.

Screening

The USPTF, IDSA, ACOG, American Academy of Pediatrics (AAP), and the American Academy of Family Physicians (AAFP) recommend screening pregnant women for ASB.[2,12,14,15] The IDSA, AAP, and ACOG recommend pregnant women be screened with a urine culture early in pregnancy,[2,14] whereas the USPTF and AAFP recommend screening with a urine culture at 12–16 weeks' gestation, or at the first prenatal visit, if this occurs later.[12,15]

If the initial culture is negative, the IDSA and others do not make a specific recommendation for or against repeated screening for ASB, because there is limited evidence to guide timing of screening.[2] Conflicting data exist on the incidence of ASB after 20 weeks' gestation.[87,107,108] However, only 1% to 2% of women with an initial negative culture obtained early in pregnancy will develop pyelonephritis later, and no data exist to date that additional screening decreases this risk.[2,84,86,109]

The gold standard screening test for ASB in pregnancy is a urine culture.[2,12] Culture should be obtained midstream.[110] Many studies have examined alternative tests because urine cultures are expensive, are labor-intensive, and require a period of 24 to 48 hours before a result is determined; however, at this time, an inexpensive, rapid, sensitive, and specific alternative to culture has not been proven. Urinalysis and urine dipstick are specific, but not sensitive, for bacteriuria, and therefore, use in screening would result in many false-negative results.[13,107,111–118] Urine dipslide, a variant method of urine culture that uses an agar-soaked plastic paddle attached to a plastic vial, is both sensitive and specific for bacteriuria in pregnancy and could be useful in countries with limited resources and microbiologist availability.[114] However, further validation is needed, especially in standard daily practice.[119] Therefore, in light of the consequences of bacteriuria and pyelonephritis in the obstetric population, and because culture data are vital to tailor appropriate antimicrobial therapy in the era of increased antimicrobial resistance, urine culture remains the recommended screening test.

Treatment

Antimicrobial treatment of ASB in pregnancy eliminates bacteriuria and significantly reduces the incidence of pyelonephritis.[96] There is insufficient evidence to recommend one specific drug over another,[34] and the ideal treatment duration also remains debatable, ranging from a single dose to 7 days of treatment. Most single-dose regimens are based on the unique pharmacokinetic properties of fosfomycin, which achieves high concentrations in the urine for up to 3 days after treatment with a single 3 g oral dose.[63,64,66–68] However, single doses of nitrofurantoin, sulfa, amoxicillin, and trimethoprim have also been examined.[34,67] A Cochrane Review of the duration of antimicrobial therapy in 13 studies reported that single-dose therapy may be less effective than a 7-day regimen.[34] The IDSA recommends a treatment duration of 3 to 7 days.[2]

Follow-up and Prevention

Options for follow-up after treatment of ASB include close surveillance or antimicrobial prophylactic therapy. Up to one-third of patients treated for ASB will have recurrent bacteriuria after treatment if prophylaxis is not instituted, and therefore, periodic screening for recurrent bacteriuria is recommended.[2,120,121] Daily prophylactic therapy with 50 to 100 mg of nitrofurantoin should also be considered. Although there is limited high-quality evidence that antimicrobial prophylaxis decreases bacteriuria in pregnancy,[122,123] this is a well-established therapy in nonpregnant patients.[124] Postcoital prophylaxis can also be considered.[125] However, nonpharmacologic prophylaxis such as cranberry juice supplementation is not recommended, because it has not been proven to reduce ASB in pregnancy and is associated with a high dropout rate, and efficacy even in nonpregnant patients remains controversial.[126]

LOWER URINARY TRACT INFECTIONS (CYSTITIS)

A symptomatic lower UTI (cystitis) is diagnosed based on the presence of symptoms such as dysuria, urgency, frequency, hematuria, and suprapubic discomfort in combination with bacteriuria. The incidence of cystitis during pregnancy is less well characterized than ASB but is estimated at 1% to 2% (**Table 3**).[98,101,127]

Diagnosis, treatment, and follow-up of symptomatic lower UTI are identical to those for ASB. Urine culture remains the diagnostic modality of choice. As with ASB, there is no evidence to support one specific antimicrobial regimen over another for treatment of symptomatic UTI, and treatment is recommended for 3 to 7 days.[35] Follow-up, including periodic screening for recurrent bacteriuria and consideration of daily antimicrobial prophylactic therapy, is also recommended after treatment.[122–125]

UPPER URINARY TRACT INFECTIONS (PYELONEPHRITIS)
Epidemiology

The incidence of pyelonephritis in the ASB screening era is 1% or less (see **Table 3**).[17,20,99,128] This incidence is decreased from an incidence of 4% or higher before routine screening and treatment of ASB was initiated.[4–6] Risk factors for pyelonephritis include ASB, young age, nulliparity, previous episodes of pyelonephritis, sickle-cell disease/trait, diabetes, and other immunosuppression.[17,20,128] Pyelonephritis occurs more often in the second and third trimesters, when stasis and hydronephrosis are most evident, and only 10% to 20% of pyelonephritis occur in the first trimester.[17,129]

Significance

As stated previously, up to 40% of pregnant women with untreated ASB develop pyelonephritis,[2,4–6] which may also be associated with preterm birth and low birth weight,[20,21,96,98–102] although this remains controversial.[103–105] In addition to the potential detrimental effects on the fetus, pyelonephritis is also associated with maternal morbidity. Maternal complications of pyelonephritis include anemia, acute kidney injury, sepsis, pulmonary insufficiency, and acute respiratory distress syndrome.[17,20,98,128–130] Maternal morbidity of pyelonephritis is similar across all 3 trimesters.[129]

Diagnosis

Pyelonephritis is a clinical diagnosis consisting of symptoms such as fever, chills, flank pain, nausea, vomiting, and costovertebral angle tenderness in the presence of bacteriuria and pyuria.[11,16,131,132] Imaging is not required to diagnose pyelonephritis. Urine culture is the diagnostic test of choice. Whether routine blood cultures should also be obtained for pregnant patients with pyelonephritis has not yet been adequately studied. Approximately 20% to 30% of blood cultures will be positive in pregnant patients with pyelonephritis.[17,133] However, discrepancies between positive blood and urine cultures are rare and excluding routine blood cultures would result in significant cost savings.[133] A recent *Cochrane Review* concluded that there was insufficient evidence at this time to conclude if routine blood cultures should be obtained in pregnant women with pyelonephritis.[134]

Treatment

Pregnant patients with pyelonephritis should be admitted and treated with intravenous antimicrobials and hydration. Initial antimicrobial therapy is empiric and should be tailored to culture results. Empiric treatment options include ampicillin plus gentamycin or a single-agent cephalosporin such as ceftriaxone.[35,132,133] Historically, these regimens have resulted in 95% or better response rates within 72 hours,[17,35,120,133,135,136] although resistance to ampicillin alone approaches 50% in contemporary studies.[133] No single-treatment regimen has been proven to be superior to others,[17,35,133,135,136] and individual treatments should be tailored to local antibiograms and susceptibility patterns.

There are no organizational guidelines on the duration of treatment of pyelonephritis in pregnant women; however, most recommend a treatment course of 7 to 14 days,[16,17,35,132,133] in line with IDSA recommendations for nonpregnant patients.[11] After treatment, follow-up cultures should be obtained, as with ASB and cystitis. Prophylactic antimicrobial therapy should be strongly considered to reduce the risk of recurrent pyelonephritis.[122–125,137] In a study of 400 pregnant patients with pyelonephritis, 2.7% of women were readmitted for recurrent pyelonephritis, all of whom were noncompliant with antimicrobial prophylaxis, reinforcing the importance of this therapy.[17]

In patients who do not respond to culture-directed treatment, alternative diagnoses should be considered and an imaging study such as a renal ultrasound should be obtained to rule out renal abscess, nephrolithiasis, or other structural abnormality, although it is important to remember that some degree of hydronephrosis is expected in pregnancy.[1,16,132] In a recent study of 105

pregnant women with pyelonephritis, 45% had right hydronephrosis, 17% had left hydronephrosis, and only 14% had a normal ultrasound, yet all patients were managed with antimicrobials alone.[99]

SUMMARY

Bacteriuria is a common complication of pregnancy that may lead to significant adverse maternal and fetal outcomes. Antimicrobial selection should reflect safety considerations for both the mother and the fetus. ASB, cystitis, and pyelonephritis should be treated promptly, and patients should be followed closely after treatment, with strong consideration of daily antimicrobial prophylaxis.

REFERENCES

1. Waltzer WC. The urinary tract in pregnancy. J Urol 1981;3:271–6.
2. Nicolle LE, Bradley S, Colgan R, et al. Infectious Diseases Society of America guidelines for the diagnosis and treatment of asymptomatic bacteriuria in adults. Clin Infect Dis 2005;40(5):643–54.
3. Roberts AP, Beard RW. Some factors affecting bacterial invasion of bladder during pregnancy. Lancet 1965;1:1133–6.
4. Kass EH. Bacteriuria and pyelonephritis of pregnancy. Arch Intern Med 1960;105:194–8.
5. Sweet RL. Bacteriuria and pyelonephritis during pregnancy. Semin Perinatol 1977;1:25–40.
6. Harris RE. The significance of eradication of bacteriuria during pregnancy. Obstet Gynecol 1979; 53(1):71–3.
7. Patterson TF, Andriole VT. Detection, significance, and therapy of bacteriuria in pregnancy. Update in the managed health care era. Infect Dis Clin North Am 1997;11(3):593–608.
8. Millar LK, Cox SM. Urinary tract infections complicating pregnancy. Infect Dis Clin North Am 1997; 11(1):13–26.
9. Romero R, Oyarzun E, Mazor M, et al. Meta-analysis of the relationship between asymptomatic bacteriuria and preterm delivery/low birth weight. Obstet Gynecol 1989;73:576–82.
10. Schieve LA, Handler A, Hershow R, et al. Urinary tract infection during pregnancy: its association with maternal morbidity and perinatal outcome. Am J Public Health 1994;84(3):405–10.
11. Gupta K, Hooton TM, Naber KG, et al. International clinical practice guidelines for the treatment of acute uncomplicated cystitis and pyelonephritis in women: a 2010 update by the Infectious Diseases Society of America and the European Society for

Microbiology and Infectious Diseases. Clin Infect Dis 2011;52(5):e103–20.

12. U.S. Preventative Services Task Force. Screening for asymptomatic bacteriuria in adults: U.S. Preventative Services Task Force reaffirmation recommendation statement. Ann Intern Med 2008;149:43–7.

13. Lin K, Fajardo K, U.S. Preventive Services Task Force. Screening for asymptomatic bacteriuria in adults: evidence for the U.S. Preventative Services Task Force reaffirmation recommendation statement. Ann Intern Med 2008;149:W20–4.

14. AAP Committee on Fetus and Newborn, ACOG Committee on Obstetric Practice. Guidelines for perinatal care. 7th edition. Elk Grove Village (IL): American Academy of Pediatrics; 2012.

15. American Academy of Family Physicians. Summary of recommendations for clinical preventative services. AAFP Policy Action November 1996. Leawood (KS): American Academy of Family Physicians; 2015.

16. Schaeffer AJ, Schaeffer EM. Infections of the urinary tract. In: Wein AJ, editor. Cambell-Walsh urology. 10th edition. Philadelphia: Saunders, an imprint of Elsevier Inc; 2012. p. 257–326.

17. Hill JB, Sheffield JS, McIntire DD, et al. Acute pyelonephritis in pregnancy. Obstet Gynecol 2005;105:18–23.

18. Macejko AM, Schaeffer AJ. Asymptomatic bacteriuria and symptomatic urinary tract infections during pregnancy. Urol Clin North Am 2007;34:35–42.

19. Jamie WE, Edwards RK, Duff P. Antimicrobial susceptibility of gram-negative uropathogens isolated from obstetric patients. Infect Dis Obstet Gynecol 2002;10(3):123–6.

20. Wing DA, Fassett MJ, Getahun D. Acute pyelonephritis in pregnancy: an 18-year retrospective analysis. Am J Obstet Gynecol 2014;210(3):219.e1–6.

21. Agger WA, Siddiqui D, Lovrich SD, et al. Epidemiologic factors and urogenital infections associated with preterm birth in a midwestern U.S. population. Obstet Gynecol 2014;124(5):969–77.

22. Gilbert GL, Garland SM, Fairley KF, et al. Bacteriuria due to ureaplasmas and other fastidious organisms during pregnancy: prevalence and significance. Pediatr Infect Dis 1986;5:S239–43.

23. Cohen I, Veille JC, Calkins BM. Improved pregnancy outcome following successful treatment of chlamydial infection. JAMA 1990;263(23):3160–3.

24. Hsia TY, Shortliffe LM. The effect of pregnancy on rat urinary tract dynamics. J Urol 1995;154(2 Pt 2):684–9.

25. Nel JT, Diedericks A, Joubert G, et al. A prospective clinical and urodynamic study of bladder function during and after pregnancy. Int Urogynecol J Pelvic Floor Dysfunct 2001;12(1):21–6.

26. Bakircioglu ME, Sievert KD, Lau A, et al. The effect of pregnancy and delivery on the function and ultrastructure of the rat bladder and urethra. BJU Int 2000;85(3):350–61.

27. Dashe JS, Gilstrap LC. Antibiotic use in pregnancy. Obstet Gynecol Clin North Am 1997;24:617–29.

28. Lamont HF, Blogg HJ, Lamont RF. Safety of antimicrobial treatment during pregnancy: a current review of resistance, immunomodulation and teratogenicity. Expert Opin Drug Saf 2014;13:1569–81.

29. Whalley PJ, Adams RH, Combes B. Tetracycline toxicity in pregnancy. Liver and pancreatic dysfunction. JAMA 1964;189:357–62.

30. Porter PJ, Sweeney EA, Golan H, et al. Controlled study of the effect of prenatal tetracycline on primary dentition. Antimicrob Agents Chemother (Bethesda) 1965;5:668–71.

31. Crider KS, Cleves MA, Reefhuis J, et al. Antibacterial medication use during pregnancy and risk of birth defects. National Birth Defects Prevention Study. Arch Pediatr Adolesc Med 2009;163(11):978–85.

32. FDA. United States FDA pharmaceutical pregnancy categories. Fed Regist 1980;44:37434–67.

33. FDA. Content and format of labeling for human prescription drug and biological products; requirements for pregnancy and lactation labeling. Fed Regist 2014;79(233):72063–103.

34. Guinto VT, De Guia B, Festin MR, et al. Different antibiotic regimens for treating asymptomatic bacteriuria in pregnancy. Cochrane Database Syst Rev 2010;(9):CD007855.

35. Vazquez JC, Abalos E. Treatments for symptomatic urinary tract infections during pregnancy. Cochrane Database Syst Rev 2011;(1):CD002256.

36. Duff P. Antibiotic selection in obstetrics: making cost-effective choices. Clin Obstet Gynecol 2002;45(1):59–72.

37. Boucher HW, Talbot GH, Bradley JS, et al. Bad bugs, no drugs: no ESKAPE! An update from the Infectious Diseases Society of America. Clin Infect Dis 2009;48(1):1–12.

38. Schito GC, Naber KG, Botto H, et al. The ARESC study: an international survey on the antimicrobial resistance of pathogens involved in uncomplicated urinary tract infections. Int J Antimicrob Agents 2009;34(5):407–13.

39. Boucher HW, Talbot GH, Benjamin DK Jr, et al. 10 x '20 Progress–development of new drugs active against gram-negative bacilli: an update from the Infectious Diseases Society of America. Clin Infect Dis 2013;56(12):1685–94.

40. CDC. Antibiotic resistance threats in the United States. 2013. Available at: http://www.cdc.gov/drug resistance/pdf/ar-threats-2013-508.pdf. Accessed February 7, 2015.

41. Pathak A, Chandran SP, Mahadik K, et al. Frequency and factors associated with carriage of multi-drug resistant commensal Escherichia coli among women attending antenatal clinics in Central India. BMC Infect Dis 2013;13:199.

42. Wagenlehner FM, Bartoletti R, Cek M, et al. Antibiotic stewardship: a call for action by the urologic community. Eur Urol 2013;64(3):358–60.

43. Weller TMA, Rees EN. Antibacterial use in pregnancy. Drug Saf 2000;22(5):335–8.

44. Nahum GG, Uhl K, Kennedy DL. Antibiotic use in pregnancy and lactation. What is and is not known about teratogenic and toxic risks. Obstet Gynecol 2006;107:1120–38.

45. Czeizel AE, Rockenbauer M, Sorensen HT, et al. Augmentin treatment during pregnancy and the prevalence of congenital abnormalities: a population-based case-control teratologic study. Eur J Obstet Gynecol Reprod Biol 2001;2001(97):188–92.

46. Dencker BB, Larsen H, Jensen ES, et al. Birth outcome of 1886 pregnancies after exposure to phenoxymethylpenicillin in utero. Clin Microbiol Infect 2002;8:196–201.

47. Czeizel AE, Rockenbauer M, Sorensen HT, et al. A population-based case-control teratologic study of ampicillin treatment during pregnancy. Am J Obstet Gynecol 2001;185:140–7.

48. American College of Obstetricians and Gynecologists Committee on Obstetric Practice. ACOG Committee Opinion No. 494: sulfonamides, nitrofurantoin, and risk of birth defects. Obstet Gynecol 2011;117(6):1484–5.

49. Czeizel AE, Rockenbauer M, Sorensen HT, et al. Use of cephalosporins during pregnancy and in the presence of congenital abnormalities: a population-based, case-control study. Am J Obstet Gynecol 2001;184(6):1289–96.

50. Duff P. Antibiotic selection in obstetric patients. Infect Dis Clin North Am 1997;11(1):1–12.

51. Zhanel GC, Wiebe R, Dilay L, et al. Comparative review of the carbapenems. Drugs 2007;67(7):1027–52.

52. Czeizel AE, Rockenbauer M, Sorensen HT, et al. A teratological study of lincosamides. Scand J Infect Dis 2000;32:579–80.

53. Bar-Oz B, Weber-Schoendorfer C, Berlin M, et al. The outcomes of pregnancy in women exposed to the new macrolides in the first trimester. A prospective, multicentre, observational study. Drug Saf 2012;35(7):589–98.

54. Czeizel AE, Rockenbauer M, Sorensen HT, et al. A population-based case-control teratologic study of oral erythromycin treatment during pregnancy. Reprod Toxicol 1999;13:531–6.

55. Christensen B. Which antibiotics are appropriate for treating bacteriuria in pregnancy? J Antimicrob Chemother 2000;46(Suppl 1):29–34.

56. Nordeng H, Lupattelli A, Romoren M, et al. Neonatal outcomes after gestational exposure to nitrofurantoin. Obstet Gynecol 2013;121:306–13.

57. Goldberg O, Koren G, Landau D, et al. Exposure to nitrofurantoin during the first trimester of pregnancy and the risk for major malformations. J Clin Pharmacol 2013;53(9):991–5.

58. Boggess KA, Benedetti TJ, Raghu G. Nitrofurantoin-induced pulmonary toxicity during pregnancy: a report of a case and review of the literature. Obstet Gynecol Surv 1996;51(6):367–70.

59. Youngster I, Arcavi L, Schechmaster R, et al. Medications and glucose-6-phosphate dehydrogenase deficiency: an evidence-based review. Drug Saf 2010;33(9):713–26.

60. Karpman E, Kurzrock EA. Adverse reactions of nitrofurantoin, trimethoprim and sulfamethoxazole in children. J Urol 2004;172(2):448–53.

61. Bruel H, Guillemant V, Saladin-Thiron C, et al. Hemolytic anemia in a newborn after maternal treatment with nitrofurantoin at the end of pregnancy. Arch Pediatr 2000;7(7):745–7 [in French].

62. Raz R. Fosfomycin: an old-new antibiotic. Clin Microbiol Infect 2012;18:4–7.

63. Keating GM. Fosfomycin trometamol: a review of its use as a single-dose oral treatment for patients with acute lower urinary tract infections and pregnant women with asymptomatic bacteriuria. Drugs 2013;73(17):1951–66.

64. Rousson N, Karageorgopoulos DE, Samonis G, et al. Clinical significance of the pharmacokinetic and pharmacodynamic characteristics of fosfomycin for the treatment of patients with systemic infections. Int J Antimicrob Agents 2009;34:506–15.

65. Krcmery S, Hromec J, Demesova D. Treatment of lower urinary tract infection in pregnancy. Int J Antimicrob Agents 2001;17(4):279–82.

66. Estebanez A, Pascual R, Gil V, et al. Fosfomycin in a single dose versus a 7-day course of amoxicillin-clavulanate for the treatment of asymptomatic bacteriuria during pregnancy. Eur J Clin Microbiol Infect Dis 2009;28(12):1457–64.

67. Usta TA, Dogan O, Ates U, et al. Comparison of single-dose and multiple-dose antibiotics for lower urinary tract infection in pregnancy. Int J Gynaecol Obstet 2011;114(3):229–33.

68. Falagas ME, Vouloumanou EK, Togias AG, et al. Fosfomycin versus other antibiotics for the treatment of cystitis: a meta-analysis of randomized controlled trials. J Antimicrob Chemother 2010;65(9):1862–77.

69. Hernandez-Diaz S, Werler MM, Walker AM, et al. Folic acid antagonists during pregnancy and the risk of birth defects. N Engl J Med 2000;343:1608–14.

70. Nogard B, Czeizel AE, Rockenbauer M, et al. Population-based case control study of the safety of

sulfasalazine use during pregnancy. Aliment Pharmacol Ther 2001;15:483–6.

71. Amann U, Egen-Lappe V, Strunz-Lehner C, et al. Antibiotics in pregnancy: analysis of potential risks and determinants in a large German statutory sickness fund population. Pharmacoepidemiol Drug Saf 2006;15(5):327–37.

72. Niebyl JR. Antibiotics and other anti-infective agents in pregnancy and lactation. Am J Perinatol 2003;20(8):405–14.

73. Paton JH, Reeves DS. Clinical features and management of adverse effects of quinolone antibacterials. Drug Saf 1991;6:8–27.

74. Schaefer C, Amoura-Elefant E, Vial T, et al. Pregnancy outcome after prenatal quinolone exposure. Evaluation of a case registry of the European Network of Teratology Information Services (ENTIS). Eur J Obstet Gynecol Reprod Biol 1996;69: 83–9.

75. Larsen H, Nielsen GL, Schonheyder HC, et al. Birth outcome following maternal use of fluoroquinolones. Int J Antimicrob Agents 2001;18:259–62.

76. Elyasi S, Khalili H, Dashti-Khavidaki S, et al. Vancomycin-induced nephrotoxicity: mechanism, incidence, risk factors and special populations. A literature review. Eur J Clin Pharmacol 2012;68(9): 1243–55.

77. Bourget P, Fernandez H, Delouis C, et al. Transplacental passage of vancomycin during the second trimester of pregnancy. Obstet Gynecol 1991;78: 908–11.

78. Reyes MP, Ostrea EM, Cabinian AE, et al. Vancomycin during pregnancy: does it cause hearing loss or nephrotoxicity in the infant? Am J Obstet Gynecol 1989;161:977–81.

79. Mercieri M, Di Rosa R, Pantosi A, et al. Critical pneumonia complicating early-stage pregnancy. Anesth Analg 2010;110(3):852–4.

80. Metexas EI, Falagas ME. Update on the safety of linezolid. Expert Opin Drug Saf 2009;8:485–91.

81. Shea K, Hilburger E, Baroco A, et al. Successful treatment of vancomycin-resistant Enterococcus faecium pyelonephritis with daptomycin during pregnancy. Ann Pharmacother 2008;42(5):722–5.

82. Kass EH. Pyelonephritis and bacteriuria: a major problem in preventive medicine. Ann Intern Med 1962;56:46–53.

83. Kass EH. Bacteriuria and the diagnosis of infections of the urinary tract. Arch Intern Med 1957; 100:709–14.

84. Norden CW, Kass EH. Bacteriuria of pregnancy - a critical appraisal. Annu Rev Med 1968;19:431–70.

85. Nicolle LE. Asymptomatic bacteriuria when to screen and when to treat. Infect Dis Clin North Am 2003;17:367–94.

86. Little PJ. The incidence of urinary infection in 5000 pregnant women. Lancet 1966;388(7470):925–8.

87. Stenqvist K, Dahlen-Nilsson I, Janson GL, et al. Bacteriuria in pregnancy. Frequency and risk of acquisition. Am J Epidemiol 1989;129:372–9.

88. Zhanel G, Harding GKM, Nicolle LE. Asymptomatic bacteriuria in diabetics. Rev Infect Dis 1991;13: 150–4.

89. Zhanel GC, Nicolle LE, Harding GKM. Prevalence of asymptomatic bacteriuria in women with diabetes mellitus. Clin Infect Dis 1995;21:316–22.

90. Kunin CM, McCormack RC. An epidemiologic study of bacteriuria and blood pressure among nuns and working women. N Engl J Med 1968; 278:635–42.

91. Turck M, Goffe BS, Petersdorf RG. Bacteriuria of pregnancy. Relation to socioeconomic factors. N Engl J Med 1962;266:857–60.

92. Hazhir S. Asymptomatic bacteriuria in pregnant women. Urol J 2007;4(1):24–7.

93. Awoleke JO, Adanikin AI, Ajayi DD, et al. Predictors of asymptomatic bacteriuria among pregnant women in a low-resource setting. J Obstet Gynaecol 2015;35(1):25–9.

94. Pastore LM, Savitz DA, Thorp JMJ. Predictors of urinary tract infection at the first prenatal visit. Epidemiology 1999;10(3):282–7.

95. Imade PE, Izekor PE, Eghafona NO, et al. Asymptomatic bacteriuria among pregnant women. N Am J Med Sci 2010;2(6):263–6.

96. Smaill F, Vazquez JC. Antibiotics for asymptomatic bacteriuria in pregnancy. Cochrane Database Syst Rev 2007;(2):CD000490.

97. Gratacos E, Torres PJ, Vila J, et al. Screening and treatment of asymptomatic bacteriuria in pregnancy prevent pyelonephritis. J Infect Dis 1994; 169(6):1390–2.

98. Gilstrap LC, Leveno KJ, Cunningham EF. Renal infection and pregnancy outcome. Am J Obstet Gynecol 1981;141:709–16.

99. Farkash E, Weintraub AY, Sergienko R, et al. Acute antepartum pyelonephritis in pregnancy: a critical analysis of risk factors and outcomes. Eur J Obstet Gynecol Reprod Biol 2012;162(1):24–7.

100. Banhidy F, Acs N, Puho EH, et al. Pregnancy complications and birth outcomes of pregnant women with urinary tract infections and related drug treatments. Scand J Infect Dis 2007;39(5):390–7.

101. Mazor-Dray E, Levy A, Schlaeffer F, et al. Maternal urinary tract infection: is it independently associated with adverse pregnancy outcome? J Matern Fetal Neonatal Med 2009;22(2):124–8.

102. Lumbiganon P, Villar J, Laopaiboon M, et al. One-day compared with 7-day nitrofurantoin for asymptomatic bacteriuria in pregnancy. A randomized controlled trial. Obstet Gynecol 2009; 113:339–45.

103. Chen YK, Chen SF, Li HC, et al. No increased risk of adverse pregnancy outcomes in women with

urinary tract infections: a nationwide population-based study. Acta Obstet Gynecol Scand 2010; 89(7):882–8.

104. Mann JR, McDermott S, Gregg A, et al. Maternal genitourinary infection and small for gestational age. Am J Perinatol 2009;26(9):667–72.

105. Schneeberger C, Kazemier BM, Geerlings SE. Asymptomatic bacteriuria and urinary tract infections in special patient groups: women with diabetes mellitus and pregnant women. Curr Opin Infect Dis 2014;27(1):108–14.

106. Kazemier BM, Schneeberger C, De Miranda E, et al. Costs and effects of screening and treating low risk women with a singleton pregnancy for asymptomatic bacteriuria, the ASB study. BMC Pregnancy Childbirth 2012;12:52.

107. McNair RD, MacDonald SR, Dooley SL, et al. Evaluation of the centrifuged and Gram-stained smear, urinalysis, and reagent strip testing to detect asymptomatic bacteriuria in obstetric patients. Am J Obstet Gynecol 2000;182(5):1076–9.

108. McIsaac W, Carroll JC, Biringer A, et al. Screening for asymptomatic bacteriuria in pregnancy. J Obstet Gynaecol Can 2005;27:20–4.

109. Elder HA, Santamarina BAG, Smith S, et al. The natural history of asymptomatic bacteriuria during pregnancy: the effect of tetracycline on the clinical course and the outcome of pregnancy. Am J Obstet Gynecol 1971;111:441–62.

110. Schneeberger C, van den Heuvel ER, Erwich JJHM, et al. Contamination rates of three urine-sampling methods to assess bacteriuria in pregnant women. Obstet Gynecol 2013;121:299–305.

111. Lumbiganon P, Laopaiboon M, Thinkhamrop J. Screening and treating asymptomatic bacteriuria in pregnancy. Curr Opin Obstet Gynecol 2010; 22(2):95–9.

112. Shelton SD, Boggess KA, Kirvan K, et al. Urinary interleukin-8 with asymptomatic bacteriuria in pregnancy. Obstet Gynecol 2001;97:583–6.

113. Eigbefoh JO, Isabu P, Okpere E, et al. The diagnostic accuracy of the rapid dipstick test to predict asymptomatic urinary tract infection of pregnancy. J Obstet Gynaecol 2008;28(5):490–5.

114. Mignini L, Carroli G, Abalos E, et al. Accuracy of diagnostic tests to detect asymptomatic bacteriuria during pregnancy. Obstet Gynecol 2009;113: 346–52.

115. Robertson AW, Duff P. The nitrite and leukocyte esterase tests for the evaluation of asymptomatic bacteriuria in obstetric patients. Obstet Gynecol 1988;71:878–81.

116. Tincello DG, Richmond DH. Evaluation of reagent strips in detecting asymptomatic bacteriuria in early pregnancy: prospective case series. BMJ 1998;316:435–7.

117. Bachman JW, Heise RH, Naessens JM, et al. A study of various tests to detect asymptomatic urinary tract infections in an obstetric population. JAMA 1993;270(16):1971–4.

118. Deville WLJM, Yzermans JC, van Duijn NP, et al. The urine dipstick test useful to rule out infections. A meta-analysis of the accuracy. BMC Urol 2003;4:4.

119. Winkens R, Nelissen-Arets H, Stobberingh E. Validity of the urine dipslide under daily practice conditions. Fam Pract 2003;20(4):410–2.

120. Cunningham FG, Morris GB, Mickal A. Acute pyelonephritis of pregnancy: a clinical review. Obstet Gynecol 1973;42(1):112–7.

121. Whalley PJ, Cunningham FG. Short-term versus continuous antimicrobial therapy for asymptomatic bacteriuria in pregnancy. Obstet Gynecol 1977; 49(3):262–5.

122. Schneeberger C, Geerlings SE, Middleton P, et al. Interventions for preventing recurrent urinary tract infection during pregnancy. Cochrane Database Syst Rev 2012;(11):CD009279.

123. Lenke RR, VanDorsten JP, Schifrin BS. Pyelonephritis in pregnancy: a prospective randomized trial to prevent recurrent disease evaluating suppressive therapy with nitrofurantoin and close surveillance. Am J Obstet Gynecol 1983;146(8):953–7.

124. Albert X, Huertas I, Pereiro II, et al. Antibiotics for preventing recurrent urinary tract infection. Cochrane Database Syst Rev 2004;(3):CD001209.

125. Pfau A, Sacks TG. Effective prophylaxis for recurrent urinary tract infections during pregnancy. Clin Infect Dis 1992;14:810–4.

126. Wing DA, Rumney PJ, Preslicka CW, et al. Daily cranberry juice for the prevention of asymptomatic bacteriuria in pregnancy: a randomized, controlled pilot study. J Urol 2008;180(4):1367–72.

127. Gilstrap LC, Ramin SM. Urinary tract infections during pregnancy. Obstet Gynecol Clin North Am 2001;28:581–91.

128. Jolley JA, Kim S, Wing DA. Acute pyelonephritis and associated complications during pregnancy in 2006 in US hospitals. J Matern Fetal Neonatal Med 2012;25(12):2494–8.

129. Archabald KL, Friedman A, Raker CA, et al. Impact of trimester on morbidity of acute pyelonephritis in pregnancy. Am J Obstet Gynecol 2009;201(4):406. e1–4.

130. McDonnold M, Friedman A, Raker C, et al. Is postpartum pyelonephritis associated with the same maternal morbidity as antepartum pyelonephritis? J Matern Fetal Neonatal Med 2012;25(9):1709–11.

131. Pinson AG, Philbrick JT, Lindbeck GH, et al. Fever in the clinical diagnosis of acute pyelonephritis. Am J Emerg Med 1997;15(2):148–51.

132. Cunningham FG, Leveno KJ, Bloom SL, et al. Renal and urinary tract disorders. In: Cunningham FG,

Leveno KJ, Bloom SL, et al, editors. Williams Obstetrics. 24th edition. New York: McGraw-Hill; 2013.

133. Wing DA, Park AS, Debuque L, et al. Limited clinical utility of blood and urine cultures in the treatment of acute pyelonephritis during pregnancy. Am J Obstet Gynecol 2000;182(6):1437–40.

134. Gomi H, Goto Y, Laopaiboon M, et al. Routine blood cultures in the management of pyelonephritis in pregnancy for improving outcomes. Cochrane Database Syst Rev 2015;(2):CD009216.

135. Millar LK, Wing DA, Paul RH, et al. Outpatient treatment of pyelonephritis in pregnancy: a randomized clinical trial. Obstet Gynecol 1995;1995(86):560–4.

136. Wing DA, Hendershott CM, Debuque L, et al. A randomized trial of three antibiotic regimens for the treatment of pyelonephritis in pregnancy. Obstet Gynecol 1998;1998(92):249–53.

137. Sandberg T, Brorson JE. Efficacy of long-term antimicrobial prophylaxis after acute pyelonephritis in pregnancy. Scand J Infect Dis 1991;23:221–3.

Bacteruria and Urinary Tract Infections in the Elderly

Keri Detweiler, DO[a], Daniel Mayers, DO[a],
Sophie G. Fletcher, MD[b],*

KEYWORDS

- Asymptomatic bacteriuria • Bacteriuria • Urinary tract infection • Cystitis • Pyuria

KEY POINTS

- Despite several consensus guidelines proposed by various interest groups in recent years, a concise definition of urinary tract infection and associated symptoms does not exist.
- Results of urinalysis are often misinterpreted and mishandled.
- Treatment of elderly patients with bacteriuria necessitates skilled history taking, examination, and complete diagnostic urine testing.
- It is now being suggested that the healthy urinary tract is not a sterile environment, but in fact is populated by a dynamic set of microorganisms that change throughout time based on environmental and behavioral factors.
- Multiple studies have shown no morbidity or mortality benefit to antibiotic therapy in either community-dwelling elderly or long-term care facility residents with asymptomatic bacteriurea.

INTRODUCTION

Both urinary tract infection (UTI) and asymptomatic bacteriuria (ASB) are common among elderly adults and represent a significant health care burden. UTIs are responsible for 15.5% of infectious disease hospitalizations in adults aged 65 or older, second only to pneumonia, and they are responsible for 6.2% of infectious disease-related deaths.[1] Despite their frequency, differentiating between ASB and true UTI remains controversial among health care providers. In light of emerging antibiotic-resistant pathogens, this distinction has become increasingly important, because although symptomatic UTI requires appropriate antibiotic therapy, ASB does not.

PURPOSE OF THIS REVIEW

This article will review proposed definitions of ASB and UTI, highlight emerging research in causes and prevention of bacteriuria and UTI in the elderly, and examine improvements in patient outcomes over the past 20 years with improved practice guidelines. The authors' search criteria for the literature review utilized the PubMed database with the following key words: urinary tract infection, asymptomatic bacteriuria, bacteriuria, urinary tract microflora, urinary tract infection treatment, urinary tract infection risk factors, and combinations thereof. For inclusion, papers must have been published after 1980 and written in English. Exclusion criteria included foreign journal articles not translated to English.

The authors have nothing to disclose.
[a] Touro University College of Osteopathic Medicine – California, 1310 Club Drive, Vallejo, CA 94592, USA;
[b] Kaiser Permanente Northern California, 401 Bicentennial Way, Santa Rosa, CA 95403, USA
* Corresponding author.
E-mail address: sophiegfletcher@gmail.com

urologic.theclinics.com

DEFINITIONS OF ASYMPTOMATIC BACTERIURIA

As defined by the Infectious Disease Society of America (IDSA), ASB is the presence of 105 colony-forming units per milliliter (CFU/mL) or more of 1 bacterial species in 2 consecutive urine specimens in women, or a single urine specimen in men, in the absence of clinical signs and symptoms of UTI. A single specimen containing greater than or equal to 105 CFU/mL of a bacteria species is sufficient when obtained by catheterization in both men and women.[2]

DEFINITIONS OF URINARY TRACT INFECTION

For the purpose of this article, UTI means infection localized anywhere along the urinary tract, manifesting as cystitis, pyelonephritis, or prostatitis. Despite several consensus guidelines proposed by various interest groups in recent years, a concise definition of UTI and associated symptoms does not exist. Conserved criteria typically include pyuria as evidenced by presence of leukocyte esterase or white blood cells on urinalysis, symptoms attributable to the urinary tract, and a urine culture confirming a pathogenic source.[2–4] Of these components, what constitutes urinary tract symptoms is most variable. Typical symptoms include fever greater than 38 C or chills, dysuria, frequency, urgency, new-onset or worsening incontinence, and suprapubic or flank pain. Clinicians often include lethargy, confusion, or a change in baseline function, but this can be particularly difficult to assess in complicated patients with baseline impaired cognition or extensive comorbidities.

CHALLENGES AND CONTROVERSY IN DIAGNOSIS

Several challenges exist in the evaluation of urinary symptoms in the elderly patient. Symptoms of UTI are highly variable, often nonspecific to infection, and can be difficult to assess in patients with limited communication abilities or poor baseline function. Additionally, problems are frequently encountered in the collection, testing, and interpretation of urine specimens. Urine specimens should be obtained midstream by clean catch, or by in-and-out catheter when controlled voiding or cooperation is problematic. Chronic indwelling catheters should be removed and a new catheter inserted prior to obtaining samples, as biofilm is ubiquitous to long-term catheters. However, explanation and adherence to these collection standards are lacking. A prospective observational study by Pallin and colleagues[5] examined

emergency department cases at a major academic hospital that included urinalysis as part of their evaluation. By postencounter interview, it was found that 57% of the 137 participants received no instruction on urine collection, and that only 6% of participants had in fact used proper midstream clean-catch technique. Improper collection leads to specimen contamination by normal genitourinary flora, increasing the likelihood of false-positive urinalysis or misinterpretation of normal flora as pathogenic infection.

Results of urinalysis are often misinterpreted and mishandled. Pyuria, for example, can be a useful laboratory component in making the diagnosis of UTI but can also lead clinicians astray. Although absence of pyuria has strong negative predictive value for ASB or UTI, presence of pyuria is poorly specific for clinically significant infection.[2] Pyuria may be present in up to 45% of chronically disabled or incontinent adults, and in up to 90% of institutionalized adults, regardless of colonization or infection status.[4,6] A retrospective review of 339 cases from 2 academic centers found that pyuria was present in 70% of cases of UTI and 42.3% of cases of ASB, but was associated with inappropriate antimicrobial treatment by an odds ratio of 3.27 (95% confidence interval [CI], 1.49–7.18).[7] Specimens that do demonstrate pyuria should reflexively be sent for urine culture for confirm presence of a pathogen, but this step remains a common struggle in many health care institutions. In the observation study by Pallin and colleagues,[5] only 59% of samples with positive urinalysis were sent for urine culture, but again positive urinalysis regardless of symptoms was associated with antibiotic treatment by an odds ratio of 4.9 (95% CI, 1.7–14). These findings highlight the necessity of skilled history taking, examination, and complete diagnostic urine testing for the appropriate treatment of elderly patients.

EPIDEMIOLOGY
Asymptomatic Bacteriuria

Prevalence of asymptomatic bacteriuria increases in both men and women with age. Although ASB is uncommon in young men and found in only 1% to 2% of young women, prevalence increases to 6% to 16% in women and 5% to 21% in men ages 65 to 90 years. The prevalence increases further with increasing comorbidities, and may be as high as 25% to 50% in institutionalized women and 15% to 35% of institutionalized men, although a significant number of these patients have been observed to spontaneously develop negative urine cultures within 3- to 6-month time frames.[8] In elderly patients with chronic indwelling catheters,

ASB is universal. Multivariate analyses have emphasized that the duration of catheterization is the most important risk factor in development of catheter-associated bacteriuria,[9–11] while other studies have estimated colonization rate after catheter placement is 3% to 7% per day.[8] However, one-third to one-half of cases of bacteriuria will clear with removal of the catheter.[12,13]

Urinary Tract Infection

Because definitions of UTI vary, it should be noted that reported incidence and prevalence across the literature can be difficult to assess. In both community-dwelling and institutionalized adults, the prevalence of UTIs varies with gender and generally increases with age. Incidence of infection in men increases from 0.05 in men ages 65 to 74 years, to 0.08 in men over 85 years.[14] Infection is more common in postmenopausal women, with an incidence of 0.07 per person–year, increasing to 0.13 per person–year after age 85.[15] UTIs are quite common in institutionalized adults, accounting for 30% to 40% of health care-associated infections,[16,17] and substantially more prevalent in patients with chronic indwelling catheters. Mean incidence of catheter-related UTI was 3.2 cases per 1000 catheter days in 1 long-term care facility, compared with only 0.57 cases per 1000 days for all residents. Bacteremia from a urinary source is anywhere from 3 to 39 times more common in patients with chronic indwelling catheters.[18–20]

MICROBIOLOGY

Although some differences in common urinary tract pathogen prevalence are noted, *Escherichia coli* remains the most commonly cultured organism in both community-dwelling and institutionalized adults. Studies examining community-dwelling women report *E coli* isolates in 75% to 82% of positive urine culture, with the majority of remaining cultures attributed to *Klebsiella, Proteus mirabilis* and enterococcus.[20] Similar organisms are responsible for both ASB and UTI in institutionalized adults. Two large cohort studies of long-term care residents found *E coli* to be the most common urinary isolate, accounting for 54.6% to 69% of positive cultures. One study found enterobacteriaceae species to account for 34.8% of remaining cultures, while the second distributed these between *Klebsiella* (12%) and *Enterococcus faecalis* (8%).[21,22] Other common hospital-associated pathogens like *Pseudomonas aeruginosa,* vancomycin-resistant enterococci, and *Candida* spp have been identified in this population as well.[23]

Patients with indwelling catheters are uniquely at higher risk for biofilm-associated organisms, polymicrobial infections, and yeast colonization and infection. Large epidemiologic studies in both Europe and North America show that *E coli* remains the most common cause of both ASB, accounting for 21.4% of positive cultures, and UTI, accounting for 31% to 35.3% of positive cultures in this population.[24] Indwelling catheters are uniquely associated with biofilm organisms, making colonization and infection by *P mirabilis, P stuarti,* and *P aeruginosa* significantly more common.[23] Candida spp are also particularly common in these patients, accounting for 12.9% of catheter-associated UTI by some estimates.[24]

RISK FACTORS

Many genetic, behavioral, and comorbid host factors have been speculated as risk factors for both ASB and UTI. Some of these represent modifiable behavioral factors, while others are more inherent to the patients overall health. Multiple studies support a history of UTI as a primary risk factor for future infection, conveying as high as a fourfold to sevenfold risk compared with patients who have never had a symptomatic UTI.[20,25,26] This, combined with the growing understanding of uropathogen virulence and patient genetic variations, seems to imply that a certain percent of the population is inherently more susceptible to UTIs. Comorbid conditions including diabetes, dementia, incontinence, and iron deficiency anemia have all been described as independent risk factors for ASB and UTI.[27–30]

In premenopausal women, lactobacilli predominate the vaginal flora and are responsible for the relatively acidic pH of the vagina. This acidic environment is lost in postmenopausal women, and is implicated in the increased colonization and infection by *E coli* and enterococcus species.[27] Sexual activity has been associated with UTI in postmenopausal women, particularly within a 2 week period after activity, although this association is less robust than in premenopausal counterparts.[27]

In men, benign prostatic hypertrophy has been established as a risk factor for UTI. Although it is reasonable to presume this association is a product of urinary stasis, the relationship may in fact be more complicated. Interestingly, a cross-sectional study by Truzzi and colleagues[31] of 196 healthy participants found an association between bacteriuria and postvoid residuals greater than 180 mL in men, but this association has not been reproducible in ambulatory postmenopausal women[27,29,30]

PATHOPHYSIOLOGY

Our understanding of urinary tract colonization and infection has greatly expanded over the past decade, and substantial new evidence has highlighted the complicated interplay between protective host factors and pathogen virulence factors that determine the likelihood of infection. In the disease-free state, the urinary mucosa acts as a protective barrier from infectious attacks. Certain bacteria can evade this protective function by binding specific mucosal receptors, which in turn may initiate a rapid inflammatory response by the host. For example, P-fimbriated E coli, responsible for the majority of symptomatic UTIs, bind a glycosphingolipid receptor on the mucosal surface, triggering various inflammatory cascades, engaging submucosal tissue, and in some cases, leading to direct invasion of deeper tissues and the blood stream.[32]

It is now being suggested that what differentiates ASB from symptomatic infection is not necessarily the virulence factors of the invading bacteria, but a combination of virulence factors and the inherent genetic makeup and immune response of the host. Multiple mouse studies have correlated various genetic variations with decreased initial inflammatory responses, and therefore increased likelihood of ASB.[33,34] Similar findings have been mirrored in human studies. Specific TLR4 mutations have been associated with ASB in children, while other polymorphisms of the same receptor seem to protect from recurrent cystitis in adults.[35–38] On the other hand, genes that exaggerate host inflammatory responses or blunt antimicrobial efforts are associated with decreased bacterial clearance, and more severe bladder and kidney infection.[35] In both mice and human studies, polymorphisms of IRF3, a component of interferon signaling, have been associated with a majority of subjects.[34,36] This concept was further highlighted by Marschall and colleagues,[30] in a prospective cohort study demonstrating that while patient comorbidities could be correlated to presence of ASB, none of 12 E. coli virulence genes tested could be associated with likelihood of ASB.

The human microbiota and its complicated, symbiotic role in maintaining health have gained substantial attention throughout many disciplines over recent years. It is now being suggested that the healthy urinary tract is not a sterile environment, but in fact is populated by a dynamic set of microorganisms that change throughout time based on environmental and behavioral factors. Routine culture media are designed to produce common uropathogens but do not support the growth of many slow-growing, fastidious, or anaerobic organisms. However, advanced detection technologies have shown many other microbiota in the urinary tract of healthy adults, bringing to question the role of bacteria outside the context of disease. A recent review by Whiteside and colleagues[39] reports multiple genera including Jonquetella, Parvimonas, Proteiniphilum, and saccharofermentas in the urinary tract of healthy patients over age 70, through polymerase chain reaction (PCR) and detection of 16s rRNA subunits. A study by Santiago-Rodriguez and colleagues [40] also demonstrated viral communities in 20 individuals, including bacteriophages and low-risk or novel strains of human papiloma virus, but flora components were unassociated with history of urinary tract health. Although the exact role of these symbiotic organisms is still poorly understood, it is postulated that their metabolic byproducts may convey antimicrobial advantages and contribute to urinary health.

TREATMENT
Asymptomatic Bacteriuria

Although antibiotic treatment is indeed necessary in the case of UTI, the current consensus among urology and infectious disease groups is that they are not for ASB. Multiple studies have shown no morbidity or mortality benefit to antibiotic therapy in either community-dwelling or long-term care facility residents with ASB. However, such treatment does expose patients unnecessarily to potential medication adverse effects.[41–45]

Community-dwelling Adults

Several studies have suggested that for community-dwelling women with nonspecific symptoms, hydration and full diagnostic work up for urinary infection may be preferable to antibiotic treatment.[46,47] For example, a 2010 study found no superior outcomes to ciprofloxacin over ibuprofen for treatment of uncomplicated UTI.[46] A separate prospective cohort study of 51 women with symptoms of an uncomplicated UTI in the Netherlands found that delaying antibiotic treatment up to 1 week resulted in spontaneous resolution of symptoms in the majority of participants, with no complications of pyelonephritis or bacteremia.[48]

In elderly adults with unambiguously symptomatic UTI, antibiotic therapy should be chosen to best target suspected causative pathogens while minimizing unwanted adverse effects or interactions in the context of a patient's other comorbidities. Urinary pathogens should be evaluated for antibiotic sensitivity, and therapy should be tailored to a sensitive antibiotic with the most narrow spectrum. If symptoms are mild, treatment may even be delayed until culture results are available. When available, previous urinary cultures and sensitivities should be reviewed for likely pathogens and possible antibiotic resistance patterns. Where applicable, local antibiograms should also be consulted for consideration of geographic resistance patterns.

For stable patients with cystitis, oral therapy with nitrofurantoin or trimethoprim-sulfamethoxazole (TMP/SMX) is often effective. In women, 3 to 5 days is typically sufficient. Therapy is typically extended to a 7- to 14-day course for men, although a recent retrospective study of male veterans suggests this may not relay any benefit in terms of early or late recurrence of infections.[49] The IDSA also deems single-dose fosfomycin to be appropriate first-line therapy, since many organisms remain susceptible, although this regimen has been associated with inferior efficacy. Fluoroquinolones like ciprofloxacin and levofloxacin are acceptable second-line therapies for patients with allergies or intolerance to first-line agents, but susceptibility should be followed given increasing resistance of common uropathogens to this class. Amoxicillin-clavulanate may be considered with close follow-up, but amoxicillin alone and ampicillin are no longer recommended due to poor efficacy and high resistance patterns.

In cases of suspected pyelonephritis not requiring hospitalization, a 14 day course of oral TMP/SMX or a 5- to 7-day course of oral fluoroquinolone can be considered. In regions where fluoroquinolone resistance is high, an initial parenteral dose of ceftriaxone or 24-hour dose of aminoglycoside prior to oral therapy is recommended. In cases of known organism resistance to oral medications, pyelonephritis requiring hospitalization, or hemodynamically unstable patients, parenteral therapy is preferred to oral. Aminoglycosides (gentamicin, tobramycin), with or without ampicillin or a cephalosporin, are useful empiric regimens, as most common pathogens remain susceptible. Response should be re-evaluated after the initial 48 to 72 hours and modified according to culture and susceptibility results. Aminoglycoside toxicity is rare within the first 48 to 72 hours of use, but renal function and drug levels should be monitored with use extended past 7 days.[23,27]

Institutionalized Adults

Both nitrofurantoin and TMP/SMX are good empiric choices for patients residing in long-term care facilities. Nitrofurantoin may in fact have lower resistance rates, but is often avoided in older adults, because it is contraindicated in renal insufficiency. In patients with a history of enterobacteriaceae or nitrofurantoin-resistant E coli infections, TMP/SMX is a reasonable alternative therapy.[21] For institutionalized women with uncomplicated cystitis, a 3-to 5-day course of TMP/SMX is likely sufficient, although a 2001 publication from the Society for Healthcare Epidemiology of America recommends 7 days.[50]

Chronic Catheterization

Indwelling catheters should be removed and replaced with a new catheter prior to collection of urine specimen and the initiation of treatment. Nitrofurantoin should be avoided in this population, as Proteus mirabilis and Pseudomonas are widely resistant. In patients who are not severely ill, empiric treatment with levofloxacin is appropriate until culture results are available. Antibiotic therapy tailored to sensitivities is especially important in this population, as frequent antibiotic exposure makes resistance particularly likely. If the patient responds rapidly to therapy, a 7-day course of antibiotic may be appropriate. For those with delayed response, treatment should be expanded to 10 to 14 days.

PREVENTION

Preventive options are of great interest for patients at high risk of infection or who suffer from frequent infection. Speculated options range from behavioral modifications to prescribed medications, but have varied bodies of evidence to support their use.

Community-Dwelling and Long-Term Care Facility Residents

Women with frequent UTIs are often told to increase fluid intake as a means of treatment. However, a 1999 study found that excessive water intake leads to dilute urine, which may actually dilute host-produced antimicrobial factors in urine that serve to prevent and fight infection. Urine from subjects with higher water intake was noted to increase deposition rates of E coli and E fecalis on silicone rubber.[51]

Cranberry supplements in a variety of forms have been long investigated in the prevention of UTI. In vitro studies have demonstrated that proanthocyanidin, a component of the fruit, inhibits P-fimbriated E coli from adhering to the bladder epithelium.[52,53] Interestingly, a randomized control study by Stapleton and colleagues[54] of 176 women with history of UTI found a reduction in colonization by P-fimbriated E coli in women taking 4 to 8 ounces daily of a well characterized, commercially available cranberry juice, but did not demonstrate statistically significant difference in infection rates. To the authors' knowledge, this is the first study to show potential in vivo evidence of the in vitro propose mechanism of proanthocyanidins. A Cochrane review in 2013 found a small trend toward fewer UTIs in people taking cranberry products, but no statistically significant benefit.[55] However, it should be noted that this review pertained to studies using cranberry juices, but cranberry concentrates or extract. D-mannose, a compound naturally found in pineapple, has been implicated in infection prevention by similar mechanism of interrupting bacterial adherence to the uroepithelium. Its efficacy, however, has not been demonstrated in the scientific literature.

Community-dwelling women who experience frequent UTIs (often defined as than 2 infections within a 6-month period) may be candidates for low-dose prophylactic antibiotic therapy. First-line therapy is typically nitrofurantoin 50 or 100 mg or half-strength TMP/SMX taken daily or every other day. An alternative is to supply short-term, self-administered courses of TMP/SMX or a fluoroquinolone to women who are familiar with their common symptoms and presentation of UTI.[47]

Although multiple studies have shown no association between oral estrogen therapy and UTI frequency, several trials have shown improvements topical vaginal estrogen, possibly through the restoration of normal vaginal flora and re-establishment of an acidic environment.[56,57]

Indwelling Catheters

There has been no evidence to support the use of antimicrobial impregnated catheters, but hydrophilic-coated catheters for clean intermittent catheterization and chlorhexidine-coated indwelling catheters have shown promising evidence of infection reduction.[12,13] In general, catheters should be placed only when absolutely indicated, and they should be removed as soon as they are no longer needed. When possible, alternatives to indwelling catheterization should be considered. Both intermittent clean catheterization and condom catheters may be associated both with increased comfort and fewer adverse outcomes.[58–61]

SUMMARY

Both UTI and ASB are common problems among elderly adults and represent a significant health care burden. Despite their frequency, differentiating between ASB and true UTI remains controversial among health care providers. Several challenges exist in the evaluation of urinary symptoms in the elderly patient. Symptoms of UTI are variable; problems are encountered in the collection, testing, and interpretation of urine specimens; and results of urinalysis are often misinterpreted and mishandled. Multiple studies have shown no morbidity or mortality benefit to antibiotic therapy in either community-dwelling or long-term care facility residents with ASB. The field is in need of research on the use of molecular tools to identify individuals at risk. Furthermore, the elucidation of host genetic factors, and how to incorporate them into clinical practice, could make a huge impact in the treatment of elderly patients.

REFERENCES

1. Curns AT, Holman RC, Sejvar JJ, et al. Infectious disease hospitalizations among older adults in the United States from 1990 through 2002. Arch Intern Med 2005;165(210):2514–20.
2. Nicolle LE, Bradley S, Colgan R, et al. Infectious Diseases Society of America guidelines for the diagnosis and treatment of asymptomatic bacteriuria in adults. Clin Infect Dis 2005;40(5):643–54.
3. Horan TC, Andrus M, Dudeck MA. CDC/NHSN surveillance definition of healthcare-associated infection and criteria for specific types of infections in the acute care setting. Am J Infect Control 2008;36(9):309–32.
4. Juthani-Mehta M, Drickamer MA, Towle V, et al. Nursing home practitioner survey of diagnostic criteria for urinary tract infections. J Am Geriatr Soc 2005;53(11):1986–90.
5. Pallin DJ, Ronene C, Kamaneh M, et al. Urinalysis in acute care of adults: pitfalls in testing and interpreting results. Open Forum Infect Dis 2014;1(1):ofu019.
6. Ouslander JG, Schapira M, Schnelle JF, et al. Does eradicating bacteriuria affect the severity of chronic urinary incontinence in nursing home residents? Ann Intern Med 1995;122:749–54.
7. Latour K, Kinross P, Moro ML, et al. Point prevalence survey of healthcare associated infections and antimicrobial use in European long-term care facilities. 2013. Stockholm (Sweden): ECDC; 2014.
8. Nicolle LE. Asymptomatic bacteriuria in the elderly. Infect Dis Clin North Am 1997;11:647–62.
9. Garibaldi RA, Burke JP, Britt MR, et al. Meatal colonization and catheter-associated bacteriuria. N Engl J Med 1980;303:316–8.
10. Platt R, Polk BF, Murdock B, et al. Risk factors for nosocomial urinary tract infection. Am J Epidemiol 1986;124:977–85.
11. Warren J, Bakke A, Desgranchamps F, et al. Catheter-associated bacteriuria and the role of biomaterial in prevention. In: Naber KG, Pechere JC, Kumazawa J, et al, editors. Nosocomial and healthcare associated

infections in urology. Plymouth (United Kingdom): Health Publications Ltd; 2001. p. 153–76.

12. Tenke P, Kovacs B, Bjerklund Johansen TE, et al. European and Asian guidelines on management and prevention of catheter-associated urinary tract infections. Int J Antimicrob Agents 2008;31(Suppl 1): S68–78.

13. Tenke P, Koves B, Johansen TE. An update on prevention and treatment of catheter-associated urinary tract infections. Curr Opin Infect Dis 2014;27(1): 102–7.

14. Griebling TL. Urologic Diseases in America project: trends in resource use for urinary tract infections in men. J Urol 2005;173(4):1288–94.

15. Caljouw MA, Den Elzen WP, Cools HJ, et al. Predictive factors of urinary tract infections among the oldest old in the general population. A population-based prospective follow-up study. BMC Med 2011;9:57.

16. Jsan L, Langberg R, Davis C, et al. Nursing home-associated infections in Department of Veterans Affairs community living centers. Am J Infect Control 2010;38(6):461–6.

17. Cotter M, Donlon S, Roche F, et al. Healthcare-associated infection in Irish long-term care facilities: results from the First National Prevalence Study. J Hosp Infect 2012;80(3):212–6.

18. Nicolle LE. Catheter-related urinary tract infection. Drugs Aging 2005;22:627–39.

19. Warren JW. Catheter-associated urinary tract infections. Infect Dis Clin North Am 1997;11:609–22.

20. Marques LP, Flores JT, Barros Junior Ode O, et al. Epidemiological and clinical aspects of urinary tract infection in the community-dwelling elderly women. Braz J Infect Dis 2012;16(5):436–41.

21. Das R, Perrelli E, Towle V, et al. Antimicrobial susceptibility of bacteria isolated from urine samples obtained from nursing home residents. Infect Control Hosp Epidemiol 2009;30(11):1116–9.

22. Sundvall PD, Ulleryd P, Gunnarsson RK. Urine culture doubtful in determining etiology of diffuse symptoms among elderly individuals: a cross-sectional study of 32 nursing homes. BMC Fam Pract 2011;12:36.

23. Nicolle LE. Resistant pathogens in urinary tract infections. J Am Geriatr Soc 2002;50:S230–5.

24. Lacovelli V, Gaziev G, Topazio L, et al. Nosocomial urinary tract infections: a review. Urologia 2014; 81(4):222–7.

25. Hu KK, Boyko EJ, Scholes D, et al. Risk factors for urinary tract infections in postmenopausal women. Arch Intern Med 2004;164(9):989–93.

26. Raz R, Gennesin Y, Wasser J, et al. Recurrent urinary tract infections in postmenopausal women. Clin Infect Dis 2000;30(1):152–6.

27. Nicolle LE. Urinary tract infections in the elderly. Clin Geriatr Med 2009;25:423–36.

28. Jackson SL, Boyko EJ, Scholes D, et al. Predictors of urinary tract infection after menopause: a prospective study. Am J Med 2004;117(12):903–11.

29. Huang AJ, Brown JS, Boyko EJ, et al. Clinical significance of postvoid residual volume in older ambulatory women. J Am Geriatr Soc 2011;59(8):1452–8.

30. Marschall J, Piccirillo M, Foxman B, et al. Patient characteristics but not virulence factors discriminate between asymptomatic and symptomatic E. coli bacteriuria in the hospital. BMC Infect Dis 2013;13:213.

31. Truzzi JC, Almeida MR, Nunes EC, et al. Residual urinary volume and urinary tract infection—when are they linked. J Urol 2008;180:182–5.

32. Godaly G, Ambite I, Svanborg C. Innate immunity and genetic determinants of urinary tract infection susceptibility. Curr Opin Infect Dis 2015;28:88–96.

33. Hagberg L, Hull R, Hull S, et al. Difference in susceptibility to gram-negative urinary tract infection between c3 h/hef and c3 h/hen mice. Infect Immun 1984;46:839–44.

34. Yadav M, Zhang J, Fischer H, et al. Inhibition of tir domain signaling by tcpc: Myd88-dependent and independent effects on escherichia coli virulence. PLoS Pathog 2010;6:e1001120.

35. Ragnarsdottir B, Lutay N, Gronberg-Hernandez J, et al. Genetics of innate immunity and UTI susceptibility. Nat Rev Urol 2011;8:449–68.

36. Fischer H, Lutay N, Ragnarsdottir B, et al. Pathogen specific, irf3-dependent signaling and innate resistance to human kidney infection. PLoS Pathog 2010;6:e1001109.

37. Ragnarsdottif B, Jonsson K, Urbano A, et al. Toll-like receptor 4 promoter polymorphisms: common tir4 variants may protect against severe urinary tract infection. PLoS One 2010;5:e10734.

38. Hawn TR, Scholes D, Li SS, et al. Toll-like receptor polymorphisms and susceptibility to urinary tract infections in adult women. PLoS One 2009;4:e5990.

39. Whiteside SA, Hasaan R, Dave S, et al. The microbiome of the urinary tract—a role beyond infection. Nat Rev Urol 2015;12:81–90.

40. Santiago-Rodriguez TM, Ly M, Bonilla N, et al. The human urine virome in association with urinary tract infections. Front Microbiol 2015;6:14.

41. Nicolle LE, Bjornson J, Harding GK, et al. Bacteriuria in elderly institutionalized men. N Engl J Med 1982; 309:1420–5.

42. Nicolle LE, Mayhew WJ, Bryan L. Prospective randomized comparison of therapy and no therapy for asymptomatic bacteriuria in institutionalized elderly women. Am J Med 1987;83:27–33.

43. Juthani-Mehta M. Asymptomatic bacteriuria and urinary tract infection in older adults. Clin Geriatr Med 2007;23:585–94.

44. Ouslander JG, Schapira M, Schnelle JF, et al. Pyuria among chronically incontinent but otherwise

asymptomatic nursing home residents. J Am Geriatr Soc 1996;44(4):420–3.

45. Abruytn E, Mossey J, berlin JA, et al. Does asymptomatic bacteriuria predict mortality and does antimicrobial treatment reduce mortality in elderly ambulatory women? Ann Intern Med 1994;120: 827–33.

46. Bleidom J, Gagyor I, Kochen MM, et al. Symptomatic treatment (ibuprofen) or antibiotics (Ciprofloxacin) for uncomplicated urinary tract infection? Results of a randomized controlled pilot trial. BMC Med 2010; 8:30.

47. Mody L, Juthani-Mehta M. Urinary tract infections in older women: a clinical review. JAMA 2014;311(8): 844–54.

48. Knottnerus BJ, Geerlings SE, Moll van Charante EP, et al. Women with symptoms of uncomplicated urinary tract infection are often willing to delay antibiotic treatment: a prospective cohort study. BMC Fam Pract 2013;14:71.

49. Drekonja DM, Rector TS, Cutting A, et al. Urinary tract infections in male veterans, treatment patterns and outcomes. JAMA Intern Med 2013;173(1):62–8.

50. Gupta K, Hooton T, Naber K, et al. International clinical practice guidelines for the treatment of acute uncomplicated cystitis and pyelonephritis in women: a 2010 update by the Infectious Diseases Society of America and the European Society for Microbiology and Infectious Diseases. Clin Infect Dis 2011;52(1): e103–20.

51. Habash MB, Van der Mei HC, Busscher HJ, et al. The effect of water, ascorbic acid and cranberry derived supplementation on human urine and uropathogen adhesion to silicone rubber. Can J Microbiol 1999;45(8):691–4.

52. Gupta K, Chou MY, Howell A, et al. Cranberry products inhibit adherence of p-fimbriated *Escherichia coli* to primary cultured bladder and vaginal epithelial cells. J Urol 2007;177(6):2357–60.

53. Howell AB, Vorsa N, Der Marderosian A, et al. Inhibition of the adherence of P-fimbriated *Escherichia coli* to uroepithelial cell surfaces by proanthocyanidin extracts from cranberries. N Engl J Med 1998; 229(15):1085–6.

54. Stapleton A, Dziura J, Hooton T, et al. Recurrent urinary tract infection and urinary *Escherichia coli* in women ingesting cranberry juice daily: a randomized controlled trial. Mayo Clin Proc 2012;87(2): 143–50.

55. Jepson RG, Williams G, Craig JC. Cranberries for preventing urinary tract infections. Cochrane Database Syst Rev 2012;(10):CD001321.

56. Raz R, Stamm W. A controlled trial of intra-vaginal estriol in post-menopausal women with recurrent urinary tract infections. N Engl J Med 1993;329: 753–7.

57. Eriksen B. A randomized, open, parallel group study on the preventive effect of an estriol-releasing vaginal ring (Estring) on recurrent urinary tract infections in postmenopausal women. Am J Obstet Gynecol 1999;180:1072–9.

58. Penrotta C, Aznar M, Mejia R, et al. Oestrogens for preventing recurrent urinary tract infections in postmenopausal women. Cochrane Database Syst Rev 2008;(2):CD005131.

59. Saint S, Kaufman SR, Rogers MA, et al. Condom versus indwelling urinary catheters: a randomized trial. J Am Geriatr Soc 2006;54:1055–61.

60. Hooton T, Bradley S, Cardenas D, et al. Diagnosis, prevention, and treatment of catheter-associated urinary tract infection in adults: 2009 international practice guidelines from the Infectious Diseases Society of America. Clin Infect Dis 2010;50:625–63.

61. Warren JW, Tenney JH, Hoopes JM, et al. A prospective microbiologic study of bacteriuria in patients with chronic indwelling urethral catheters. J Infect Dis 1982;146:719–23.

Index

Note: Page numbers of article titles are in **boldface** type.

Urol Clin N Am 42 (2015) 569–575

http://dx.doi.org/10.1016/S0094-0143(15)00108-1

urologic.theclinics.com

United States Postal Service

Statement of Ownership, Management, and Circulation
(All Periodicals Publications Except Requestor Publications)

1. Publication Title	2. Publication Number	3. Filing Date
Urologic Clinics of North America	0 0 0 - 7 1 1 1	9/18/15

4. Issue Frequency	5. Number of Issues Published Annually	6. Annual Subscription Price
Feb, May, Aug, Nov	4	$355.00

7. Complete Mailing Address of Known Office of Publication (Not printer) (Street, city, county, state, and ZIP+4®)

Elsevier Inc.
360 Park Avenue South
New York, NY 10010-1710

Contact Person
Stephen R. Bushing

Telephone (Include area code)
215-239-3688

8. Complete Mailing Address of Headquarters or General Business Office of Publisher (Not printer)

Elsevier Inc., 360 Park Avenue South, New York, NY 10010-1710

9. Full Names and Complete Mailing Addresses of Publisher, Editor, and Managing Editor (Do not leave blank)

Publisher (Name and complete mailing address)

Linda Belfus, Elsevier Inc., 1600 John F. Kennedy Blvd., Suite 1800, Philadelphia, PA 19103

Editor (Name and complete mailing address)

Kerry Holland, Elsevier Inc., 1600 John F. Kennedy Blvd., Suite 1800, Philadelphia, PA 19103-2899

Managing Editor (Name and complete mailing address)

Adrianne Brigido, Elsevier Inc., 1600 John F. Kennedy Blvd., Suite 1800, Philadelphia, PA 19103-2899

10. Owner (Do not leave blank. If the publication is owned by a corporation, give the name and address of the corporation immediately followed by the names and addresses of all stockholders owning or holding 1 percent or more of the total amount of stock. If not owned by a corporation, give the names and addresses of the individual owners. If owned by a partnership or other unincorporated firm, give its name and address as well as those of each individual owner. If the publication is published by a nonprofit organization, give its name and address.)

Full Name	Complete Mailing Address
Wholly owned subsidiary of	1600 John F. Kennedy Blvd. Ste. 1800
Reed/Elsevier US holdings	Philadelphia, PA 19103-2899

11. Known Bondholders, Mortgagees, and Other Security Holders Owning or Holding 1 Percent or More of Total Amount of Bonds, Mortgages, or Other Securities. If none, check box. ☐ None

Full Name	Complete Mailing Address
N/A	

12. Tax Status (For completion by nonprofit organizations authorized to mail at nonprofit rates) (Check one)
The purpose, function, and nonprofit status of this organization and the exempt status for federal income tax purposes:
☐ Has Not Changed During Preceding 12 Months
☐ Has Changed During Preceding 12 Months (Publisher must submit explanation of change with this statement)

PS Form 3526, July 2014 (Page 1 of 3 (Instructions Page 3)) PSN 7530-01-000-9931 PRIVACY NOTICE: See our Privacy policy in www.usps.com

---

13. Publication Title	14. Issue Date for Circulation Data Below
Urologic Clinics of North America	August 2015

15. Extent and Nature of Circulation			Average No. Copies Each Issue During Preceding 12 Months	No. Copies of Single Issue Published Nearest to Filing Date
a. Total Number of Copies (Net press run)			1097	884
b. Legitimate Paid and/Or Requested Distribution (By Mail and Outside the Mail)	(1)	Mailed Outside-County Paid/Requested Mail Subscriptions stated on PS Form 3541. (Include paid distribution above nominal rate, advertiser's proof copies and exchange copies)	469	339
	(2)	Mailed In-County Paid/Requested Mail Subscriptions stated on PS Form 3541. (Include paid distribution above nominal rate, advertiser's proof copies and exchange copies)		
	(3)	Paid Distribution Outside the Mails Including Sales Through Dealers And Carriers, Street Vendors, Counter Sales, and Other Paid Distribution Outside USPS®	273	321
	(4)	Paid Distribution by Other Classes of Mail Through the USPS (e.g. First-Class Mail®)		
c. Total Paid and/or Requested Circulation (Sum of 15b (1), (2), (3), and (4))			742	660
d. Free or Nominal Rate Distribution (By Mail and Outside the Mail)	(1)	Free or Nominal Rate In-County Copies included on PS Form 3541	94	78
	(2)	Free or Nominal Rate In-County Copies included on PS Form 3541		
	(3)	Free or Nominal Rate Copies mailed at Other classes Through the USPS (e.g. First-Class Mail®)		
	(4)	Free or Nominal Rate Distribution Outside the Mail (Carriers or Other means)		
e. Total Nonrequested Distribution (Sum of 15d (1), (2), (3) and (4)			94	78
f. Total Distribution (Sum of 15c and 15e)			836	738
g. Copies not Distributed (See instructions to publishers #4 (page #3))			261	146
h. Total (Sum of 15f and g)			1097	884
i. Percent Paid and/or Requested Circulation (15c divided by 15f times 100)			88.76%	89.43%

* If you are claiming electronic copies go to line 16 on page 3. If you are not claiming Electronic copies, skip to line 17 on page 3.

16. Electronic Copy Circulation	Average No. Copies Each Issue During Preceding 12 Months	No. Copies of Single Issue Published Nearest to Filing Date
a. Paid Electronic Copies		
b. Total paid Print Copies (Line 15c) + Paid Electronic copies (Line 16a)		
c. Total Print Distribution (Line 15f) + Paid Electronic Copies (Line 16a)		
d. Percent Paid (Both Print & Electronic copies) (16b divided by 16c X 100)		

☐ I certify that 50% of all my distributed copies (electronic and print) are paid above a nominal price

17. Publication of Statement of Ownership
☐ If the publication is a general publication, publication of this statement is required. Will be printed in the **November 2015** issue of this publication.

18. Signature and Title of Editor, Publisher, Business Manager, or Owner

Stephen R. Bushing

Stephen R. Bushing – Inventory Distribution Coordinator

Date
September 18, 2015

I certify that all information furnished on this form is true and complete. I understand that anyone who furnishes false or misleading information on this form or who omits material or information requested on the form may be subject to criminal sanctions (including fines and imprisonment) and/or civil sanctions (including civil penalties).

PS Form 3526, July 2014 (Page 3 of 3)

Moving?

Make sure your subscription moves with you!

To notify us of your new address, find your **Clinics Account Number** (located on your mailing label above your name), and contact customer service at:

Email: journalscustomerservice-usa@elsevier.com

800-654-2452 (subscribers in the U.S. & Canada)
314-447-8871 (subscribers outside of the U.S. & Canada)

Fax number: 314-447-8029

Elsevier Health Sciences Division
Subscription Customer Service
3251 Riverport Lane
Maryland Heights, MO 63043

*To ensure uninterrupted delivery of your subscription, please notify us at least 4 weeks in advance of move.

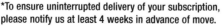
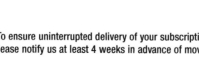

ELSEVIER

Printed and bound by CPI Group (UK) Ltd, Croydon, CR0 4YY

03/10/2024

01040381-0014